The Wounded Warrior Handbook

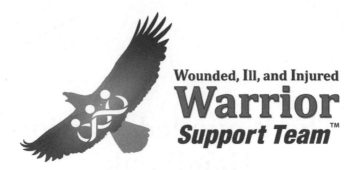

Wounded, Ill, and Injured

Warrior
Support Team™

Please accept this book as a token of our support.

OUR MISSION: Provide resources, support, fellowship, and social events to wounded, ill, and injured troops, and veterans, including those living with combat operational stress and/or post-traumatic stress; provide resources and support to caregivers and family members.

For additional information visit
www.wiiwarrior.com
Phone (573) 449-2003
Email: wiiwst@marineparents.com

an outreach program of

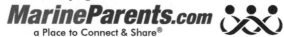

MarineParents.com
a Place to Connect & Share®

The Wounded Warrior Handbook

A Resource Guide for Returning Veterans

Special Edition

Janelle Moore
Cheryl Lawhorne
and
Don Philpott

ROWMAN & LITTLEFIELD
Lanham • Boulder • New York • London

Published by Rowman & Littlefield
A wholly owned subsidary of The Rowman & Littlefield Publishing Group, Inc.
4501 Forbes Boulevard, Suite 200, Lanham, Maryland 20706
www.rowman.com

Unit A, Whitacre Mews, 26-34 Stannary Street, London SE11 4AB

Copyright © 2012 by Government Institutes
First Rowman & Littlefield edition 2014
Updated Rowman & Littlefield second edition 2015

British Library Cataloguing in Publication Information Available

The hardback edition of this book was previously cataloged by the Library of Congress as follows:

Hill, Janelle.
    The wounded warrior handbook : a resource guide for returning veterans / Janelle Moore, Cheryl Lawhorne, and Don Philpott. — 2nd ed.
       p. cm. — (Military life ; 6)
    Includes index.
    1. Disabled veterans—Services for—United States—Handbooks, manuals, etc.
    2. Veterans—Services for—United States—Handbooks, manuals, etc. 3. Disabled veterans—Rehabilitation—United States. 4. Veterans—United States—Handbooks, manuals, etc. 5. Veterans' families—United States—Handbooks, manuals, etc.
    I. Lawhorne, Cheryl, 1968– II. Philpott, Don, 1946– III. Title.
    UB363.P55 2012
    362.1086'970973—dc23   2011044808

ISBN 978-1-60590-738-3 (hbk. : alk. paper)
ISBN 978-1-4422-5196-0 (pbk. : alk. paper)
ISBN 978-1-4422-5243-1 (electronic)

♾™ The paper used in this publication meets the minimum requirements of American National Standard for Information Sciences—Permanence of Paper for Printed Library Materials, ANSI/NISO Z39.48-1992.

Printed in the United States of America

Contents

Foreword

As a nation we owe our serving men and women an enormous debt of gratitude for the magnificent job they have done and continue to do on our behalf under the most challenging conditions. Their courage, valor, strength and commitment are an inspiration to us all.

However, it is difficult to find the words to express our thanks and admiration for those men and women who have been severely wounded, while serving to uphold the principles that we hold so dear. Their sacrifice must never be forgotten. As a nation we must do everything in our power to provide them with what they need to speed their medical recovery and return them to active duty or transition into civilian life.

For our wounded warriors and their families and loved ones these are understandably very challenging times. A family is suddenly told that their loved one has been wounded in a combat zone and their lives are thrown into chaos. The military goes to exceptional lengths to provide immediate comfort, support and assistance. However, families sometimes have more questions than there are answers. How is their wounded warrior being treated and where? Can they travel to be with their wounded warrior? Are they entitled to time off work without fear of losing their job?

There are many questions that overwhelm families in the early days. Help is available both from the military and the many support organizations dedicated to helping our wounded warriors and their families. There are hundreds of websites that can be visited and even more documents, leaflets and brochures are available packed with good advice and information.

This sheer wealth of information can be completely overwhelming, especially at a time when a family has so many other issues both practical and emotional to deal with.

The authors of this book provide an easy-to-understand yet comprehensive guide to what our wounded warriors and their families need to know about their medical treatment, rehabilitation, counseling, support and transition.

If you have questions this book should help you to find the answers. You will have enough information to make you better informed and able to make better decisions. If you require more information the book provides a comprehensive resource guide.

Our wounded warriors and their families rightly deserve all the help and support they can get. *The Wounded Warriors Handbook* is an important tool to assist and empower them.

General Barry McCaffrey
U.S. Army (Ret.)

Preface

This handbook has been written as an easy-to-use reference guide for wounded warriors, as well as for their families and loved ones. There is a huge and growing amount of literature available from the military and others; there are scores of support organizations involved in this arena and there are hundreds of websites offering information and help.

All of these do a magnificent job in their respective areas, but it can be a daunting task to pull together all this information, especially at a time of crisis. The information here has been gathered from literally hundreds of these sources in the public domain.

A lot of the information included in this book comes from the Department of Veterans Affairs (VA) and the Department of Defense (DoD) and we acknowledge their cooperation. However, this in no way implies any endorsement in any way from either the VA or DoD in respect to the materials contained in this book. We have made every effort to be as up-to-date and accurate as possible, but there are constant changes in this field and we could not have covered all of them.

Our aim is to provide a comprehensive framework that will allow you to quickly access information that you need regarding medical treatment, rehabilitation, counseling, support, and transition. We also deal with important financial, legal, and tax matters. However, this book is a guide only and is not a legal, claims, or medical handbook. If you have detailed questions in these and other specialist areas you must seek the advice of an appropriate expert.

While we cannot go into great detail in all these matters, we hope that there is sufficient information to give you a better understanding of procedures, processes, and policies so that you know what is going on, what your rights are, and how you can exercise them. Further detailed information is included in the appendices at the end of this book.

Note: Benefit amounts, per diem rates, and other figures mentioned in this book were, to the best of our ability, correct at the time of going to print but they should be used as guides only, as they do change. Also, because of the present economic climate, it is expected that there will be major federal budget cuts. How this might impact services provided by the VA and DoD is uncertain at this time.

1

Introduction:
Pre-Battlefield Injury to Recovery

The patriots who have volunteered to serve in our armed services have no equal in the world. I made a solemn commitment to the Congress, to the nation, and to you to keep the welfare of men and women in uniform uppermost in my mind at all times.

—Defense Secretary Robert M. Gates

When battlefield injury occurs far from home, the road to recovery may be long and difficult to navigate. Even with the dedicated support of medical professionals, loved ones, military leadership, and brothers and sisters-in-arms this pathway from injury to home requires caring over time and over miles. Differences in the type of injury, in the nature of support available along the way, and the types of resources and responsibilities waiting at home may dictate different stops along the way for different service members.

Movement from care at the point of battlefield injury—physical, psychological, or combined—through levels of care abroad and within the U.S. and ultimately homeward is a complex process involving the interplay of personal endurance, military and medical leadership, technology and communications and networks of civilian and military caregivers, supporters, and communities.

The modern evacuation and movement of injured provides new opportunities for care, necessary tracking and communications and needs for protection from additional health burdens, both physical and administrative.

Programs and policies that must integrate and synthesize the efforts of command, community, and family resources have to consider the following areas at each stop along the route from hazardous duty to adaptive home life. All these issues are dealt with in greater detail in later sections. They include:

Chapter 1

- Over one million service members have sustained injury in the wars in Iraq and Afghanistan. Approximately half of these have been serious enough that the service member has been unable to continue to function in theater and has required a medical evacuation back to the continental United States. The injuries include but are by no means limited to traumatic amputations, loss of sight, and traumatic brain injury. Almost 270,000 service members have been diagnosed with brain injuries since 2001 and it is estimated that 1 in 5 veterans have PTSD. The emotionally injured may also be evacuated. Importantly, even severe emotional injuries may not be readily apparent on the battlefield and occur in greater numbers as home approaches and the challenges of return meet the worries of lost health and function. Sometimes this might not be apparent for many months or even years.
- The "invisibility" of psychological injury and traumatic brain injury presents a complex medical situation in which denial, stigma, fear of re-exposure to painful memories and lack of knowledge of treatment options and efficacy impede help-seeking and strain an already stressed system of care resources. Administrative procedures can become part of secondary injury. While on the other hand, when health systems create opportunities to miss care, the combination of fears, stigma and emotional pain can enhance missed opportunities for psychological and behavioral care.
- Most serious combat injuries powerfully impact the children and families of service members. Data suggest that problems do not immediately resolve and commonly worsen during the course of the first year after hospitalization. Difficulty in readjusting to life back home may alter family relationships and support, contributing to a vicious cycle of psychosocial challenges for both the injured service member and the family. The family should be seen as care collaborators in all health interventions and planning.
- Returning combat veterans, even those not psychologically injured, experience a variety of behavioral and emotional responses secondary to their war experience and combat occupational stress. Distress symptoms are common and may include insomnia, nightmares or other forms of sleep disorder; hyper vigilance, jitteriness or overexcitement; and avoidance or social withdrawal. Reintegration with family and life is both a goal and can be a challenge.
- Systems of care must address not only disorders, but the many emotional and behavioral manifestations of distress which require a holistic, comprehensive approach. They must incorporate health care provided by military, VA, and civilian treatment facilities; facilitate family participation in health care and treatment planning; and engage traditional community resources (e.g., churches and schools) as well as employee and local, state, and federal programs implemented specifically to provide assistance to returning veterans.

- Secondary injury can result from the induced helplessness, overwhelming stress and indignities and self-medication resulting from administrative delays, errors and omissions, which may unnecessarily complicate recovery.
- Variability in the time and emotional availability and responsiveness of family members requires resources and flexibility in order to identify and establish care advocates for each injured service member.
- People returning from combat deployment can sometimes initiate or increase the frequency of risk and/or addictive behaviors that compromise their health and the health and safety of those around them. Excessive alcohol use may develop as a misguided attempt to reduce stress. Irritability or anger (common symptoms on return home) may turn into violence, at times directed to one's family, in the context of excessive alcohol use or the decreased emotional control that can accompany traumatic brain injury and other issues such as post-traumatic stress disorder or alcohol addiction.
- Medical advances and current practice have altered the amount of time an individual may remain in a specific care environment. Rarely in the modern world of war is the injured now in theater or even overseas for long periods of time. Yet healing and administrative processes still take time and hold patients in new settings where family may or may not be present and resources have to be constantly adjusted to meet needs. Resources have to be sufficient and flexibly assigned to meet each level of care in order to sustain the recovery process and be responsive to the cultural context of the injured and geographical considerations (i.e., those residing in rural or remote locations).
- Current processes of medical evacuation generally provide for superb initial stabilization and management of physical and psychosocial injuries to service members within the military medical system. However, they do not address well the longer-term challenges associated with care across boundaries of community, family, VA and civilian medical services. The care of injured from battlefield to home must be re-engineered to incorporate the new health care available, the technology and transport and the varied effects of injury on family members, the subsequent impact on the nature and availability of family resources to the injured service member, and the range in available resources during evacuation and at home station over time and in transition through the separation process.
- Navigating the complexities of ongoing medical care and disability evaluation is in and of itself a health challenge and a health burden. It can be an impediment to the intrinsically human process of adaptation to serious physical or emotional injury. Navigating this complex road requires acknowledging the injury's impact on one's identity, one's future, one's family and one's livelihood. Such knowledge changes how we view ourselves and our family, and can change how our family and friends view us and our future. This adaptation, recovery and return requires time and community to sustain the process.

For more information visit: www.usuhs.mil/csts and www.centerforthestudy oftraumaticstress.org.

BE PREPARED

Being able to quickly locate important documents during a crisis is very important. That means talking a little time beforehand to make sure they have been gathered together and deposited in a safe but convenient place.

These documents should include birth and marriage certificates, legal documents such as wills and financial power of attorney, medical documents such as health care advance directives, insurance documents, beneficiary designation forms, and travel documents such as passports. You should have the original of each document safely stored in one location and several copies stored in a second location. Both sets of documents should be easily accessible if needed in a hurry. When you gather everything together, check all expiry dates and renew if necessary. Information on how to get these documents, how to renew them and so on, will be explained in later sections.

The importance of these documents, however, is that they will enable the service member to have his or her wishes carried out immediately—especially if they are not in a position to express their wishes themselves.

Important documents are:

A health care advance directive, sometimes called a health care proxy medical power of attorney, is a form that designates someone as an agent to make health care decisions on behalf of a person in the event that he or she becomes unable to do so. A servicemember may also use a health care advance directive to list limitations regarding which types of treatment he or she is willing to receive. Health care advance directives often become important in situations when a service member is unconscious and a physician requires authorization to perform certain procedures. In the absence of a health care advance directive, these decisions will fall to a service member's spouse, parents or next of kin, depending on state law. Signing a health care proxy may avoid conflict in situations when state law is unclear or family members might disagree on the appropriate course of action.

A living will is a document directing a physician to refrain from taking lifesaving measures (such as CPR), or to remove life-sustaining treatment (such as a feeding tube) under certain conditions, such as a permanent coma following brain death. In the absence of a living will or other intervention, doctors are bound to use all available life-sustaining and lifesaving measures to keep a patient alive.

A last will and testament governs the distribution of a person's property after he or she dies. The laws about what constitutes a valid will are complex,

SOME STATISTICS

- Troops who have served in OEF/OIF since 2001: about 2.5 million
- U.S. killed in action, all branches: 6,838 (as of October 19, 2014)
- U.S. wounded: 51,972 (as of October 19, 2014)
- U.S. wounded, time to receive other-continent, state-of-the-art critical care: 13 hours (Vietnam: 15 days)
- Combat troops exposed to bomb blasts who may suffer at least mild TBI: 11–28%
- OEF/OIF troops diagnosed with mild/moderate/severe TBI: 30%
- Portion of total OIF bomb blast victims with TBI: 60%
- Forms the typical wounded soldier is required to file: 22
- The VA's biggest and most important challenge remains the caring for the onslaught of veterans returning from 12 years of war. At the end of 2013, the VA reported that more than half of all returning veterans required treatment.

and they vary by state. A service member who wishes to create a will or modify an existing will should consult a qualified legal professional.

Creating these documents often involves making difficult personal decisions and also requires legal expertise. Service members who wish to create a will or sign a power of attorney, health care advance directive or living will should consult a qualified legal professional.

A financial power of attorney is a legal document by which one person gives another person the authority to act in his or her place regarding financial affairs. Service members are often encouraged to grant powers of attorney prior to deployment to enable a spouse or other family member to manage their affairs while they are away. A financial power of attorney can be general—giving the attorney-in-fact unlimited authority over the principal's affairs—or limited to specific actions, such as filing tax returns or signing insurance forms. Powers of attorney may be limited to a specific period of time or may extend until the death of the principal or until revocation. A power of attorney must be "durable," however, in order to remain valid if the principal becomes incapacitated—for example, if the principal falls into a coma or suffers severe brain damage. Most powers of attorney become effective immediately when signed by the principal.

Rules regarding powers of attorney vary by state and some banks and financial institutions require an original power of attorney, so it is advisable to execute multiple original documents. Service members and their families should consult a legal professional when preparing a power of attorney.

Traumatic Injury Insurance under Service Members' Group Life Insurance (TSGLI) Policy document. This insurance is organized as part of the Servicemembers' Group Life Insurance (SGLI) and is designed to provide financial assistance to service members during their recovery period from a serious traumatic injury. TSGLI is intended to provide immediate (pending the review process, which can be lengthy) cash assistance to cover the expenses associated with the changes that accompany a traumatic injury, for example, constructing a ramp for wheelchair access to a home or adapting an automobile with hand controls. TSGLI pays a lump-sum benefit that is based on the severity of the service member's injury.

The program is not disability compensation and has no effect on entitlement for compensation and pension benefits provided by the Department of Veterans Affairs or disability benefits provided by the Department of Defense.

All members eligible for SGLI automatically became insured for traumatic injury protection of up to $100,000 unless they decline SGLI coverage. The benefit provides payouts of a tax-free lump-sum payment ranging from $25,000 to $100,000, depending on the extent of a service member's injury, for service members who have lost limbs, eyesight, or speech or received other traumatic injuries as a direct result of injuries received during operations Iraqi Freedom or Enduring Freedom.

To be eligible for payment of TSGLI, you must meet all of the following requirements:

- You must be insured by SGLI when you experience a traumatic injury
- You must incur a scheduled loss and that loss must be a direct result of a traumatic injury
- You must have suffered the traumatic injury prior to midnight of the day that you separate from the uniformed services
- You must suffer a scheduled loss within 2 years (730 days) of the traumatic injury
- You must survive for a period of not less than seven full days from the date of the traumatic injury (The 7-day period begins on the date and time of the traumatic injury, as measured by Zulu [Greenwich Meridian] time and ends 168 full hours later)

Effective October 1, 2011, the Veterans' Benefit Improvement Act of 2010 removed the requirement that injuries during the retroactive period be incurred in Operations Enduring or Iraqi Freedom. http://benefits.va.gov/insurance/tsgli.asp

For more information about the program, service members should contact their Service TSGLI Representative. The Air Force POC for TSGLI is the Casualty Assistance Representative (CAR). For the other services, contact the Service Injured Support Program (Army AW2, Marine M4L, and Navy Safe Harbor). See the following section for information about these programs. To read about the TSGLI program, go to: www.insurance.va.gov/sgliSite/legislation/TSGLIFacts.htm.

2

Medical Issues:
Things to Know

Severely injured service members often require prolonged treatment, time to heal, and rehabilitative care before a decision can be made on their medical ability to remain on active duty or medically separate. The Military Health System (MHS) is meeting this challenge by improving coordination of health care for service members and veterans with Veterans Affairs (VA). MHS is dedicated to ensuring that service members are provided outstanding clinical care and streamlined administrative processes to return them to duty status or to transition them from MHS care to the VA health care system in an effective and timely manner.

Wartime demands and a surge in emerging technologies have contributed to the historic overhaul of the $18 billion defense health care system, according to Army Maj. Gen. Elder Granger, deputy director and program executive officer of TRICARE Management Activity. "We're dedicated to what we do," Granger said, and emphasized that the 135,000-strong medical system staff "works around the clock around the world in support of the war, families and veterans."

Central to the changes was the creation of a senior oversight committee staff made up of senior officials from both DoD and Veterans Affairs. It includes all service secretaries and is co-chaired by the deputy secretaries of both departments, according to the statement. Officials hope that hundreds of proposed actions will make the system more patient-focused.

Key on the health care front, DoD has created the Defense Center of Excellence for Psychological Health and Traumatic Brain Injury. Officials expect it to become a literal worldwide web of clinicians, researchers, educators and leaders from both within the military system and outside, including private practice and academia.

DoD and VA, mandated by the former President's Management Agenda, have created a joint federal recovery coordinator program. These coordinators are charged with managing needs of severely injured service members and their families and "are really starting to make a difference" in ensuring military veterans are getting the best health care available, according to then Defense Secretary Robert Gates.

Also high on the department's list of reforms are improving the disability evaluation system and improving data sharing between DoD and VA. The departments already have switched to a single disability rating system.

Military bodies responsible for assisting injured service members and wounded transitioning veterans:

Army—Wounded Warrior Transition Brigades
Navy—Safe Harbor Program
Marine Corps—Marine for Life and Wounded Warrior Regiment
Air Force—Palace HART (Helping Airmen Recover Together).

THE MEDEVAC PROCESS

Current military strategies mandate that the medical force structure be joint, agile and interoperable to ensure optimal responsiveness in diverse operations.

Components of MHS's Deployable Medical Capability include:

First Responder Care is the ability to provide initial medical care at or near the point of injury by the individual, medical and/or non-medical personnel. This may include preparing the casualty for transportation to the next medical capability as required.

Essential Care (Forward Resuscitative Care) is the ability to provide capabilities required by medical personnel to salvage life, limb, or eyesight and to relieve pain.

Definitive Care In-Theater (Theater Hospitalization) is the ability to provide capabilities required by medical personnel to repair, restore, stabilize, or rehabilitate casualties within the theater. These include preparation for strategic transport, return to duty, or processes for rehabilitation, as appropriate. This includes the utilization of telemedicine in this setting as a force multiplier.

En Route Care is the ability to provide a systematic evacuation capability of critically injured/ill patients accompanied by trained medical providers from one medical capability to another.

Patient Movement within a Joint Operational Area (JOA) (Intra-Theater) is the ability to conduct the efficient joint movement of patients to appropriate levels of care. Effective patient regulation and transport ensures that troops receive definitive care quickly and only at the level required. Those troops with less severe injuries/conditions are returned to duty in minimal time, while those with significant injuries are efficiently transported to higher levels of care, thus reducing mortality rates and maximizing recovery chances.

Patient Movement Outside of a Joint Operational Area (Inter-Theater) is the ability to conduct effective coordination and movement from a joint operational area to an appropriate definitive care facility (with en route care provided). Critical patients must be rapidly identified for replacement in the joint operational area. These processes allow commanders to project forces more accurately and maintain maximum troop strength where needed.

Joint Medical Logistics and Infrastructure Support (JMLIS) is the ability to work in conjunction with service force management and force de-sign organizations to ensure the medical supplies, material and equipment with which our medical forces deploy include the latest technologies and advances in the medical field. It also ensures medical supplies, material and equipment are delivered to the right person, at the right place, at the right time.

Joint Theater Medical Command and Control (JTMC2) is the ability to leverage the concurrent transformation of joint and service education and training, joint medical logistics in enterprise-wide support, common infor-mation management, information technology, operating architectures, and environments. Joint medical information systems must be fully networked and interoperable among services (line and medical) at the tactical and opera-tional levels.

FEDERAL RECOVERY COORDINATORS

Federal recovery coordinators ensure the appropriate oversight and coordina-tion is provided for care of active duty service members and veterans with major amputations, severe traumatic brain injury, spinal cord injury, severe sight or hearing impairments and severe multiple injuries. The coordinators also work closely with family members to take care of services and needs. The aim is to ensure that life-long medical and rehabilitative care services and other federal benefits are provided to seriously wounded, injured and ill ac-tive duty service members, veterans and their families.

The first 10 coordinators were located at Walter Reed Army Medical Cen-ter in Washington, DC; the Naval Medical Center in Bethesda, MD; the Brooke Army Medical Center at Fort Sam Houston, TX; and Balboa Park Naval Medical Center in San Diego. A further ten have been added and further re-covery coordinators will be appointed as needs are determined.

The coordinators have a background in health care management and work closely with the clinicians and case management teams to develop and execute plans of services needed across the continuum of care, from recovery through rehabilitation to reintegration to civilian life.

These federal recovery coordinators are in addition to patient advocates the VA has hired, trained and put in place. These advocates, most of them veterans of combat in Iraq and Afghanistan, ensure a smooth transition of wounded service members through the VA's health care system, while also cutting red tape for other benefits.

YOUR SUPPORT TEAM

Wounded service members have case managers assigned to work with them during their recovery period. The job of these individuals is to provide information and help assist the service member and family during the recovery period and the Physical Evaluation Board (PEB) and Medical Evaluation Board (MEB) process (discussed in detail in chapter 3). These individuals also provide information on Veteran Service Organizations (VSOs). Many military hospitals serving wounded or injured service members also have Family Assistance Centers. Families can also seek assistance from the installation chaplains, social workers, and family center: Army Community Services, Marine Corps Community Services, Air Force Family Support Center, Navy Fleet and Family Support Center, and Coast Guard Work Life Offices.

LEVELS OF CARE

Inpatient

While your service member is on inpatient status, meaning they are occupying a bed within the hospital, there is a multidisciplinary team which cares for them and oversees their recovery. Membership of this team is determined based on the injuries received and needs of the individual service member. There are some common components on these teams.

To ensure that medical treatment is continuing as smoothly as possible, a "medical case manager" is assigned to your service member. Given the large numbers of providers and support personnel who may be caring for a patient, the composition of the medical team can be confusing for family members (and patients!). The case manager "directs traffic" and is a resource for family members who may have questions about their loved one's medical care. However, case managers can be under a lot of pressure themselves. That is why it is important to have someone act as the advocate for the wounded warrior who is able to handle the flow of information and discuss issues with the case manager.

A licensed professional social worker is assigned to all service members when they arrive at the Military Treatment Facility (MTF). They act as a liaison between the medical treatment team and the service member and family. The social worker provides psychosocial assessment and intervention for both the service member and family. The social worker can provide medical crisis counseling and supportive counseling. They will assist in meeting the needs of the family, whatever they may be, by linking the family with the appropriate agencies and resources. The social worker is a linchpin in the system of wounded care as they provide a continuity factor for the service member/family from arrival at the MTF until discharge. While other members of the team will change, the social worker normally remains throughout the inpatient process.

The social worker is an integral part of discharge planning, which begins the moment the service member arrives at the MTF. The social worker ensures a smooth transition to the next level of care. The next level of care could be the VA, another military treatment facility, a treatment facility near the service member's family, outpatient status at the MTF, or a complete discharge from medical care. The social worker incorporates the needs of the family during this transition, to include coordinating for home health care, equipment, etc. If the service member returns at some point in the future to inpatient status at the MTF, the Department of Social Work Services will try to assign the same social worker to the service member and family.

Be actively involved with the social worker and establish contact when you arrive. Ask for what you need.

The medical team often includes doctors, nurses, social workers, various therapists, technicians, and numerous other supporting staff members. When a patient is treated by several different medical services (or specialties), the number of "team members" can increase dramatically.

The following is a partial listing (and brief description) of the various personnel who may comprise a multidisciplinary medical team. Families will encounter many of these healthcare professionals during your service member's hospital stay.

Care Team Roles and Definitions

Attending physician/surgeon: The senior doctor directing medical care.

Resident or resident physician: A doctor at any level in a graduate medical education program, including subspecialty programs. Other terms used to refer to these individuals include interns, house officers, house staff, trainees or fellows.

The term "fellow" is sometimes used to denote physicians in subspecialty programs (versus residents in specialty programs) or in graduate medical education programs that are beyond the requirements for eligibility for first board certification in the discipline.

The term "intern" is sometimes used to denote physicians in their first year of training.

Staff physician: A fully trained doctor who is a member of the medical/surgical staff.

Staff nurse: A fully trained registered nurse (RN) assigned to a particular service or ward. RNs care for patients at the hospital bedside, in private clinics, and in the patient's home. Nurses may also work to help prevent disease, to educate the public about health issues, to enhance public health, and to support ill patients both physically and mentally.

A nurse may also be the case manager for your service member.

Nurse Practitioner: A nurse practitioner (NP) is a registered nurse (RN) who has completed advanced education and training in the diagnosis and management of common medical conditions, including chronic illnesses. Nurse practitioners provide a broad range of health care services.

Licensed Practical Nurse/Licensed Vocational Nurse: LPNs/LVNs perform duties that may include giving injections, taking vital signs, performing basic diagnostic tests, observing patients, dressing wounds, and administering medication. They also assist patients in daily living activities such as eating, dressing, exercising, and bathing.

Physician assistant: Physician assistants (PAs) practice medicine under the supervision of physicians and surgeons. They should not be confused with medical assistants, who perform routine clinical and clerical tasks. PAs are trained to provide diagnostic, therapeutic, and preventive health care services, as delegated by a physician.

Social worker: Social workers help people function the best way they can in their environment and solve personal and family problems. Social workers often see clients who face life-threatening medical conditions or social problems. Social Workers, who are generally RNs, often serve as case managers.

Respiratory therapist: Respiratory therapists evaluate, treat, and care for patients with breathing or other cardiopulmonary disorders. Practicing under the direction of a physician, respiratory therapists assume primary responsibility for all respiratory care therapeutic treatments and diagnostic procedures, including the supervision of respiratory therapy technicians.

Occupational therapist: Occupational therapists (OTs) help people improve their ability to perform tasks in their daily living and working environments. They work with individuals who have conditions that are mentally, physically, developmentally, or emotionally disabling. They also help them to develop, recover, or maintain daily living and work skills.

Physical therapist: Physical therapists (PTs) provide services that help restore function, improve mobility, relieve pain, and prevent or limit permanent physical disabilities of patients suffering from injuries or disease. They restore, maintain, and promote overall fitness and health.

Variety of essential supportive personnel: Clergy, medical assistants, laboratory, dietary/nutrition, clerical staff, etc. Variety of students: Medical, nursing, dental, physical therapy, etc. Other non-medical personnel interacting with the family during the inpatient stay may include Service member Family Management Specialist (SFMS), Service member Family Assistance Center (SFAC), Service member Family Liaison, chaplains, representatives from the Medical Hold/Holdover Company, and unit liaisons.

The SFMS can work many issues for the severely wounded service member and family. They can assist with awards (Purple Heart), pay issues (such as receiving the full measure of hostile fire pay), employment, legal issues and issues dealing with the Medical and Physical Evaluation Boards. The SFMS can continue to interact with the service member and family for up to five years after leaving the MTF.

The SFAC is a valuable resource for families. They can provide shuttle and public transportation schedules, as well as emergency taxi vouchers. The SFAC can assist with obtaining a letter granting permission to use the commissary (grocery store) and PX (department store).

Chaplains provide spiritual support for the service member and the family. There are chapels located within the hospital.

Representatives from the Medical Hold and Holdover Companies usually make contact with the service member and family within five days of the service member's arrival at the MTF. These companies are military units that the service members are often assigned to or attached to while at the MTF. Unit liaisons are representatives from the military unit that your service member belonged to while in theater (Iraq or Afghanistan). These liaisons are there to support the service member and can help with issues regarding locating possessions left in theater, unit awards, and other administrative issues as well as assisting in any way that they can. Check to see if your service member's unit has a liaison at the MTF. If there is no unit liaison at the MTF, stay in touch with the Rear Detachment Commander (member of your service member's unit left behind to care for families). Not only can they provide you with information and support, they can also update the members of your service member's unit still deployed and keep them current on your service member's condition.

Your service member may be transferred to the VA system as an inpatient. There is a VA liaison inside the MTF to facilitate this transfer. Please confer with the liaison and remember that your T&TOs at the MTF will have to be closed out, and the travel voucher filed, before leaving.

OPERATION WAR FIGHTER

The purpose of this program is to provide service members with meaningful activity outside the hospital environment, and to offer them a formal means of transition back into the work force. This is a voluntary program and has orientation sessions at the MTF.

Call the Military Severely Injured Center for details: 888-774-1361.

Description

- A voluntary program
- Identifies recuperating military service members interested and medically cleared to work in the Pentagon
- Matches their military and non-military skills/interests with the support needs of the various Pentagon offices—priority given to matching participants with parent military service, OSD, & Joint Staff offices
- Provides the logistical support necessary for them to get to work and return to the medical center on a regularly scheduled basis
- Provides a core project staff to coordinate the program and assist participants (military and employing offices) in resolving work-related issues
- Provides recognition of participation (e.g., certificate) to each individual upon completion
- The program is designed to provide temporary augmentation and assistance, not to fill permanent, continuing requirements
- Focused primarily, but not exclusively, on administrative support functions

A danger during the outpatient phase is the amount of unscheduled time that a service member has. If you are functioning as an NMA, then you are aware of this time. The Operation Warfighter Program helps provide structure and purpose to some of that time. There sometimes are barriers that can develop that inhibit the service member from taking full advantage of programs offered. The next program can assist with encouraging the service member to advocate on their own behalf and overcome barriers or behaviors that impede forward progress.

Warrior Outreach Wellness Program

This is a program offered by the Department of Psychiatry at the MTF. This program empowers service members to take responsibility for their own health and well-being physically, emotionally, mentally, and spiritually. It educates them about the issues they face, and the impact these issues have on their functioning. It encourages service members to seek out services and appropriately advocate for their needs. The program holds a weekly "orientation" group in collaboration with the Medical Holding Company. The program offers Lunch and Learn initiatives with a series of groups and interactive discussions. The program assists with connections to services both on and off post, and meets service members where they live in on-post housing. It also assists service members with the management of medical treatment through education on "the system."

Your service member may also be transferred to another military treatment facility, usually in an effort to either get the service member closer to home, · or to connect the service member to a specific type of care. Work with your liaison to determine if someone can travel with the service member and how the T&TOs will change during this time.

Outpatient

When a service member reaches the point of no longer requiring inpatient hospital care but still requires treatment at the MTF, the service member may be moved to on-post accommodation and become an outpatient. At that point in time, a number of things happen. Most significantly to the family, the T&TOs that the family has been using will be terminated.

Unless a physician determines that the service member needs assistance with daily needs, the family will be encouraged to return home to await the return of their service member. The T&TOs that the family had must be closed out and the travel voucher submitted before leaving the MTF.

Non-Medical Attendant Orders

If a physician determines that the service member needs a non-medical attendant (NMA), the service member is allowed to designate one person to stay and help with daily needs. The request must be approved by the Deputy Commander of Clinical Services (DCCS) and orders will be issued by the military treatment facility (MTF). Non-medical attendant orders cover per diem only. The family member shares a room with the service member and thus would not require lodging.

If NMAs are requested and approved, the NMA order is then issued by the calendar month. This means that if your service member becomes an outpatient on November 15, the first set of NMA orders would expire on November 30. Start working on the extension immediately with a new memorandum from your service member's doctor. Submit the memorandum to the Casualty Affairs Office. NMAs are then issued for thirty-day cycles until the doctor determines that assistance with daily living is no longer necessary. Each 30 day extension requires a new memorandum from the doctor, so pay close attention to the dates.

Just like T&TOs, you must file a travel voucher for NMAs to be reimbursed for per diem.

The travel voucher should be filed the next business day after the NMA expires. In the above example, the first voucher would be filed on December 1. The next set of NMA orders would be issued for December 1 through December 31 and the voucher submitted on the next business day after the 31st.

The Finance Office is the place to file the voucher; they will help you with the paperwork. You will need a copy of the NMA orders and all extensions to file your voucher.

If you need to take a break and hand over the responsibilities of being the non-medical attendant to another person designated by your service member, you can do that. As long as there is a memorandum requiring an attendant, the duties can be shifted. This means that new orders would have to be issued to the new designee, and your orders would need to be closed out and a travel voucher filed.

There is support available at all times for the service member as well as the family. Reach out to the SFAC social worker, chaplain, Service member Family Management Specialist or any of the other professionals there to answer the call. Your emotional well-being is important, as is the emotional well-being of your service member. Most of us do not have experience dealing with this level of trauma or a long recuperative process. The support community at the MTF can provide insight and assistance in regaining or maintaining a positive mental outlook during this difficult time.

PATIENT'S BILL OF RIGHTS

Rights

Quality Care: You have the right to quality care based on your health care needs regardless of race, creed, sex, national origin or religion.

Respect and Dignity: You have the right to considerate and respectful care, with recognition of your family's religious and cultural preferences.

Privacy and Confidentiality: You have the right to privacy and confidentiality concerning medical care. This includes expecting any discussion or consultation about your care to be conducted discreetly and privately. You have the right to expect that only people involved in your care of the monitoring of its quality will read your medical record. Other individuals can read your record only when authorized by you and your legally authorized representative.

You have the right to wear appropriate personal religious or symbolic clothing as long as it does not interfere with treatment or procedures.

You have the right to consent prior to any recording or filming for teaching or research purposes. You have the right to designate family members or loved ones to be informed of your condition. Photographing and recording (including digital telephones and PDAs) are not permitted without your permission.

You have the right to a chaperone upon request.

Personal Safety and Security: You have the right to a safe, secure environment while in the hospital. You have the right to access protective and advocacy services. Contact numbers and/or points of contact are available upon request.

Identity: You have the right to complete and current information about your diagnosis, treatment, medications, and the expected outcomes in terms that you can understand.

Consent: You have the right to be informed and to consent to all procedures, treatments and admissions.

Communication: You have the right to expect that your needs will be communicated to the health care team, including access to an interpreter when language barriers are a problem.

Pain Management: You have the right to have a complete evaluation of any pain you may have, as well as the right to be treated appropriately for that pain.

Refusal of Treatment: You have the right to refuse care, treatment, and services in accordance with applicable law and regulations.

Advance Directive: You have the right to formulate an advance directive (living will and/or medical durable power of attorney), and to take part in ethical issues pertinent to your care. An advanced directive from another facility will be honored if you provide a copy to the treatment team.

Transfer and Continuity of Care: You have the right to information if you are transferred to another facility. Discharge information about your condition and ongoing health care needs will be provided to you when you are discharged from the hospital.

Hospital Rules and Regulations: You have the right to information about hospital rules and regulations that apply to you.

You and Your Child: You have the right to know the treatment plan for your child and to have answers to all your questions and concerns about your child's treatment.

Research: You have the right to a second opinion with a specialist at your own request and expense.

Responsibilities

Providing Information: You are responsible for providing accurate and complete information about present complaints, illnesses, hospitalizations, medications, and other matters relating to your health. You should report unexpected changes in your condition to your doctor. You must tell your health care team if you do not clearly understand the plan of care and what is expected of you. You must tell your health care team if you have any concern over the safety and care you are receiving.

Compliance with Instructions: You should follow the treatment plan given to you by your doctor, nurses or other health care workers. This includes keeping your appointments, and notifying the clinic when you are unable to do so.

Maintain Positive Health Practices: You have the responsibility to develop and maintain healthy habits, including good nutrition and adequate sleep and rest, and routine exercise.

Refusal of Treatment: You are responsible for you own actions when you refuse treatment or do not follow the doctor's or other health care worker's instructions.

Hospital Rules: You are responsible for following hospital rules and regulations affecting patient care and conduct. Any suspicious activity should be reported to the hospital staff.

Hospital Charges: You are responsible for paying hospital bills as soon as possible.

Respect and Consideration: You are responsible for treating our staff and other patients with respect and consideration.

Protecting Others from Illness or Infection: Do not let friends or family visit if they are sick, or have been exposed to a communicable disease, such as chicken pox. You and your visitors should wash your hands frequently.

Smoking Policy: You may not smoke while in the facility. You may smoke only in the designated smoking areas located outside the buildings.

Medical Records: You must return your outpatient medical records to your assigned medical treatment facility after all medical consultation or other appointments are finished. All medical records are the property of the U.S. government and must be returned to the appropriate Military Treatment Facility so that a complete record of your care can be maintained.

Reporting of Patient Complaints: Any concerns, questions, and complaints should be given to the SFAC. This will help the commander provide the best possible care for all patients. After duty hours, the Administrative Officer of the Day will receive calls and refer them to the appropriate office.

Important

1. Make a list of the names and contact numbers of all of the people involved in the care of your wounded warrior and keep it current.
2. Create an appointment log so that you can keep detailed notes about meetings and treatments.

This enables you to keep track of everyone involved and what their roles are as well as what is being done. It also means you can pass on these notes should the need arise.

> **PATIENT SAFETY: "SPEAK UP"**
>
> **S**peak up if you have questions or concerns.
> **P**ay attention to the care you are receiving.
> **E**ducate yourself about your health conditions.
> **A**sk a family member or friend to be your advocate.
> **K**now what medications you take and why you take them.
> **U**se a health care organization that is certified by JCAHO.
> **P**articipate in all decisions about your care.

INJURIES

Brain Injuries

Traumatic Brain Injury (TBI)

TBI has been called the signature wound of the Global War on Terror (GWOT). It has previously been reported that TBI could reach as high as 50% among combat-related casualties. One of the reasons our service members have been surviving injuries that in earlier conflicts would have been fatal is the technology now available. The advances in protective equipment and in battlefield medicine have played a pivotal role in service members surviving their injuries.

The long-term impact of TBI on a veteran attempting to enter the workforce is significant. In many cases, it really is a "silent injury." These veterans may look just like they did before the injury, but they have significantly different cognitive challenges. Some of the symptoms are: forgetting details; trouble concentrating and multi-tasking; and becoming more agitated and angry than normal. Some service members with TBI are disciplined or demoted prior to their diagnosis because of the changes in their behavior and inability to do their job.

One of the greatest needs for employers is education and awareness about the nature of brain injury, its effects on a person, and how it can be accommodated on the job.

Depending on the nature and severity of the injury—mild, moderate, severe or penetrating—the person may have challenges in attention, concentration, general awareness, learning, memory, speed and efficiency of thinking, reasoning, judgment, insight, problem solving, and awareness of the significance of their cognitive problems. Many will have cognitive communication problems such as speaking well but not staying on topic, talking about inappropriate subjects or using inappropriate words, rude behavior, difficulty understanding jokes or puns, seeming uninterested or talking non-stop, and

Common Symptoms of Brain Injury	
▶ Difficulty organizing daily tasks	▶ Trouble with memory, attention or concentration
▶ Blurred vision or eyes tire easily	▶ More sensitive to sounds, lights or distractions
▶ Headaches or ringing in the ears	▶ Impaired decision making or problem solving
▶ Feeling sad, anxious or listless	▶ Difficulty inhibiting behavior - impulsive
▶ Easily irritated or angered	▶ Slowed thinking, moving speaking or reading
▶ Feeling tired all the time	▶ Easily confused, feeling easily overwhelmed
▶ Feeling light-headed or dizzy	▶ Change in sexual interest or behavior

forgetting what has already been said. Other impacts can be not feeling motivated to get started on a task, leaving things half done, and not knowing their strengths and weaknesses. There can also be associated depression and problems with anger and impulsivity.

While it is technology that has contributed to their survival rate, it is also advanced technology that can assist them in coping and dealing with their challenges. There is now equipment available that essentially is a cognitive prosthetic device. Personal Directory Assistants (PDAs) can be programmed with such tools as the PEAT (Planning Executive Assistance and Trainer) system to assist them in their scheduling, cueing them for important tasks, and monitoring performance. Digital pictures and names of the people they want to remember can also be entered into their PDA. It is not unrealistic to imagine an application of this technology in the workplace to accommodate individuals with TBI. In particular, the younger veterans are very technologically savvy and comfortable with this type of equipment.

Mild Traumatic Brain Injury

The key factors in a case of mTBI include an injury event—such as a blow to the head—which causes an alteration of consciousness. Such "alteration" can be losing consciousness, seeing stars or simply being temporarily disoriented.

Testing programs use "automated neuropsychological assessment metrics" to identify affected service members. The screening is intended to take pre-deployment measurements for a baseline, then retest after the deployment to measure for differences.

Service members identified as at risk for mTBI are then recommended for follow-up treatment. Doctors will be able to monitor recovery in such a way as to ensure service members are not returned to the fight until their recovery is complete. The good news is that it is a treatable condition. Patience, time and understanding are the keys to coping with and treating an mTBI through to full recovery.

Once service members return from deployment, family members may begin noticing irritability, sleeplessness, chronic headaches, clumsiness, and mem-

FLOW CHART FOR SCREENING AND EVALUATION OF POSSIBLE TRAUMATIC BRAIN INJURY (TBI) IN OPERATION ENDURING FREEDOM (OEF) AND OPERATION IRAQI FREEDOM (OIF) VETERANS

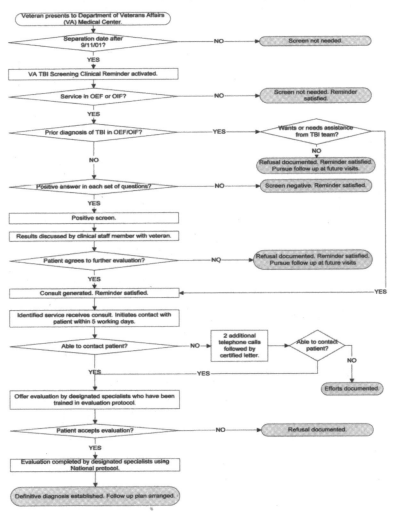

ory problems. This five-symptom cluster is a common sign of mTBI, with families often the first to notice such changes.

It is important for families to understand what the recovery process is and what they can do to help. You have to understand that they are going to forget things and they're going to be irritable, but once the headaches stop and the sleeplessness ends, there will be improvement.

Other Brain Injuries

If the head is hit or violently shaken (such as from a blast or explosion), a "concussion" or "closed head injury" can result. Concussion is seldom life-threatening, so doctors often use the term "mild" when the person is only dazed or confused or loses consciousness for a short time. However, a concussion can result in serious symptoms. People who survive multiple concussions may have more serious problems. People who have had a concussion may say that they are "fine" although their behavior or personality has changed. If you notice such changes in a family member or friend, suggest they seek medical care. Keep in mind that these are common experiences, but may occur more frequently with TBI. If in doubt, ask your doctor.

Post-Traumatic Stress Disorder (PTSD)

PTSD is an anxiety disorder that can occur after you have gone through an extreme emotional trauma that involved the threat of injury or death. Most survivors of trauma return to normal given a little time. However, some people have stress reactions that don't go away on their own, or may even get worse over time. These individuals may develop PTSD. People who suffer from PTSD often suffer from nightmares, flashbacks, difficulty sleeping, and feeling emotionally numb.

These symptoms can significantly impair your daily life. In addition, PTSD is marked by clear physical and psychological symptoms. It often has symptoms like depression, substance abuse, problems of memory and cognition, and other physical and mental health problems. The disorder is also associated with difficulties in social or family life, including occupational instability, marital problems, family discord, and difficulties in parenting. People with PTSD have three kinds of experiences for weeks or months after the event is over and the individual is in a safe environment.

People who have PTSD have experiences from all three of these categories that stay with them most of the time and interfere with their ability to live their life or do their job. If you still are not sure if this is a problem for you, you can take a quick self-assessment through the Mental Health Self-Assessment Program at www.militarymentalhealth.org.

Most service members do not develop PTSD. It also is important to remember that you can experience some PTSD symptoms without having a diagnosis of PTSD. PTSD cases often resolve on their own in the first 3 months, but even without the full diagnosis, if you have symptoms, you can benefit from counseling or therapy.

The good news: PTSD is treatable. You do not need to suffer from the symptoms of PTSD alone. Therapy has proven to be very effective in reducing and even eliminating the symptoms. Self-medication is common, and if it

RE-EXPERIENCE THE EVENT OVER AND OVER AGAIN
You can't put it out of your mind no matter how hard you try You have repeated nightmares about the event You have vivid memories, almost like it was happening all over again You have a strong reaction when you encounter reminders, such as a car backfiring
AVOID PEOPLE, PLACES, OR FEELINGS THAT REMIND YOU OF THE EVENT
Your work hard at putting it out of your mind You feel numb and detached so you don't have to feel anything You avoid people or places that remind you of the event
FEEL "KEYED UP" OR ON-EDGE ALL THE TIME
You may startle easily You may be irritable or angry all the time for no apparent reason You are always looking around, hyper-vigilant of your surroundings You may have trouble relaxing or getting to sleep

appears someone may be self-medicating to cope, please consult a licensed, trained healthcare professional immediately. Early treatment leads to the best outcomes. So, if you think you or someone in your family may have PTSD, please seek treatment right away.

What Happens in Treatment for PTSD?

Treatment for PTSD focuses on helping the trauma survivor reduce fear and anxiety, gain control over traumatic stress reactions, make sense of war experiences, and function better at work and in the family. A standard course of treatment usually includes:

- Assessment and development of an individual treatment plan.
- Education of veterans and their families about post-traumatic stress and its effects.
- Training in relaxation methods, to help reduce physical arousal/tension.
- Practical instruction in skills for coping with anger, stress, and ongoing problems.
- Detailed discussion of feelings of anger or guilt, which are very common among survivors of war trauma.
- Detailed discussions to help change distressing beliefs about self and others (e.g., self-blame).
- If appropriate, careful, repeated discussions of the trauma (exposure therapy) to help the service member reduce the fear associated with trauma memories.
- Medication to reduce anxiety, depression, or insomnia.
- Group support from other veterans often felt to be the most valuable treatment experience.

If you or a loved one experiences distress associated with combat trauma, see your primary care manager. If you need counseling or help locating services, call Military One Source at 800-342-9647.

Mental health professionals in VA medical centers, community clinics, and Readjustment Counseling Service Vet Centers have a long tradition of working with family members of veterans with PTSD. Couples counseling and educational classes for families may be available. Family members can encourage the survivor to seek education and counseling, but should not try to force their loved one to get help. Family members should consider getting help for themselves, whether or not their loved one is getting treatment.

Self-Care Suggestions for Families

- Become educated about PTSD.
- Take time to listen to all family members and show them that you care.
- Spend time with other people. Coping is easier with support from others, including extended family, friends, church groups, or other community groups.
- Join or develop a support group.
- Take care of yourself. Family members frequently devote themselves totally to those they care for and, in the process, neglect their own needs. Pay attention to yourself. Watch your diet and exercise, and get plenty of rest. Take time to do things that feel good to you.
- Try to maintain family routines, such as dinner together, church, or sports outings.
- If needed, get professional help as early as possible, and get back in touch with treatment providers if things worsen after treatment has ended.

For more information about PTSD, please visit the VA website: www.va.gov. A PTSD guide for families can be found at the following web address: www.ptsd.va.gov.

Online PTSD Resources

National Center for Post-Traumatic Stress Disorder (PTSD). A special center within Veterans Affairs created to advance the clinical care and social welfare of America's veterans through research, education, and training in the science, diagnosis, and treatment of PTSD and stress-related disorders: www.ptsd.va.gov.

Ameriforce Deployment Guide. Fact sheets and information for service members and their families on post-deployment, including home, finances, career, and more. www.ameriforce.net/deployment.

Courage to Care. A site created by Uniformed Services University for the Health Sciences, which belongs to the Center for Traumatic Studies and includes a wealth of additional information. Courage to Care is an electronic health campaign for military and civilian professionals serving the military community, and for military men, women and families. www.usuhs.mil/psy/courage.html.

The "Courage to Care: Helping National Guard and Reserve Reenter the Workplace" fact sheet is specific to reservists returning to the workplace and can be found at: www.usuhs.mil/psy/GuardReserveReentryWorkplace.pdf.

Military OneSource. This free 24-hour service, provided by the Department of Defense, is available to all active duty, Guard, and Reserve members and their families. Masters-level consultants provide 24/7 information and make referrals on a wide range of issues. You can reach the program by telephone at 800-342-9647 or through the website at www.militaryonesource.com.

Blast Injuries

The Army is aggressively diagnosing and treating soldiers who suffer concussive injuries and stress related to blast attacks, says the Army's surgeon general, Lt. Gen. (Dr.) Eric B. Schoomaker.

"We know the importance of prevention of these injuries and illnesses; we know the importance of timely diagnosis and treatment of both concussive and post-traumatic stress symptoms," Schoomaker said. "And we are aggressively executing programs that are designed to educate, to prevent, to screen and to provide the appropriate care in a timely fashion for all of these deployment-related stresses and injuries."

While screenings performed immediately after returning from deployment might be successful in identifying physical symptoms, the process might allow gaps in detecting latent symptoms related to context. Because certain emotional symptoms related to concussive injuries or combat stress emerge later than their physical counterparts, Schoomaker said, he advocates an additional screening three to six months after deployments. Identifying the root of emotional symptoms may help affected service members avoid family, social, alcohol or other problems resulting from a lack of proper diagnosis and treatment.

Combat Occupational Stress Syndrome/Combat Stress Reaction

Combat stress reaction is generally short-term and should not be confused with acute stress disorder, post-traumatic stress disorder, or other long-term disorders attributable to combat stress, although any of these may commence as a combat stress reaction.

Post-Concussive Syndrome (PCS)

PCS is a specific set of neuropsychological (thinking, behavioral, and emotional) disorders caused by traumatic brain injury, aka concussion. PCS results from actual, physical, damage, or injury to the brain caused by an external force. A brain subjected to such violent forces can be torn or sheared, crushed, or displaced, or simply destroyed. It can bleed, swell, and occasionally, it might even shut down. PCS affects the ability to think, do, and know. Memory, mood and attention are the top three complaints of brain injury patients. Intellectual dullness and mental rigidity are apparent signs of brain injury. Personality changes are common, and rapid mood swings alternate with waxing and waning energy levels. Taken individually, such impairments might not amount to much. However, such impairments usually appear in groups or clusters. In many cases the impairments are widespread and disrupt many brain systems. The overall effect can be profoundly disabling.

Generalized Anxiety Disorder (GAD)

A condition characterized by 6 months or more of chronic, exaggerated worry and tension that is unfounded or much more severe than the normal anxiety most people experience. People with GAD usually expect the worst. They worry excessively about money, health, family, or work, even when there are no signs of trouble. They are unable to relax and often suffer from insomnia. Sometimes the source of the worry is hard to pinpoint. Simply the thought of getting through the day provokes anxiety. Many people with GAD also have physical symptoms, such as fatigue, trembling, muscle tension, headaches, irritability or hot flashes. People with GAD may feel light-headed or out of breath. They also may feel nauseated or have to go to the bathroom frequently.

Recovery Following TBI

Some symptoms may be present immediately; others may appear much later. People experience brain injuries differently. Speed of recovery varies. Most people with mild injuries recover fully, but it can take time. In general, recovery is slower in older persons. People with a previous brain injury may find that it takes longer to recover from their current injury. Some symptoms can last for days, weeks, or longer. Talk to your health care provider about any troubling symptoms or problems.

TO PROMOTE HEALING & MANAGE SYMPTOMS	
Things That Can Help	*Things That Can Hurt*
• Get plenty of rest and sleep • Increase activity slowly • Carry a notebook—write things down if you have trouble remembering • Establish a regular daily routine to structure activities • Do only one thing at a time if you are easily distracted—turn off the TV or radio while you work • Check with someone you trust when making decisions	• Avoid activities that could lead to another brain injury—i.e. contact sports, motorcycles, skiing • Avoid alcohol as it may slow healing of the injury • Avoid caffeine or "energy-enhancing" products as they may increase symptoms • Avoid pseudoephedrine-containing products as they may increase symptoms—check the labels on cough, cold and allergy medicines • Avoid excessive use of over-the-counter sleeping aids—they can slow thinking and memory
Resources for More Information & Help: Centers for Disease Control www.cdc.gov/ncipc.tbi Defense and Veterans Brain Injury Center www.dvbic.org Brain Injury Association www.biausa.org	

DEPRESSION

Our nation's war on terror affects the health of our military and their families. Deployment, redeployment, single parenting, long absences, as well as losses sustained from injury or death are stressors that impact our community's physical and mental health. While most service members and their families are resilient, some may experience mental health problems that require medical attention.

Depression, one of the most common and treatable mental disorders, often presents itself during a primary care visit. This can be in the form of unexplained fatigue and vague aches and pains.

Primary care providers play an important role in early detection and intervention of mental disorders, which can often prevent and mitigate long-term health consequences. Due to concerns around stigma and one's career, primary care is often the setting of choice for service members and families to address mental health issues. Early identification and intervention is very important.

Upon return from duty, a mental health screen called the PDHA (post-deployment health assessment) is administered; the PDHRA (post-deployment health reassessment) is administered 90–180 days after returning home.

Signs of Depression

The signs of depression are often obvious. It is important to observe changes in demeanor and in mood of patients with whom one is familiar. Depression can also manifest in fatigue, problems with concentration and sleep, and weight loss. Unexplained pains and headaches may also be symptoms that warrant exploration.

There may be a sense of "I can handle it on my own," or a sense of shame about having feelings that could indicate depression. Being there and listening can be of the greatest assistance. Help seeking begins with self-awareness and a sense of safety, which can be facilitated by your presence and interest.

Treatment is effective. The majority of individuals who seek and receive treatment will get better. Depression also affects one's family. Taking care of one's self protects the health and cohesion of one's family. Adherence to prescribed medication is important. As with many health issues, medication adherence is a challenge. A primary care visit can be a "teachable moment" to reinforce the progress a patient has made and the benefits to self and family of adhering to treatment.

Depression does not mean discharge or medical separation. Many on active duty can receive treatment for depression and continue to work effectively.

Depression Resources

www.psych.org
www.nimh.nih.gov
www.militaryonesource.com
www.usuhs.mil/psy/CourageToCarePatientFamilyDepressionFactSheet.pdf

Common Reactions to Trauma

Most people who directly experience a major trauma have severe problems in the immediate aftermath. Many people then feel much better within three months after the event, but others recover more slowly, and some do not recover enough without help. Becoming more aware of what you've undergone since your trauma is the first step toward recovery.

Some of the most common problems after a trauma are:

- Fear and anxiety. Anxiety is a common and natural response to a dangerous situation. For many it lasts long after the trauma has ended. This happens when views of the world and a sense of safety have changed. You may become anxious when you remember the trauma. But sometimes anxiety may come from out of the blue. Triggers or cues that can cause anxiety may include places, times of day, certain smells or noises, or any situation that reminds you of the trauma. As you begin to pay more attention to the times you feel afraid, you can discover the triggers for your anxiety. In this way, you may learn that some of the out-of-the-blue anxiety is really triggered by things that remind you of your trauma.

- Re-experiencing of the trauma. People who have been traumatized often re-experience the traumatic event. Some people have flashbacks, or very vivid images, as if the trauma were occurring again. Nightmares are also common. These symptoms occur because a traumatic experience is so shocking and so different from everyday experiences that you can't fit it into what you know about the world. So in order to understand what happened, your mind keeps bringing the memory back, as if to better digest it and fit it in.
- Increased arousal is also a common response to trauma. This includes feeling jumpy, jittery, shaky, being easily startled, and having trouble concentrating or sleeping. Continuous arousal can lead to impatience and irritability, especially if you're not getting enough sleep. The arousal reactions are due to the fight or flight response in your body.
- Avoidance is a common way of managing trauma-related pain. The most common is avoiding situations that remind you of the trauma, such as the place where it happened. Often situations that are less directly related to the trauma are also avoided, such as going out in the evening if the trauma occurred at night. Another way to reduce discomfort is trying to push away painful thoughts and feelings. This can lead to feelings of numbness, where you find it difficult to have both fearful and pleasant or loving feelings. Sometimes the painful thoughts or feelings may be so intense that your mind just blocks them out altogether, and you may not remember parts of the trauma.
- Many people who have been traumatized feel angry and irritable. If you are not used to feeling angry this may seem scary as well. It may be especially confusing to feel angry at those who are closest to you. Sometimes people feel angry because of feeling irritable so often. Anger can also arise from a feeling that the world is not fair.
- Trauma often leads to feelings of guilt and shame. Many people blame themselves for things they did or didn't do to survive. Feeling guilty about the trauma means that you are taking responsibility for what occurred. While this may make you feel somewhat more in control, it can also lead to feelings of helplessness and depression.
- Grief and depression are also common reactions to trauma. This can include feeling down, sad, hopeless or despairing. You may cry more often. You may lose interest in people and activities you used to enjoy. You may also feel that plans you had for the future don't seem to matter anymore, or that life isn't worth living. These feelings can lead to thoughts of wishing you were dead, or doing something to hurt or kill yourself.
- Many people find it difficult to feel sexual or have sexual relationships after a traumatic experience.
- Some people increase their use of alcohol or other substances after a trauma.

AMPUTEES

The high kinetic energy delivered by modern munitions causes extensive soft-tissue zones of injury and results in wounds that are subject to more complications and may take longer to heal.

These munitions focus destructive forces on the extremity, creating a particularly complex wound with fragments of the weapon and other debris driven into it.

Battlefield wounds are initially left open because of the high risk of infection, and a staged approach to amputation surgery is necessary to obtain wound closure and a residual limb that can provide the best function. Because of the severe nature of the wounds, reconstructive procedures are often done later, even months or years after the injury.

Advances in surgical techniques, prosthetic technology and physical rehabilitation are producing some astonishing results; however, the loss of a limb or limbs and the effects of other blast-related injuries are life-altering events. Technological, emotional and pain-related needs will be long-term for these young servicemen and women, many of whom have multiple amputations and other injuries.

Any patient who undergoes an amputation, whether it is caused by a traumatic injury or disease, can develop phantom pain, the sensation of pain in a limb which is no longer part of the body, or residual limb pain, known as stump pain, in the part of the limb that has not been amputated. In addition, musculoskeletal pain in the opposite limb, back and neck is often reported. Some studies suggest that if a patient has pain in the area about to be amputated before the amputation, there is a greater likelihood of developing phantom pain.

The actual cause of phantom pain is not known. Many authorities believe that when a body part is amputated, the region of the brain responsible for perceiving sensation from that area begins to function abnormally, leading to the perception that the body part still exists.

Residual limb pain, unlike phantom pain, occurs in the body part that still exists, in the stump that remains. It typically is described as a "sharp," "burning," "electric-like," or "skin-sensitive" pain. It is also called nerve pain or neuropathic pain. Untreated or undertreated pain can devastate a person's quality of life and emotional well-being.

To learn more about chronic pain in veterans and amputees, visit the Amputee Coalition of America online at www.amputee-coalition.org and www.partnersagainstpain.com.

The Walter Reed Hospital closed its doors in July 2011 and moved to new and upgraded facilities at the National Naval Medical Center in Bethesda,

BIG ADVANCES IN PROSTHETICS RESEARCH

A Defense Department program is tapping into the realm of science fiction to develop life-like, functional prosthetic devices for wounded combat troops so they can go on to live normal lives.

Army Col. Geoff Ling, manager of the Defense Advanced Research Projects Agency's (DARPA) Revolutionizing Prosthetics programs, said the agency is making tremendous headway in advancing technology considered unimaginable just a few years ago.

Researchers at DEKA Research and Development Corp. in Manchester, NH, have developed what Ling calls a "strap-and-go arm" that users activate with the flick of a switch.

"All you have to do is strap it on, and you're ready to go," he said. "It requires no surgery or any of that stuff. All you do is literally wake up in the morning and put it on like you could a jacket, and you just go."

Three volunteers in the test program reported strong acceptance for the device that comes in three models: one for amputees who have lost a complete arm and others for those with amputations above and below the elbow.

"These arms are working just beyond anyone's wildest imagination," Ling said.

Embedded electronics enable users to activate a switch, either with a foot or their chin, to activate it. By flicking the switch, they can cycle through five different gripping actions to match the task at hand, whether it's using a pen, picking up a key, lifting a coffee cup or using a power drill.

"It's very easy to master," Ling said. "Guys who have it will tell you they can master the use of the arm in an hour or two."

All were able to "perform remarkably" with the device, he said. One tester who lost his arm at the shoulder was able to field strip and reassemble an M-16 rifle using the prosthesis. An above-the-elbow amputee was able to grab a root beer bottle off a shelf, open it with a bottle opener and drink it. Another, who lost both hands in combat, reported he now feels able to take on a civilian job.

As this effort advances, DARPA is pushing forward with even more ambitious Revolutionizing Prosthetics programs that will enable a user to control the prosthesis through thought. The limb, as envisioned, would enable users to move as they normally do, without having to think about the actual process to make it happen.

MD, and at Fort Belvoir, VA. The new facilities have cost $2.6 billion. The hospital in Bethesda is being renamed the Walter Reed National Military Medical Center. One if its facilities is the Military Advanced Training Center, a 31,000-square-foot, $10 million center which offers some of the most state-of-the-art care found anywhere in the world.

The facility combines office and counseling space with workout facilities, data gathering, high-tech simulators, and even a family lounge with a full kitchen. It is designed to bring together all the hospital's elements of advanced amputee care, but much of it also will benefit other patients, such as those suffering from traumatic brain injuries or post-traumatic stress disorder.

The gait lab has nearly doubled its size in the new building. The lab electronically records patients' movements while wearing prosthetic devices to give feedback to the patients and specialists on rehabilitation efforts. It can now record movements from 23 camera angles, up from eight, and has six force plates, up from four, that measure pressure put on the ground as steps are taken. It also added a treadmill built into the floor that will allow specialists, for the first time, to collect force-plate data from wounded warriors while running.

One of only three in the world, a high-tech computer-assisted rehabilitation environment was added to the center to help amputee soldiers adapt to real-life scenarios.

In front of a large projection screen, soldiers stand on an elevated, multi-axis platform that rocks and sways as the computer-driven scenario changes. In one scenario, the patients stand as if in a boat as it moves through a course. In other scenarios, patients are required to raise their hands while moving to hit objects that appear to be flying by. This helps patients become more stable and confident using their prosthetic devices.

Most of the equipment is standard fitness-center equipment to allow soldiers to transition from the center to a gym in their hometown or Army installation with no adjustment to their workouts, officials said.

Also among the treatment rooms is a weapons simulator to get soldiers back to shooting, a vehicle simulator to help them relearn to drive using prostheses, and areas that offer practice walking on uneven terrain features, such as sand, gravel and cobblestone.

Spinal Cord Injury (SCI)

The spinal cord is the main pathway for transmitting information between the brain and the nerves that lead to muscles, skin, internal organs and glands. Injury to the spinal cord disrupts movement, sensation and function. Paraplegia results from injury to the lower part of the spinal cord, causing paralysis of the lower part of the body, including the bowel and bladder. Tetraplegia (sometimes called quadriplegia) results from injury to the spinal cord in the neck

A new prosthesis gives service member amputees more flexibility and helps them better perform their military jobs if they choose to stay on active duty.

In 2006, Otto Bock HealthCare, a global provider of prosthetic components that started out providing devices for German World War I veterans in 1919, began developing a prosthetic knee system that is an upgrade to its already popular C-Leg. It was awarded a three-year, $1 million contract to develop a leg that will allow more service members to stay on active duty if they choose to.

The prosthesis is for above-the-knee amputees and uses a microprocessor to control the knee's hydraulic functions and anticipate the wearer's actions and make changes in real time. This gives service members greater flexibility to change speeds or directions without sacrificing stability.

Mobility is improved, allowing more movement without the user having to concentrate on the knee, said Hans-Willem van Vliet, the program manager.

The new system has more sensors, a faster hard drive, more memory, and provides smooth transitions between movements such as level-ground walking, climbing stairs, and running.

It also allows service members the ability to turn around while walking and walk backward in one fluid movement, something that is not possible with the current C-Leg. It adapts automatically between walking speeds and gaits, Vliet said. He emphasized that engineers have not simply improved the C-Leg, but have completely rebuilt the technology on the inside. Engineers are working to stretch battery life to 50 hours on one charge. This will give service members on long road marches the duration they need to reach a power supply for recharging.

Requirements also called for making the system saltwater resistant, a difficulty with the onboard computer systems. They also are planning a remote control, about the size of a car-lock remote, that will allow the user to switch among as many as 10 modes with the click of a button.

The current C-Leg allows service members two operating modes: one for walking and one for bicycling or another activity. To switch between modes, the wearer has to swing the leg forward in a jerky fashion. In some instances the user may not be able to switch modes because of limited movement. Reprogramming a mode requires a visit to a technician.

Air Force Lt. Col. Andrew Lourake, a pilot at Andrews Air Force Base, MD, was the first above-the-knee amputee to return to active duty as a pilot. He was fitted with a C-Leg five years ago. Lourake said he could not do his job without the C-Leg because it allows him to switch between walking and flying modes. Still, he said, he is impressed with the new design. The new system costs about $30,000.

area, causing paralysis to the lower body, upper body and arms. SCI requires ongoing management of impairments and prevention of related problems.

Veterans with SCI may receive monthly disability compensation. They may receive additional compensation if the injury resulted in loss of use of hands or feet or in other disabilities. The rating may include other service-connected disabilities not related to their spinal injury. Many veterans with service-connected disabilities are also entitled to vocational counseling, grants for adapted housing and automobiles, a clothing allowance and payment for home and attendant care.

The VA has the largest single network of SCI care in the nation. It provides a full range of care to over 26,000 veterans with spinal cord injuries and disorders and specialty care to about 13,000 of these veterans. The VA integrates vocational, psychological and social services within a continuum of care and addresses changing needs throughout the veteran's life.

VA services are delivered through a "hub and spoke" system of care, extending from 24 regional SCI centers offering primary and specialty care by multidisciplinary teams to the 135 SCI primary care teams or support clinics at local VA medical centers. Each primary care team has a physician, nurse and social worker, and those with support clinics may have additional team members. Newly injured veterans and active-duty members are referred to a VA SCI center for rehabilitation after being stabilized at a trauma center.

National Recreational Events

Staying active is as important to the physical and emotional well-being of people with SCI as it is to other people. The VA sponsors two annual athletic events that offer camaraderie with other SCI veterans and the opportunity to enjoy and participate in competitive sports. These are the National Veterans Wheelchair Games, which is cosponsored with the Paralyzed Veterans of America (PVA), and the National Disabled Veterans Winter Sports Clinic, cosponsored with the Disabled American Veterans.

Spinal Cord Injury and Disorders (SCI&D) Extended Care Services

SCI&D LTC Centers provide: LTC, long-stay services beyond 90 days; chronic ventilator care; skilled nursing or rehabilitation care for specific conditions or interventions; respite care; hospice care; palliative care (comfort care, death not a predicted outcome); restorative time limited care; rehabilitation therapies; psychological assessment and treatment; social work services; and age-appropriate programs for transportation, therapeutic recreation (including outings), and peer support.

SCI&D Home Care (HC) is provided through the SCI&D Center to veterans, identified by the SCI&D interdisciplinary team, in need of this care and living within a 100-mile radius of the SCI&D Center. Goals of care include maintaining health and fostering independent living.

SCI&D Respite Care is recognized as an important consideration for families and caregivers of physically dependent veterans. Each veteran using attendant care is offered respite care on the SCI&D unit in a VA medical center having an SCI&D center, unless a veteran requests its provision in another setting. The duration of any respite care admission, absent complicating medical factors, is not to exceed 14 days. However, the total of all respite care for a veteran in a year, absent complicating factors, generally does not exceed 30 days.

SCI&D Referral Guidelines recommend the conditions for treatment by each element of the SCI&D Hub and Spoke system. It is important that individuals get the right care, at the right time, in the right place. What may be a relatively minor symptom, or problem in the person without SCI&D, may indicate a grave and even life-threatening problem for the individual with SCI&D. Greater awareness of the specialized health care issues facing persons with SCI&D and guidance about the most appropriate sites of care for various health issues is needed to ensure therapeutically appropriate clinical processes.

VA Extended Care Services

VA extended care services include:

VA Nursing Home Care Unit (NHCU) provides care for veterans who have a primary diagnosis of SCI&D when eligible for care or are difficult to place in the community. Primary resources for care include skilled nursing, physical therapy, occupational therapy and recreational therapy, as well as lifetime care for veterans who are unable to be managed at home.

Contract Nursing Home Care. The VA may provide institutional LTC to mandatory veterans through contracts with community nursing homes. Contract nursing home care is provided on a limited basis to all other enrolled veterans with SCI&D in need of nursing home care while pay arrangements are pursued through federal, state, community, or personal payer methods.

State Veterans Homes Program is a grant program between the VA and the state where the VA contributes to the costs of construction and a portion of the per diem. A state veterans home is a nursing home or domiciliary for veterans owned and operated by the state in which it provides service. The admission requirements of state veterans homes vary from state to state. VA social workers at the VA medical center where the veteran is being treated can provide information about state veterans homes.

Domiciliaries are VA facilities that provide care on an ambulatory self-care basis for veterans disabled by age or disease who are not in need of acute

Table 2.1. VA Regional SCI Centers

State	Address	Telephone Number
California	VA Long Beach 5901 E. 7th St. Long Beach, CA 90822	562-826-5701
	VA Palo Alto Health Care System 3801 Miranda Ave. Palo Alto, CA 94304	650-493-3000, ext. 65870
	VA San Diego Health Care System 3350 La Jolla Village Dr. San Diego, CA 92161	858-642-3117
Florida	VA Medical Center 1201 NW 16th St. Miami, FL 33125	305-575-3174
	James A. Haley 13000 Bruce B. Downs Blvd. Tampa, FL 33612	813-972-7517
Georgia	Augusta VA Medical Center One Freedom Way Augusta, GA 30904	706-823-2216
Illinois	Edward Hines VA Hospital 5th & Roosevelt Rd. PO Box 5000-5128 Hines, IL 60141	708-202-2241
Massachusetts	VA Boston Healthcare System Brockton/West Roxbury Campuses 1400 VFW Pkwy. West Roxbury, MA 02132	857-203-5128
Minnesota	VA Medical Center 1 Veterans Dr. Minneapolis, MN 55417	612-725-2000
Missouri	Jefferson Barracks Division 1 Jefferson Barracks Dr. St. Louis, MO 63125	314-894-6677
New Jersey	VA New Jersey Healthcare System 385 Tremont Ave. East Orange, NJ 07018	973-676-1000, ext. 11302
New Mexico	VA Medical Center 1501 San Pedro SE Albuquerque, NM 87108	505-256-2849
New York	VA Medical Center 130 West Kingsbridge Rd Bronx, NY 10468	718-584-9000, ext. 5423

Table 2.1. Continued

State	Address	Telephone Number
	VA Healthcare System Castle Point, NY 12511	845-831-2000, ext. 5128
Ohio	VA Medical Center 10701 East Blvd. Cleveland, OH 44106	216-791-3800, ext. 5219
Tennessee	VA Medical Center 1030 Jefferson Ave. Memphis, TN 38104	901-577-7373
Texas	VA Medical Center 4500 South Lancaster Rd. Dallas, TX 75216	214-857-1757
	VA Medical Center 2002 Holcombe Blvd. Houston, TX 77030	713-794-7128
	South Texas Veterans Health Care System Audie L. Murphy Division 7400 Merton Minter Blvd. San Antonio, TX 78229	210-617-5257
Virginia	VA Medical Center 100 Emancipation Dr. Hampton, VA 23667	757-722-9961
	Hunter Holmes McGuire VA Medical Center 1201 Broad Rock Blvd. Richmond, VA 23249	804-675-5282
Washington	VA Puget Sound Health Care System 1660 South Columbian Way Seattle, WA 98108	206-764-2332
Wisconsin	Clement J. Zablocki Medical Center 5000 W. National Ave. Milwaukee, WI 53295	414-384-2000, ext. 41288
Puerto Rico	VA Medical Center 10 Casia St. San Juan, PR 00921	787-641-7582

hospitalization and who do not need the skilled nursing services provided in a nursing home.

Community Residential Care Homes. Any veteran placed in a VA-approved residence in the community is under the oversight of the CRC program. These programs provide health care supervision to veterans not in need of hospital or nursing home care, but who are not able to live independently and have no suitable family or significant others to provide the needed supervision and supportive care. The veteran must be capable of self-preservation with minimal assistance. Examples of CRC's enriched housing may include, but are not limited to: medical foster homes, assisted living homes, group living homes, family care homes, and psychiatric CRC homes.

Care must consist of room, board, assistance with activities of daily living and supervision as determined on an individual basis. The cost of residential care is financed by the veteran's own resources. Placement is made in residential settings inspected and approved by the appropriate VA facility, but chosen by the veteran.

Skilled Home Care is provided by VA or through contract agencies to veterans who are home bound with chronic conditions, such as SCI&D.

Home Care Services such as colostomy bag changes, dressing changes, medication administration, prosthetic device assistance, turning in bed, and transfers are defined as medical services for persons with SCI&D and may be authorized as fee-basis home health services when lack of support within the home requires institutional care and/or these services facilitate discharge from VA to community living.

Fee-Basis Bowel and Bladder Care (B&B) care is considered a supportive medical service when provided to quadriplegic and paraplegic veterans who are unable to manage these functions independently. This program is essential to allowing these veterans to reside in a non-institutional setting, improving quality of life and optimizing the health of this population. A family member or other caregiver may receive reimbursement for provision of B&B care when they have been trained and certified by SCI&D trained personnel as being competent to provide this care. Aside from family members, veterans may also recruit individuals who are willing to receive training from VA to provide these health services at a low cost.

Homemaker and/or Home Health Aide (H/HHA) program provides services as an "alternative" to nursing home care. The facility H/HHA coordinator along with the interdisciplinary team makes a clinical judgment that the veteran would, in the absence of H/HHA services, require nursing home equivalent care.

Respite Services. Respite care services provide caregivers a planned period of relief from the physical and emotional demands associated with providing care. These services may be provided by VA SCI&D Centers, VA NHCUs, purchased by VA through contract services or arranged through a community service.

Home-based Primary Care (HBPC) is available in many VA facilities and the HBPC director is responsible for planning and coordinating admission to HBPC. The SCI&D Primary Care Teams at non-SCI&D Center facilities are to be consulted to assist in planning the care and treatment of the veteran with SCI&D.

VISION LOSS

Blindness has been considered one of the most devastating disabilities that can affect an individual. The term legal blindness is, however, a deceiving one. Approximately 85 percent of people classified as legally blind have some kind of usable remaining vision.

The impact of blindness is individualized and the serviceperson who is rendered totally blind by traumatic injury requires individualized, specialized care and treatment suited to the cause of blindness, physical and medical condition, age, ability to cope with frustrating situations, learning ability, and the overall needs and lifestyle of the veteran.

Indeed a person confronted with blindness may feel limited and frustrated in performing a variety of everyday activities previously taken for granted. Such tasks as dressing, eating, writing, reading and traveling may become quite difficult to do independently. Communication with other people by ordinary means is hampered, as is the ability to keep up with the daily news and current events. Social interaction, recreation, and hobbies may be drastically limited or curtailed.

It is not uncommon for the newly blinded individual to undergo a period of personal stress, serious doubts of self-worth and self-esteem, the feeling of being less of a person, or believing the future holds little promise. Pressure and strain may then be placed on the veteran, spouse, and family.

Loss of sight affects each person differently and is capable of hindering overall functioning, including employment, recreation, social and family life, and communications. To help the service member cope with these problems, the Department of Veterans Affairs has established within the Veterans Health Administration, the Blind Rehabilitation Service to provide a wide variety of services to veterans who are blind. The Blind Rehabilitation Program is designed to improve the quality of life for veterans who are blind or severely visually impaired through the development of skills and capabilities needed for personal independence, adjustment, and successful re-integration into the community and family environment.

Elements of the Blind Rehabilitation Coordinated Services Program include: 10 Blind Rehabilitation Centers, Visual Impairment Services Teams (VIST) located at many medical centers and outpatient clinics, Blind Rehabilitation Outpatient Specialists (BROS), National Consultants and a Computer Access Training (CAT) program. In addition, there are a variety of low vision services and blind rehabilitation service delivery models within the Veterans Administration, e.g., Visual Impairment Services Outpatient programs (VISOR) and Visual Impairment Centers to Optimize Remaining Sight (VICTORS) programs.

Blind Rehabilitation Service has developed a continuum-of-care model encompassing alternative rehabilitative service delivery. The following will describe in some detail the programs offered in Blind Rehabilitation Service as well as low vision services available at local VA medical centers and outpatient clinics.

The Blind Rehabilitation Centers

The Blind Rehabilitation Centers (BRCs) provide rehabilitation to legally blind veterans. Comprehensive individualized blind rehabilitation services are provided in an inpatient medical center environment by a multidisciplinary team of providers. A specialized Computer Access Training program (CAT) is offered as a specialized inpatient rehabilitation option. BRC attendance requires ongoing daily participation in the rehabilitation process. The veteran must be able to meet travel requirements to an appropriate facility and any medical condition must be stable enough to participate in the daily classes. Blind rehabilitation services are offered on site, and throughout the local community. The management of chronic medical conditions is addressed as part of the training regime and may be improved during the stay. The many years of experience by Blind Rehabilitation staff has shown that a program of comprehensive rehabilitation is usually the best course to follow for those who are legally or totally blind. An experienced professional staff member acts as a Team Coordinator and guides the individual through a process that eventually leads to maximum adjustment to the disability, re-organization of the person's life, and return to a contributing place in the family and community. To achieve comprehensive rehabilitation, the Blind Rehabilitation Centers offer a variety of classes designed to help the veteran achieve a realistic level of independence.

In Blind Rehabilitation Centers, the veterans participate in the following courses:

Orientation and Mobility

Principles of independent travel for both low vision and totally blind veterans are taught, using a "long cane" for safe and effective travel. Maximum use of any remaining vision as an aid to travel is evaluated, low vision devices are fitted and their use is made an integral part of mobility training. Sensory training classes teach the veteran how to use remaining senses, particularly hearing, as an effective aid in travel and exercises in mental mapping show the veteran how to maintain orientation while traveling through different kinds of environments.

Instruction ranges from relatively simple routes to the increasingly complex, and gradually builds the veteran's confidence in the ability to travel independently. By the completion of the instruction, the veteran should have a realistic picture of his or her travel capacity and be able to travel independently in both familiar and unfamiliar areas.

Living Skills

This phase of the rehabilitation program generally consists of several areas: communications, activities of daily living and independent living program.

Communications: Instruction in this area is designed to replace or restore the ease of written and spoken communication. Opportunities to learn and utilize Braille, typing, handwriting, telling time, management of financial records, and use of tape recorders and other electronic equipment are all provided to the veteran. These courses equip the veteran with the means to help keep up with current events, correspondence, personal files, and maintain, as far as possible, normal means of communications with other people.

Activities of Daily Living: The veteran is also taught various techniques, methods and use of devices that can aid in doing countless daily tasks. The area ranges from such simple things as shining shoes or making a cup of coffee, to complex situations such as arranging an entire wardrobe, shopping, kitchen organization, and preparation of complete meals. The emphasis is on learning by doing; techniques and methods are taught and then integrated into the veteran's daily routine. By the completion of the program, the veteran should be capable of handling these various tasks with much greater, or complete, independence. A fringe benefit is increased independence in the home situation, lessening the burden of care for the family and easing tensions that may have arisen.

Independent Living Program: Each Blind Rehabilitation Center has established an independent living program in the living skills department, designed primarily for those veterans who will be living alone after rehabilitation. After extensive instruction, the veteran is afforded the opportunity to practice the acquired skills under minimal or no supervision. Thus the veteran can experience on a practical basis the problems encountered in living independently and can provide solutions to these problems.

The Living Skills instructors arrange consultation with the medical center dietetic service, so that each veteran has the opportunity for ongoing meetings on a one-to-one basis with a dietitian. This is especially important for those veterans who require special diets; they can be educated concerning these diets and the need to follow them as closely as possible. Detailed instructions in preparation of special diets can be provided.

Manual Skills

This area provides the veteran the means to develop organizational skills, awareness of the environment, safe and efficient work habits, spatial relationships, and an understanding of tactile ability.

The manual skills area is not vocational training, although some veterans have developed vocational interests or hobbies from it. Frequently, manual skills training enables a veteran to resume performing home repairs in a workshop at home, or other related activities, thus further adding to the person's self-confidence and quality of life.

Visual Skills

Approximately 85 percent of all veterans entering a Blind Rehabilitation Center have some remaining vision that may be useful in many situations. For these veterans, a thorough visual skills evaluation is performed. Each veteran is given a comprehensive eye exam shortly after admission.

An important goal of the visual skills area is to help the veterans develop a realistic assessment and understanding of their visual capability and limitations so that they may better use their vision in daily life.

Computer Access Training Section (CATS) for the Blind

Training encompasses comprehensive instruction on access hardware/software, computer literacy, and familiarization with the computer keyboard, fundamentals of operating systems and fundamentals of word processing as well as Internet access and email.

Physical Conditioning

The onset of visual loss may interrupt or stop completely a pattern of exercise or activities that many veterans have incorporated into their daily lives, thus causing a decrease in muscular tone and stamina. Under medical supervision, each center offers a physical conditioning area.

Exercises and activities can range from the relatively sedentary to relatively vigorous, depending on the ability and need of the veteran. The exercise programs are usually self-directed by the individual veterans. Even a moderate program of regular exercise can assist many veterans in management of complicated medical situations.

Recreation

A broad array of recreational activities and interests is offered, for groups and for individuals.

Adjustment to Blindness

The difficult area of emotional and behavioral adjustment to blindness is the chief role of the clinical psychologist, social worker and the rehabilitation team.

Through individual counseling sessions, group meetings, and a variety of information techniques, they help each veteran deal with blindness and learn to cope with it. The entire rehabilitation program attempts to develop a therapeutic environment in which the total staff assists the veteran in coming to grips with the reality of visual loss.

Life at the Rehabilitation Center

Teaching activities at the Blind Rehabilitation Center follow the usual government work routine, 8 hours per day, 5 days a week. Classes of varying duration are scheduled throughout the workday. The veteran is expected to participate in a full day of training each day unless contraindicated due to physical limitations. After the workday is completed, each veteran is permitted to go on pass, subject to medical and administrative clearance. Families, friends, or relatives are welcome to visit in the evenings or on weekends, but not during the workday. All the Blind Rehabilitation Centers require that veterans remain in the center for the first weekend so that they may quickly adapt to the rehabilitation environment.

Length of the Rehabilitation Program

The length of the rehabilitation program varies from veteran to veteran. In addition to visual levels, the veteran's general health, emotional condition, learning ability and motivation will determine the length of stay. The first week of the program is spent evaluating the veteran's overall condition and assessing the veteran's general and specific needs. After a team assessment, which includes the veteran, intensive rehabilitation begins and a projection of length of training made. This projection can be updated as circumstances and the veteran's need warrant. Veterans should remember that rehabilitation is a dynamic process and cannot be rushed. This is required to thoroughly learn skills and incorporate them into the lifestyle.

Blind Rehabilitation Centers

American Lake Blind Rehabilitation Center
VA Puget Sound Health Care System
Tacoma, WA 98493-5000
Phone: 253-582-8440

Augusta Blind Rehabilitation Center
VA Medical Center
1 Freedom Way
Augusta, GA 30904-6285
Phone: 706-733-0188

Central Blind Rehabilitation Center
Edward Hines Jr. VA Medical Center
5th & Roosevelt Road
P.O. Box 5000
Hines, IL 60141
Phone: 708-202-8387

VA Connecticut Healthcare System
West Haven Campus VA Medical Center
950 Campbell Avenue
West Haven, CT 06516
Phone: 203-932-5711

Puerto Rico Blind Rehabilitation Center
VA Medical Center
10 Casis Street
San Juan, PR 00921-3201
Phone: 787-641-8325

Southeastern Blind Rehabilitation Center
VA Medical Center
700 South 19th Street
Birmingham, AL 35233
Phone: 205-933-8101

Southwestern Blind Rehabilitation Center
Southern Arizona VA Health Care System
3601 South 6th Avenue
Tucson, AZ 85723
Phone: 520-629-4643

Waco Blind Rehabilitation Center
VA Medical Center
4800 Memorial Drive
Waco, TX 76711
Phone: 254-297-3755

Western Blind Rehabilitation Center
VA Palo Alto Health Care System
3801 Miranda Avenue
Palo Alto, CA 94304-1290
Phone: 650-493-5000

West Palm Beach
VA Medical Center
7305 N. Military Trail
West Palm Beach, FL 33410-6400
Phone: 561-422-8425

Department of Veterans Affairs
Blind Rehabilitation Service
810 Vermont Ave., NW
Washington, DC 20422
Phone: 202-273-8483
VA website: www.va.gov/blindrehab

BURNS

Burns constitute between 5% and 20% of combat casualties during conventional warfare, and are particularly common in combat involving armored fighting vehicles. Even relatively small burns can be incapacitating.

Brooke Army Medical Center in San Antonio, TX, is the Defense Department's premier burn treatment center. It has a remarkable success record because burn victims get there quickly—often just 36 hours from injury in Iraq to the U.S. military hospital in Landstuhl, Germany, and then to Texas. Doctors there have treated many hundreds of patients with severe burn injuries from the wars in Iraq and Afghanistan.

On arrival, burn victims go through debridement, a process to remove any blisters or dead skin. Once the patient's condition is stable they go to the operating room where doctors cut away dead tissue to prevent infection. Then, exposed areas are covered with skin grafts.

COMPUTER AND ELECTRONIC ADAPTIVE PROGRAM (CAP) SUPPORTS WOUNDED SERVICE MEMBERS

Our service members, sailors, airmen and marines are returning every day from deployment in Operation Enduring Freedom and Operation Iraqi Freedom. Yet, many of them are not returning to their duty assignments. Instead, they are recovering at various Military Treatment Facilities (MTFs) because of injuries they sustained in the global war on terror.

CAP is committed to providing assistive technology and support to returning wounded service members. Accommodations are available for wounded service members with vision or hearing loss, upper extremity amputees as well as persons with communication and other disabilities to access the computer and telecommunication environment. CAP is available to provide accommodations to service members in the following phases.

Recovery and Rehabilitation

By working directly with staff in the intensive care units, physical and occupational therapist, audiologist and ophthalmologist, CAP can begin to introduce service members to assistive technology and accommodation support, reducing frustration and providing encouragement. One example of this technology is an augmentative communication device which enables easy communication between the patient and medical staff as well as family members.

Transition

In our efforts to ensure a smooth transition from patient to independent living, CAP is working to integrate assistive technologies into housing facilities and employment training centers at the MTFs to support the reemployment process. This technology includes alternative pointing devices, assistive listening devices, voice recognition software and Closed Circuit Televisions. The technology is being introduced to wounded service members to use at their living quarters, allowing them to email family and friends, improve their quality of care and begin the process of finding employment opportunities.

Employment

CAP is working with the Department of Defense (DoD) and the Department of Veterans' Affairs to assist in the "reemployment process." If a service member remains on active duty or becomes a civilian within DoD or another Federal agency, CAP can provide the work-related accommodation to the agency free of charge for internship and/or permanent employment.

Resources (see also chapter 10)

Military Severely Injured Center: www.military.com/support
U.S. Army Wounded Warrior Program (AW2): wtc.army.mil/aw2
Returning Service Members: www.oefoif.va.gov
REALifelines: www.dol.gov/vets/programs/Real-life/main.htm
www.careeronestop.org/militarytransition

Without skin, burn patients cannot maintain their core body temperatures, so patients' rooms and the operating room are kept between 90 and 100 degrees. The center uses two freezers as a tissue bank. Grafts are taken from the patient—if there is enough unburned tissue. If not, they use synthetic skin, pig skin or skin from cadavers. Sometimes, epicells are grown in the lab from biopsies of the patient's skin. Doctors also must control the patient's pain. Patients endure excruciating pain. The recovery process is lengthy and may involve many operations and skin grafts.

When a person experiences a burn injury or an amputation, life changes for that person. Most people undergo the grieving process. The first stage of the grieving process is shock and disbelief, then depression, anger, and finally, acceptance.

Psychological as well as physical support is essential as part of the recovery process and cognitive therapy is important in helping burn patients deal with how they view their appearance and how others react to it.

3

From the First Day

Let us strive on to finish the work we are in; to bind up the nation's wounds; to care for him who shall have borne the battle, and for his widow, and his orphan.

—Abraham Lincoln, second inaugural address

Each service handles the notification of the primary next of kin (PNOK) and secondary next of kin (SNOK) differently based on the degree of injury. It is, therefore, advisable for service members before they deploy to make families aware of the notification and transition process that will take place should they become wounded.

WHAT IS A CASUALTY?

According to the DoD, a casualty is "any person who is lost to the organization by reason of having been declared beleaguered, besieged, captured, dead, diseased, detained, duty status whereabouts unknown, injured, ill, interned, missing, missing in action, or wounded."

When a service member is killed, injured, gets sick, or is hospitalized, he or she becomes a "casualty." The service member is then further categorized according to his/her casualty type and the casualty status.

There are seven casualty statuses:

1. Deceased
2. Duty status-whereabouts unknown (DUSTWUN)
3. Missing
4. Very seriously ill or injured (VSI)

5. Seriously ill or injured (SI)
6. Incapacitating illness or injury (III)
7. Not seriously injured (NSI)

Some Basic Definitions

Wounded in Action (WIA). A service member who has incurred an injury due to an external agent or cause, other than the victim of a terrorist activity, is classified as WIA.

    Disease and Non-Battle Injury (DNBI). A person who is not a battle casualty, but who is lost to the organization by reason of disease or injury. It also includes service members who are missing due to enemy action or internment. When someone is wounded they will be further categorized in one of the following statuses:

    Very Seriously Injured (VSI). The casualty status of a person whose injury/illness is classified to be of such severity that life is imminently endangered.

    Seriously Ill or Injured (SI). The casualty status of a person whose illness or injury is classified to be of such severity that there is cause for immediate concern, but no imminent danger to life.

    Incapacitating Illness or Injury (III). The casualty status of a person whose illness or injury requires hospitalization, but medical authority does not classify as very seriously ill or injured or seriously ill or injured; the illness or injury makes the person physically or mentally unable to communicate with the next of kin.

    Not Seriously Injured (NSI). The casualty status of a person whose injury or illness may or may not require hospitalization but not classified by a medical authority as very seriously injured (VSI), seriously injured (SI), or incapacitating illness or injury (III); the person is able communicate with the Next of Kin (NOK).

    Duty Status-Whereabouts Unknown (DUSTWUN). A transitory casualty status that is used when the responsible commander suspects the member may be a casualty whose absence is involuntary, but does not feel sufficient evidence currently exists to make a definite determination of missing or deceased.

HOW TRAUMATIC STRESS REACTIONS CAN AFFECT FAMILIES

- Stress reactions may interfere with a service member's ability to trust and be emotionally close to others. As a result, families may feel emotionally cut off from the service member.

A WOUNDED WARRIOR'S VIEWPOINT

From the point of injury on the battlefield, the service member has been moved quickly through an array of treatment facilities based on the geographic location where he or she was injured and the type of injury sustained. Most service members are treated at the scene of injury by a combat life saver or field medic, then moved to an aid station awaiting evacuation to a combat support hospital (CSH).

Once at the CSH, stabilizing measures were taken and the service member given medical treatment based on the injury. The doctors at the CSH determined what the extent of injury was and began the procedure to evacuate the service member to the United States. From the CSH the service member was transported to the aircraft and began the journey back to the U.S. with a stopover in Germany. At each point along the way the service member was re-evaluated. Sometimes a delay occurs in Germany if the service member required further stabilization before travel. After days of travel and transport, the service member arrived at the MTF.

Throughout this evacuation process the service member may have been heavily medicated or unconscious. The speed of transition from the battlefield to safety in the U.S. is disorienting for anyone, but with the addition of injury and medication, it can take on a surreal quality for the service member. For those who were unconscious, their last recollection is from the point of injury or before and they awaken to find themselves in unfamiliar surroundings and seriously wounded.

At times, communication is hampered by the injury itself, pain medications, or attached medical equipment. The service member who was just days before performing duties in a hostile environment is now a patient in a hospital bed awaiting an uncertain fate. Even the unit the service member belongs to may change if the service member is assigned to the Medical Holding Company at the MTF. Service members strongly identify with their unit and may feel abandoned by their unit or in turn may feel they, even though injured, have abandoned the unit.

The service member has received both a physical trauma and a psychological/emotional trauma. As with any serious injury, there lies ahead a road to recovery that is full of challenge and uncertainty that taxes both the body and the spirit. The service member may be facing a changed physical appearance, changed physical abilities, damaged mental processes from traumatic brain injury, and the resulting emotional trauma. In addition, the service member is undergoing the readjustment from the battlefield to home.

- A returning war veteran may feel irritable and have difficulty communicating, which may make it hard to get along with him or her.
- A returning veteran may experience a loss of interest in family social activities.
- Veterans with PTSD may lose interest in sex and feel distant from their spouses.
- Traumatized war veterans often feel that something terrible may happen "out of the blue" and can become preoccupied with trying to keep themselves and family members safe.
- Just as war veterans are often afraid to address what happened to them, family members are frequently fearful of examining the traumatic events as well. Family members may want to avoid talking about the trauma or related problems. They may avoid talking because they want to spare the survivor further pain or because they are afraid of his or her reaction.
- Family members may feel hurt, alienated, or discouraged because the veteran has not been able to overcome the effects of the trauma. Family members may become angry or feel distant from the veteran.

THE IMPORTANT ROLE OF FAMILIES IN RECOVERY

The primary source of support for the returning service member is likely to be his or her family.

Families can help the veteran not withdraw from others. Families can provide companionship and a sense of belonging, which can help counter the veteran's feeling of separateness because of his or her experiences. Families can provide practical and emotional support for coping with life stressors.

If the veteran agrees, it is important for family members to participate in treatment. It is also important to talk about how the post-trauma stress is affecting the family and what the family can do about it. Adult family members should also let their loved ones know that they are willing to listen if the service member would like to talk about war experiences. Family members should talk with treatment providers about how they can help in the recovery effort.

THE NOTIFICATION PROCESS

In the event of a service member's injury or illness, only the primary next of kin (PNOK) will be notified. This notification may be by telephone. All notified families will have ready access to information as it becomes available. In all death and missing cases, the PNOK and secondary next of kin (SNOK), and any other person listed on DD Form 93 (Record of Emergency Data), will be notified in person.

The notification will be made as a matter of highest priority, taking precedence over all other responsibilities the notifier has. Whenever possible, the notifier's grade is equal to or higher than the grade of the casualty. When the PNOK is also a service member, the notifier's grade will be equal to or higher than the grade of the PNOK. Personal notification will generally be made between 0600 and 2200 hours local time and the PNOK is always notified first.

Although each service's notification process is slightly different, in general the process is as follows:

- The service will notify all PNOK and SNOK as soon as possible, generally within 24–48 hours
- In injury cases deemed to be VSI or SI, the PNOK is normally notified by telephone
- For minor injuries, notification generally comes through other channels (i.e., the hospital or directly from the service member)

The service member who does the "official" notification is not a health care professional, and they cannot offer explanations of injury or medical terms. A "Needs Assessment" checklist is done within hours of official notification to help coordinate travel for the family if necessary. It takes an average of four to five days to move the service member from the battlefield to most major army medical centers, although a longer delay could occur. This means that there will be time between the notification of the family and actual travel.

The Primary Next of Kin (PNOK)

The person most closely related to the casualty is considered the PNOK for notification and assistance purposes. This is normally the spouse for married persons and the parents for unmarried service members/individuals. The precedence of NOK with equal relationships to the casualty is governed by seniority (age). Equal relationship situations include divorced parents, children, and siblings. Minor children's rights are exercised by their parents or legal guardian. The adult NOK is usually the first person highest in the line of succession who has reached the age of eighteen. Even if a minor, the spouse is always considered the PNOK.

Delays in Notification of Family Members

The number one reason causing a delay in notification to families that the service member has been wounded or injured is incorrect phone numbers provided on the emergency information data card. It is **essential** that the service member keeps this information updated. Precious time is wasted when military officials have to track down correct notification numbers for family members. Delays are also common when the family member leaves the area without notifying the unit Rear Detachment Commander or Family Readiness Point of Contact. The number one rule of thumb is to let someone in the unit know that you are leaving the area and to provide them with a working phone number where you can be reached should they need to contact you.

Receiving Updates

The service will pass information to PNOK as it becomes available. Since the PNOK will be notified of updates, families/friends should use the PNOK as a focal point for sharing information internally. In the first hours after the incident, information may be limited. If there is no solid evidence a particular service member was involved in the incident, but military officials have reason to believe the service member was involved, families will be given a "believed to be" notification. This simply tells the family that the military has good reason to believe their loved one was involved and that they will be provided updates as they become available. This type of notification will be delivered only when there is overwhelming reason to believe their service member was involved. If it is "believed to be killed" or "believed to be missing," PNOK and SNOK will be notified in person. If it is "believed to be injured," only the primary next of kin will be notified by telephone. All family members who have been notified originally will be kept informed of developments in their cases.

Visiting

For very seriously injured/ill (VSI) or seriously injured/ill (SI) patients, the primary next of kin (PNOK) can be issued Invitational Travel Orders (ITOs) if the attending physician determines it is essential to the recovery of the patient and it is verified by the hospital commander. The services can provide transportation for up to three family members when a service member is classified as Very Seriously Ill/Injured (VSI) or Seriously Ill/Injured (SI), as determined by the attending physician and hospital commander upon injury. ITOs will be offered to immediate family members (spouse, children, mother, father, siblings [including step] OR those acting in loco parentis. The service point of contact/notifier or hospital will provide information concerning travel regulations. Transportation and lodging are provided for up to three family members in two week increments. Wounded service members' cases are evaluated every two-weeks and at the discretion of the attending physician, family members may be authorized additional time at the bedside.

Travel and Transportation Orders (T&TOs) are prepared for the family members and flight reservations are made for them. They must have approved travel orders issued before departing to the designated MTF for the government to pay for the airline tickets, per diem (allowance for food) and lodging.

Each family member's T&TOs include only one round-trip ticket from the home of that family member to the military treatment facility and back to the home. If traveling by car, the government reimburses the mileage from the family member's home to the MTF and back home. T&TOs do not cover mileage incurred while at the designated MTF.

T&TOs for family members of patients will cover the cost of travel, lodging and per diem for a pre-determined period of time, usually 30 days.

Occasionally, in the case of a non-serious injury, the time could be 15 days. The dates of coverage are listed on the orders. It is important to note that the period of time the orders are issued for may change. Minor children are put on orders for a period of five days only. If children stay past the five-day period, the cost is the responsibility of the family.

If the service member is still an inpatient at the hospital at the end of the orders, the attending physician can request an extension which must be approved. If approval is given, another set of orders is then issued for a set number of days, again usually 15 or 30 days. This process occurs repeatedly while the service member is an inpatient at the MTF. While the service member is an inpatient, the DA WIA is the issuing authority on the T&TOs. Family members should be aware of the end date on the travel orders and contact their MTF liaison to ensure the extension and new orders have been received.

Make sure you get a copy of each set of new orders and keep them in a safe place.

Orders can be terminated if it is determined that the service member no longer requires the family's assistance, or if the presence of the family is negatively impacting the service member; the service member is discharged from the hospital; or the service member is transferred to another treatment facility.

T&TOs are terminated when the service member is discharged from the hospital. At the time of discharge, if the service member needs to receive further treatment as an outpatient and is unable to function independently, a competent medical authority will make a determination if the service member needs a non-medical attendant (NMA) for assistance with daily living. If an attendant is needed and the request is approved, orders will be issued at the MTF and are for one person requested by the service member.

If this determination is made, then the T&TOs are closed out and the NMA orders are issued with no lapse in per diem. Discharge planning begins the day the service member arrives at the MTF.

The care team assigned to the service member will keep the family informed of any upcoming change in status such as moving to another treatment facility

FISHER HOUSE FOUNDATION AND HERO MILES

Fisher House Foundation is best known for the network of 54 comfort homes on the grounds of military and VA major medical centers—more are planned. The houses are 18,000 to 20,000 square foot homes, with up to 20 suites, donated to the military and VA by the Fisher family of New York through the Fisher House Foundation. The Foundation provides support to families of patients receiving care at the nearby medical center and has ensured that families of service men and women wounded or injured in Operation Iraqi Freedom and Operation Enduring Freedom do not pay for their stay at a Fisher House or other base facility if they are on a wait list.

Reservations for the Fisher House are for a minimum of 5 days and maximum of 30 days, and must be coordinated through the Department of Social Work. The maximum stay is subject to re-evaluation for medical reasons and space availability. The ongoing presence of a waiting list prevents Fisher House arrangements from being made prior to arrival at the MTF.

Each family is entitled to ONE bedroom, and most bedrooms hold a maximum of 3 people. You must keep the staff informed of who is staying with you, or if there are any changes following your check-in.

Grandparents and other relatives are welcome, provided space is available. If space is especially limited, the room must be vacated each morning with key returned to Guest House. Reservations for non-immediate family members will be handled on a day-by-day basis.

If you plan to be away from the Fisher House for more than four nights, you must check out completely so that your room is available to other families. It is recommended that you keep the staff informed of your plans every two to three days so that they may better accommodate others.

No medical services or procedures of any type are provided by Fisher House staff.

Most importantly, you should be aware that Fisher House is a volunteer operation, and while you are here, you are one of the volunteers! We appreciate your cooperation and any extra help you can give.

General Living: Linens are provided in your room. Free washers, dryers, and other cleaning supplies are in the laundry room. You will also find cleaning supplies under your sink in your bathroom. Rollaway beds and portable cribs/playpens may be checked out from the manager.

Kitchen: Prompt and thorough clean-ups of the kitchen and dining area are vital, in fairness to those who use these areas after you. Mark your own food with your name and date, and store in your assigned food locker and a designated area in the refrigerator.

Cooking must occur in the kitchen and food should only be eaten in the dining room or kitchen.

Hero Miles Program

This program has provided more than 10,000 tickets to Iraqi Freedom and Enduring Freedom hospitalized service members and their families, worth more than $12 million.

Fisher House™ is proud to partner with Hero Miles in support of our wounded and injured service men and women and their families. Hero Miles has partnerships with the following airlines:

- AirTran Airways
- Alaska Airlines
- American Airlines
- Continental Airlines
- Delta Air Lines
- Frontier Airlines
- Midwest Airlines
- Northwest Airlines
- United Airlines
- US Airways

Please note program agreements with individual airlines only permit airline tickets for military hospitalized as a result of their service in Iraq, Afghanistan, or surrounding areas, and their families. These tickets cannot be used for R&R travel or emergency leave.

Tickets will be issued to service members with ordinary leave for five or more days. It is important that you understand that you must comply with all terms and conditions, to include payment of the September 11 security fee (normally not to exceed $10 per round trip). Reservation and ticket agents are not authorized to make exceptions to the stated terms and conditions.

For more information, go to www.fisherhouse.org.

Other Options

Air Charity Network (formerly Angel Flight America) is a charitable organization that operates a network of several independent member organizations coordinating free or discounted air transportation to patients and their families to and from distant medical care and treatment facilities in the United States.

Short distance trips: A network of volunteer pilots using their own light aircraft provide transportation for patients and their families traveling less than 1,000 miles. These trips are coordinated through 6 regional organizations.

Discount air ambulance: The "Air Compassion America" program (ACAM) assists in arranging air ambulance transportation, sometimes at a discount, for patients, and their families, requiring stretcher transportation with medical monitoring or other en route care services. ACAM does not provide transportation directly. For more information call (866) 270-9198, or visit the ACAM website at www.aircompassionamerica.org.

Commercial flights: MercyMedical Airlift (MMA) provides access to a variety of charitable airline ticket programs for ambulatory outpatients traveling more than 1,000 miles. For more information call (800) 296-1217.

The Red Cross works with the military aid societies (Army Emergency Relief, Navy Marine Corps Relief Society, Air Force Aid Society and Coast Guard Mutual Assistance) to provide financial assistance for emergency travel. Local Red Cross chapters are listed in local telephone directories and online at www.redcross.org, under "Find Your Local Red Cross."

The various military relief or aid societies can provide interest-free loans, grants or a combination of loans and grants to cover emergency travel expenses for the families of injured or ill service members. If a service member's family is not near an installation for the service member's service branch, the family may seek assistance at an installation.

or moving from an inpatient to an outpatient status. When the time has come to return home, the Tactical Surgeon's Liaison Office will arrange travel. The family must close out the last set of travel orders before leaving the MTF.

Reimbursement

Each set of travel orders must be closed out and the travel voucher for reimbursement submitted to the Finance Office. There is a liaison located at the hospital to assist with all questions about T&TOs and this liaison will assist the family with the forms necessary to submit travel vouchers as will the Finance Office. You will need your bank account number and the bank routing number for reimbursement of the T&TOs which is done by direct deposit. This information is usually found on a check. Bring your receipt for lodging if staying at a local hotel. The receipt must show a zero balance.

Each set of travel orders will be reimbursed. For example if the first set of orders is from June 1 to June 30, on July 1st you submit your voucher for reimbursement. If the next set of orders is for July 1 to July 30, then on July 31 you submit another voucher for reimbursement.

The reimbursement rate (per diem) is in addition to the cost of lodging, up to the allowable government nightly rate. For family members staying in on-post lodging on T&TOs, the cost of lodging is billed directly to the government. There is no reimbursement for telephone calls, taxis in and around the area, rental cars, or mileage in and around the area.

Advances or travel advances are allowed on the first set of travel orders. Once you arrive at the MTF, tell the liaison that an advance is needed. A finance representative will come to you. You will need a copy of your orders and a picture ID. Advances are given in cash. They must be repaid either by being deducted from the travel voucher reimbursement at the end of the travel orders **or** taken from your bank account if the advance is greater than the amount to be reimbursed. Before getting an advance, make sure your service member is going to remain at the MTF for the period of time you are receiving the advance. The advance should be budgeted for the length of the orders. For example, you can request a 15-day advance against a set of 30-day travel orders. The amount received will need to last until the end of the 30-day period and for the amount of time it takes to receive reimbursement once the voucher is filed. In the above example, if receiving a 15-day travel advance against a 30-day set of travel orders, the reimbursement for that 30-day period would be the 30-day amount minus the 15-day travel advance.

You may return to your home for a period of up to 7 to 10 days to take care of business without losing your travel orders. You will not receive the per diem for the days you are at home nor will the government pay for your travel home. You will need a form granting you permission to leave and retain orders. Get a copy of that form when it is signed. Before booking your flight check to see if you qualify for Hero Miles, a program that offers free airline travel. You will have to check out of your local hotel if you are being reimbursed for the room, then check back in when returning for your trip home.

Traveling Without T&TOs

If you travel without T&TOs, you are responsible for your own lodging, food, and transportation. When T&TOs are not authorized, there are other avenues of receiving free airline tickets to visit your service member. The nonprofit Fisher House Foundation has teamed up with Operation Hero Miles to provide eligible service members undergoing treatment at a military medical center incident to their service in Iraq, Afghanistan, or the surrounding areas with a complimentary, round-trip airline ticket. The tickets are available to eligible family and friends as well. Please note that the Hero Miles are not subject to the same regulations on who may travel as the T&TOs. The request form is available for pick up at the Service member Family Assistance Center (SFAC). The request must come from the patient. Ticket eligibility is determined by the Fisher House Foundation.

There are multiple ticket restrictions. Restrictions may differ based on your MTF location. In addition, if you are going to try to use Operation Hero Miles, get approval through the Fisher House Foundation first. Don't pay for

TAKING CARE OF YOU

A Family Member's Trauma

From the moment you were informed that your service member was deploying into a combat zone, your life altered. The normal routine shifted to include the underlying concern felt when a loved one is in harm's way. The day you received notification that your service member was wounded, you were wounded as well. Families are connected: what happens to one member affects all the other members of the family. While attention is focused on supporting your service member, time needs to be spent as well acknowledging your own traumatic experience, and the ongoing effects this experience will have on you and your life.

Notification can be a traumatic experience in and of itself. Even when you know that your service member is in a combat zone and anything can happen, it is still a shock when you receive a phone call stating that something has. That phone call triggered a series of events that eventually led you to travel from the comfort of your home to the unfamiliar hospital bedside of your service member. Travel, even under the best of circumstances, is a stressful event. When combined with reuniting with your seriously wounded service member it becomes even more so. All these experiences in such a short amount of time can be overwhelming, and then you begin to factor in the reality of the injuries and condition of your service member. Life can suddenly feel out of control.

the tickets using your credit card. The foundation will provide you with the information on how to make reservations.

If you are a military family member with an ID card, check the surrounding area for all nearby military installations that might have lodging. On-post lodging at the MTF is obviously a first choice. However, be aware that families traveling on T&TOs will have priority as will wounded service members on outpatient status. Make contact with the Service member Family Assistance Center (SFAC) for information about availability of lodging and suggestions for local hotels. Also, make use of your own sources for discounts, such as motor clubs, retirement associations, non-profits, etc. Utilize every resource that you can to avoid incurring a financial burden at an already stressful time.

Once you are at the MTF, immediately check in with the SFAC so that they can assist you. There are resources available for all families, not just those who travel on orders. The SFAC has access to various resources. Army Community Service has a welcome packet that can orient you to the area. If you choose to travel on your own, without orders from DA WIA, then understand that you will not have the same privileges as those who have traveled under

Whether you are a spouse, parent, child or other relative of the service member, your life has been irrevocably changed by the events that brought you here. Change is a challenging thing and often uncomfortable while you adapt to the new reality the change has brought to your life. With change, something of the old way of life is lost, and as with all loss, there is a normal period where grieving occurs. No one can know what your loss is. Each of us is unique, and what may be significant to one person may not be to another. Your grieving process is personal. Take some time to think about what you have lost.

Understand that the extent of your own loss is not fully apparent now. It will take time to realize how much your life will be changed by this experience. Be patient with yourself while you come to grips with the shift in your life.

Your trauma is real. While you might tell yourself it is nothing compared to what your service member is enduring, it will have an effect on you. Being aware of that gives you some measure of control to lessen that effect. You have the right to feel pain and sorrow. Take care of yourself. Focus on what you have the power to do: that is, to change your own actions or reactions. Actively pursue stress management. Utilize the resources available to you. Seek out and utilize support services for yourself and your children. The social worker assigned to your service member is there for you as well. Your entire family has been wounded along with your service member, and it deserves the same care and concern as you are giving your service member.

orders. The military operates under laws and regulations, and organizations associated with the military are bound to follow those laws and regulations.

DEPRESSION

There are some common signs that might indicate depression, but getting a doctor's opinion is the first step to evaluation. Signs and symptoms include:

Symptoms of Adult Depression

- Persistent sad or empty mood
- Loss of interest or pleasure in ordinary activities
- Changes in appetite or sleep
- Decreased energy or fatigue
- Inability to concentrate, make decisions

COPING WITH STRESS

Physical signs of a stress response include:

- Rapid heartbeat
- Headaches
- Stomachaches
- Muscle tension

Emotional signs of stress can be both positive and upsetting:

- Excitement, frustration, anxiety
- Exhilaration, nervousness, anger
- Joy, discouragement

MANAGING STRESS

Stress management involves relaxing as well as tensing up. Relaxation actually is a part of the normal stress response.

When faced with life's challenges, people not only tense up to react rapidly and forcefully, but they also become calm in order to think clearly and act with control.

Techniques for managing stress include:

- Body and mental relaxation
- Positive thinking
- Problem solving
- Anger control
- Time management
- Exercise
- Responsible assertiveness
- Interpersonal communication

Physical benefits of managing stress include:

- Better sleep, energy, strength, and mobility
- Reduced tension, pain, blood pressure, heart problems, and infectious illnesses

Emotional benefits of managing stress include:

- Increased quality of life and well-being
- Reduced anxiety, depression, and irritability

- Feelings of guilt, hopelessness or worthlessness
- Thoughts of death or suicide

Symptoms of Adolescent Depression

- Loss of interest in school and regular activities; drop in school performance
- Withdrawal from friends and family
- Negative thoughts of self and future
- Difficulty making decisions

YOU AS YOUR SERVICE MEMBER'S ADVOCATE

If you have traveled to the MTF on travel and transportation orders (T&TOs), then the medical team has determined it is in your service member's best interest to have you by their side during this initial phase of the recovery process. You may have made the trip to the MTF without T&TOs at your service member's request. Everyone involved in this recovery effort, from the medical staff to supporting agencies, has the service member's best interest at heart and yours as well.

Your service member came to be at the MTF as a result of sustaining an injury that requires medical treatment that may tax the limits of their physical and emotional resources.

- Engage the care team from the beginning and establish a relationship that is both open and honest to best benefit your service member. Make sure that you thoroughly understand both the diagnosis (what medically has occurred and is occurring) and the prognosis (the impact this will have on your service member, the outcome) so that you are aware of the optimal outcome and the plan to achieve that outcome. Be aware that your service member's condition can change and both the diagnosis and prognosis may change accordingly.
- Maintain harmony with the care team, especially during the difficult times. Expect that some information may be unpleasant to hear. Remind yourself that everyone is focused on the same thing, working toward the best outcome for your service member. When things get tough, your service member needs the unified support the most. Be a positive team member.
- Know when the daily rounds are made and be there to take notes each time the care team assesses the status of your service member. Write down the terms used (spelling counts) and what those terms mean. Write down the treatment plan, and update it when necessary. Become familiar with the daily routine of care for your service member. Be aware of shift changes and times

when the staff is less available. The medical team takes care of many patients, but you are there to take care of one: your service member.

- Ask questions and identify who your primary point of contact is. Write down questions as they occur to you between rounds, so that you remember them for the next time. The focus of the health care team is on the service member during these visits. Being organized and prepared by having your questions written and taking notes will maximize the exchange of information. Remember, the care team has other patients to see and time is limited, so prepare beforehand. Keep a written copy of the treatment plan and daily routine with you at the hospital.
- Know when your service member is scheduled to undergo medical procedures such as diagnostic testing, procedures, or therapies. Be aware of any requirements that must be met before a test, such as no eating or drinking for a certain number of hours, and make sure your service member sticks to it. If the schedule changes or a test does not occur, check in with the care team to find out why.
- Know what medications are given, when, and possible side effects. If a medication is missed, ask about it. If you notice a possible side effect, bring it to the attention of the medical staff. Your observations of your service member's overall level of comfort and behaviors are important to enhancing the care received. You may notice your service member having side effects from medication, showing discomfort before pain medication is due, becoming restless while sleeping, not eating, having difficulty while eating, or other issues that concern you.
- Write down your observations that you would like to bring to the notice of the medical care team. Be specific about when the issue arose, how long it lasted, and the intensity of the event. This applies to the emotional state of your service member as well. The healing process involves both the physical and emotional, so speak up about behavioral changes you notice. You will spend more time with your service member than the health care team can, and your insight is valuable.
- You can help protect your service member from infection by being a vigilant hand washer as a first line of defense. Wash your hands throughout the day as you enter the room. Make sure visitors do the same, to include anyone who touches your service member. Bring disinfecting wipes and wipe down the surfaces your service member may come in contact with, such as bed rails, TV remote, etc. The hospital does all it can to prevent infection and you should as well. If you are not feeling well, let the staff know. They will give you a mask so that you do not spread your germs to your service member or others at the hospital. If you have an open wound or rash, keep it covered. Not only are you protecting your service member and the other patients, you are protecting yourself as well.

- Be patient with your service member and with yourself. This is a stressful time for you both, and the bottom line is to get your service member to the best possible outcome. It will take time to adjust to the situation. Expect some peaks and valleys to occur. Reunions are stressful under the best of circumstances. Crisis can play havoc with family relationships. Stay positive to benefit you both.
- Utilize all support services so that you can then support your service member to the best of your abilities. You cannot help your service member if you don't take care of yourself. There are many resources available to you. Please see chapter 10: Resources.

PRACTICAL ADVICE

Travel Preparation Considerations

Documents

- Copies of your T&TOs (keep one with you at all times).
- Military ID or government-issued ID such as driver's license.
- Power of Attorney (if your service member left you one).
- Living Will (if your service member has one, many do not).
- Immunization records for children in need of child care services (this is a MUST)
- Name and phone number of Point of Contact for the service member's unit (the DA WIA is able to tell you what the unit is if you do not know).
- Valid Passport if overseas travel is involved.
- Original prescription for any medications that you may need.
- Health insurance information for traveling family members.*

Travel Money

- Major credit card (maintain copy of front and back of card in case of loss)
- Cash or Traveler's Checks
- Checkbook and/or account number and bank routing number†

Household Considerations

- Stop the mail, or arrange for someone to pick up and forward mail to you.
- Arrange for pet care.

---

* For military dependents: If staying out of the TRICARE region for longer than 30 days, consider changing your TRICARE area.

† If staying at the MTF for an extended period of time, consider opening an account at a bank there to avoid ATM charges.

- Schedule bill payment.
- Consider changing cell phone plan to include extra minutes or unlimited long distance as needed.
- Inform trusted friend or family of travel plans and leave spare key to access house.
- Stop newspaper delivery.
- Empty all trash cans and refrigerator of perishable foods.
- Set thermostat to cost saving level.
- Arrange lawn care if necessary.
- Coordinate time off from work.
- Inform Rear Detachment Command of travel.
- Ensure car is locked and windows rolled up.

Things to Pack for Yourself

- Glasses/contacts/associated supplies.
- Prescription medication for up to 30 days plus refill information.
- Toiletries (if you forget something, check with the American Red Cross or SFAC at the MTF).
- Comfortable clothing/sleepwear/shoes/socks/belt.
- Light sweater or jacket for use in hospital.
- Cell phone/charger
- Calling card
- Handheld recorder
- Small digital or disposable camera
- Seasonally appropriate outerwear/umbrella.
- Book/journal.
- Phone numbers of key people (family, friends, creditors, employer, school, etc.).
- Comfort items (pillow, blanket, whatever provides you with special comfort).
- Hand sanitizer/disinfecting wipes.

Things to Pack for Your Service Member

Bring clothes for your service member from home, if possible. It is a good idea to pack a pair of sweat pants and shirt (can be cut for casts, etc.), underwear, shoes/sneakers, and jacket/hat if weather is cold. If you do not have clothes for your service member, ask the Red Cross or SFAC at the MTF for assistance. Service members are allowed a $200 one-time Army Emergency Relief (AER) clothing payment while on inpatient status. Ask the SFAC for assistance. Most MTFs will have a donation center which provides comfort items. Contact your local SFAC for more information.

Special Considerations for Children of Wounded Service Members

When deciding whether or not to take your children to the MTF, there are special considerations. Depending on your service member's medical status, children may not be allowed in the room, such as in the case of intensive care patients. Child care is very limited.

Minor children are only covered by T&TOs for a period of five days, and then the cost is on the family. Children will be exposed to a wide variety of traumatic injuries, many of which are visible, though it may not be their service member who is affected. The purpose of bringing the family to the service member's bedside is to support the service member during the healing process. The focus is being available to that service member at the bedside. The ultimate decision rests with the family.

Keep in mind that not all children respond positively to group child care settings. Child care is not available inside the hospital proper. Additionally, all children must be supervised in the waiting areas within all MTFs. Once the service member is considered an outpatient, pending outprocessing, the families are encouraged to go home. Families traveling on T&TOs have priority. Childcare services are available at most military installations. Parents must have their child's current shot record and complete some paperwork.

Packing for Your Child

- Clothing/shoes/outerwear
- Diapers/Wipes/Diaper Ointment
- Bottles/Sippy Cups/Formula
- Toys/Activities
- Comfort Item (favorite stuffed animal or blanket)
- Immunization Records (military dependents intending to use the Child Development Center)
- Medications (prescriptions as well), thermometer
- Toothbrush/paste/special bath items
- Car seat/stroller
- Review information on preparing child to see injured service member

Considerations for Children Not Traveling with Parent

- Arrange transportation for children to/from school/activities.
- Give Medical Power of Attorney to children's caregiver.
- If moving child out of normal TRICARE region, call TRICARE to change region.
- Give TRICARE card (or medical insurance information) to caregiver with instructions on how to procure medical appointments for child.

- Inform school and other activities about who will be acting as caregiver.
- If living on post, procure gate pass for caregiver.
- Coordinate financial support for children's necessities.
- Make list of scheduled activities for caregiver.
- Make list of allergies, medications, likes and dislikes, bedtimes, routines, etc., for caregiver.
- Leave caregiver with contact information for you and another support person in the area.
- Consider who needs to know about this injury to better support your child during this stressful time (teacher, minister, scout leader, counselor, etc.).
- Review information on talking to child about wartime injury.

Accommodation and Lodging

If the family members are traveling on ITOs, the services arrange for family member's lodging before traveling to be with the wounded service member. Families are housed in local hotels, guest lodging at a military installation, or, if available, a Fisher House, which is "a home away from home" for families of patients receiving medical care at major military and VA medical centers. The homes provide comfortable, temporary housing for families of service members recovering from serious medical conditions. Families pay $10.00 per night to stay in a Fisher House; however, this fee is waived for families of wounded service members. The homes are normally located within walking distance of the treatment facility or have transportation available. For more information on the Fisher Houses, go to: www.fisherhouse.org.

For those traveling on T&TOs, upon arriving at the airport, a service representative with transport van will meet the family and take the family to either the MTF or a local hotel. In some cases the family will have to arrange transportation from the airport. Taxis are the most direct route to most MTFs. Keep the taxi receipt to file for reimbursement.

If lodging on the installation is filled to capacity, then the T&TOs will be stamped by the on-post lodging office and you will be referred to a local hotel (referred to as "off campus" lodging) and placed on a waiting list for on-post lodging. Family members on T&TOs will be able to submit off campus hotel receipts, up to the allowable government nightly rate, for reimbursement at the end of each set of their travel orders. Direct billing is only available for on-post lodging, so you will be required to pay your bill at the off campus hotel in full prior to reimbursement. Travel advances are allowed if paying the hotel bill will be a financial burden. See the DA WIA liaison for assistance. Family members who are NOT traveling on T&TOs will be responsible for paying all room charges accrued.

If you have been placed on the waiting list for on-post lodging, you will be notified when a room becomes available. IMPORTANT: If you do not accept the room, your per diem will be terminated that day.

Note: Many hotel and motel associations offer free rooms for wounded warriors and their families i.e. members of the San Diego Hotel and Motel Association provide hundreds of free rooms every year.

CARE FOR YOURSELF AS WELL AS YOUR LOVED ONE

Caring for a loved one is exhausting work. Your own health and well-being may be the last thing on your mind, but if you're feeling drained, you may become impatient, run down, or at risk of making poor decisions. Taking care of yourself is the best thing you can do for yourself and your spouse.

- Know your strengths and weaknesses. You may enjoy preparing your loved one's meals, but dread helping them bathe. If that's the case, take the stress off of yourself by asking someone more skilled with the razor to take over that chore for you if possible. There are also professionals who will make home visits to attend to your spouse's needs, such as beauticians, podiatrists, and therapists.
- Take breaks. Caregiving is all-consuming and demanding work. Give yourself down time to restore your energy and refresh your attitude. Even a long walk or a night out at the movies will take the edge off. But also look for longer getaways, such as a day or weekend away if possible. Ask trusted family members to take over care, or look into respite care (provided for a weekend, a week or even more). Your MSI Center care manager should be able to help you locate resources for respite care.
- Take care of your own health needs. Make appointments (and keep them) for check-ups or when you're feeling sick. Sometimes it can be hard to take care of yourself when you're so focused on someone else's needs. If you become sick yourself, your situation can only become more complicated.
- Learn to lift properly. If lifting is part of your caregiving routine, have someone show you how to do it without damaging your back.
- Create a team of professionals to help you. To the extent that you can, assemble a team of professionals (health care professionals, financial and legal planners, clergy, family, friends, and co-workers) to rely on. A team approach can help you feel more prepared and better able to handle the challenges of care giving, which in turn can help reduce your own stress.
- Accept help. Neighbors, friends, co-workers, or people from your faith community may have asked how they can help you with your spouse's care.

Accept their offers and give them specific tasks, such as cooking meals, picking up groceries, doing laundry, or even spending an afternoon with your spouse while you take a break.

- Hold a family meeting. Call together children and other family members, even if they live far away, to discuss your spouse's needs. Determine how each family member can contribute, either through direct care or by taking on specific household chores and responsibilities. This way no one person is shouldering the entire load alone. If someone lives far away, they can be given the task of making phone calls and following up so they can feel included in the process. They can also make tapes and send pictures if they can't visit.
- Set realistic expectations for your spouse and yourself. No one is able to do anything "perfectly" at all times, which is also true for caregiving and recovery. When you realistically adjust to your "new normal" and lower your own and others' expectations, your stress level can be greatly reduced.
- Subscribe to care giving newsletters and magazines. Two helpful magazines and websites are Caring Today (www.caringtodaymagazine.com) and Today's Caregiver (www.caregiver.com).
- Connect with other caregivers. Whether it's a formal support group or an informal network of other caregivers, having people to turn to will ease feelings of isolation and help you get through this challenging time. People in similar situations can truly understand what you're going through as well as what might be ahead. Talking with them will help you vent your frustrations, learn caregiving tips, and gain insider's information about resources and services. Ask your MSIC care manager to put you in touch with other spouses of severely injured service members. You can also ask your health care provider or visit online resources such as: the National Family Caregivers Association at www.nfcacares.org and the Family Caregivers Alliance at www.caregiving.org.
- Get professional assistance. It is very important that you're able to get objective help for your ongoing stress, frustrations and sadness. There are even therapists who specialize in dealing with being a spouse's caregiver. You can get a referral through your care manager.
- Find out about alternatives to home care. Caring for your spouse may prove too difficult for you, even with assistance. You may want to ask your MSIC care manager for information about Department of Veterans Affairs hospitals, nursing homes, assisted living facilities, and other alternatives to home care.

Written with the help of Marjorie Dyan Hirsch, L.C.S.W., C.E.A.P. Ms. Hirsch is a certified employee assistance professional and a board-certified expert in traumatic stress. She is a corporate consultant and CEO of The

Full Spectrum in New York City. © 2005 Ceridian Corporation. All rights reserved.

CHILDREN'S SECTION: HELPING YOUR CHILDREN

What support agencies are available for wounded service members and their families?

Several DoD, other government agencies, and non-profit organizations have programs in place to support wounded/injured service members and their families. Here are a few of them:

Air Force Palace HART: The Air Force Palace HART (Helping Airmen Recover Together) program follows Air Force wounded in action until they return to active duty, or are medically retired. It then provides follow-up assistance for 5–7 years post-injury. The Air Force works to retain injured service members on active duty, if at all possible; however, if unable to return an airman to active duty, work to get them civilian employment within the Air Force. The Air Force also ensures counseling is provided on all of the benefits to which an individual service member may be entitled within the Department of Defense, Department of Veterans Affairs, and Department of Labor.

For immediate, 24-hour response, the Military Severely Injured Center can direct you to an Air Force point of contact. It can be reached toll free at 888-774-1361 or you can e-mail severelyinjured@militaryonesource.com.

U.S. Army Wounded Warrior (AW2) Program (formerly the Army Disabled Service members Support System [DS3]): Through the U.S. Army Wounded Warrior Program (AW2), the Army provides its most severely

---

CHILD CARE WHILE VISITING

Hourly child care slots are often hard to access on military installations and so families should not assume there is child care available. Child care is an added expense for families and is not covered in the ITO reimbursement. The individual who notifies you about your service member's injury can direct you to the installation child development center to help you determine if you can make child care arrangements. There may be community resources available to assist with child care. Do not forget to bring a copy of the child's shot record as you will need this to register your child at any child care facility. Some medical facilities have Family Assistance Centers (FACs) that provide assistance to the families of wounded service members once they arrive at the MTF. The FACs should be able to provide child care information.

(continued)

PREPARING A CHILD TO SEE AN INJURED FAMILY MEMBER FOR THE FIRST TIME

You've spoken with your child about your service member's severe injury and now it's time for the first visit. Whether your child will be seeing your loved one at home or in the hospital, the experience will go more smoothly if you make some preparations ahead of time. You can rehearse the visit by describing what your child will see, hear, and smell.

It's also important to reassure your child that it's OK to feel frightened or sad and allow him or her to act on these emotions at home, where children feel safest.

Although no one can predict how your child will react when first seeing a severely injured family member, planning ahead and supporting your child before, during, and after the visit will set the tone for visits to come.

What Your Child May Be Concerned About

Children often have fears that parents may not be aware of. It's possible that your child may have concerns such as these:

- That the family member will no longer be able to care for or play with the child, especially if it's a parent who was injured. It's a good idea to talk about what the family member can still do, such as read books out loud and play board games. You can also come up with specific ways the injured parent can participate in your child's activities, routines, and accomplishments. The parent might call every night at bedtime to say goodnight or read a story. Or maybe the parent can help coach next season's softball team.
- That the injury is punishment for being bad. Explain that the family member was not doing anything wrong, but that sometimes in times of war, bad things happen to good people.
- That he or she will "catch" the family member's injury. Younger children especially may need to be reassured that the injury is not contagious.

Before the Visit

There are concrete steps you can take to help your child prepare for the first visit to an injured family member. It can be a good idea to:

- Explain in age-appropriate language what to expect during the visit. If the family member is in the hospital, describe the scene for your child ahead of time. Be sure to talk about the medical apparatus and what everything does. ("There will be a tube in Daddy's arm so his body gets plenty of fluids.") For very young children, you might demonstrate with a doll or draw a sketch showing the placement of IVs and other equipment.

- Use accurate language when describing the family member's injury. This is especially important with young children, who tend to take things literally. If you say the loved one "lost a limb," the child may think it was simply misplaced. Describe how the family member looks. This is especially important if his or her appearance has changed—for instance, a shaved head, a lost limb, or severe burns. Try to use simple, age-appropriate language when discussing the changes.
- Reassure your child that the family member is still the same person, even though he or she may look different. Again, it's important to use simple, age-appropriate language. ("Mommy's face looks different now. But she is still your same Mommy, and she still loves you very much, and she likes to hear you sing.")
- Prepare your child for how he or she may feel upon seeing the family member. Your child may be frightened, sad, or angry. Let your child know that all of these feelings are perfectly acceptable. Tell your child that it's OK to leave the room if she becomes too upset, and that you'll be right there for extra hugs. Be sure to prepare the injured service member for strong emotions from your child, as well.
- Teach your child the vocabulary of the injury. Knowing words such as "prosthesis," "rehabilitation," and "physical therapy" can help take the mystery out of the experience for your child, and help him feel more in control.
- Arrange for your child to meet with the family member's medical team. This can happen either just before or after the visit. Your child may have questions about the injury or rehabilitation process that the team can answer in age-appropriate ways.

A great resource is Shannon Maxwell's book "Our Daddy Is Invincible!" http://www.amazon.com/Our-Daddy-Invincible-Shannon-Maxwell/dp/1617510033. The book talks about what happens when a parent becomes traumatically injured and talks about the recovery process, love, new adventures, and new ways to find enjoyment as a family.

During the Visit

Here are some steps you can take during the visit to help ease the stress for your child:

- Schedule the visit for a time when there is no other business to take care of. That way, if your child becomes frightened or bored, you can cut the visit short.
- Let your child know that it's OK to touch or hug the family member (assuming that it is).

(continued)

- Take your cues from your child. If your child doesn't want to go near the family member, don't force her to. Depending on your child's age and personality, it could take a while for her to adjust to the change.
- Give your child something to bring. A drawing to tape to the wall, a photograph to keep next to the bedside, or flowers for the bedside table can help your child feel as though he's doing something to make the loved one feel better.
- Fill the time as much as possible. It will be easier for the family to relax during the visit if you bring a book for you or your child to read out loud; a board game, such as checkers; completed schoolwork; or a photo album to look through. Doing these activities together and with the injured service member can help everyone feel more comfortable and reinforce the relationships among family members.
- Keep the visit short. Younger children may become bored and older children may feel uncomfortable if the visit seems to go on too long.
- Give your child a way to opt out of a visit. Your child may not be ready for the visit, but feel guilty saying so. Tell your child that it's OK not to go just yet, but suggest that she make a special drawing or write a letter for you to bring. The gesture will help your child feel better about staying home. Find ways to keep the connection between your child and the family member alive—through e-mail, telephone calls, and letters. It's important for the service member to stay involved in the child's routines as much as possible.

After the Visit

Even if you prepare your child thoroughly beforehand, he or she may still react intensely to the visit. Often these reactions are unpredictable and changeable. After the visit, make sure to:

- Keep an eye on your child for signs that she was overly disturbed by the experience and is not coping well.
- Watch out for behavior changes. Keep in mind that younger children may become clingy and return to old habits and behaviors, such as bedwetting or thumb sucking.
- Older children may suffer physical symptoms, including headaches and stomachaches; becoming irritable or aggressive; doing poorly in school; and engaging in risk-taking behaviors. If any of these behaviors continue for several weeks, seek out the advice of a professional who can help your child cope with the changes in your child's life.
- Let your child know that it's OK to talk about his feelings. Do this by talking about your own feelings. If you notice behavioral changes, be sure to encourage younger children to draw pictures of how they feel inside, and reassure your child that you are there to provide help and support.

Common Reactions to Learning about Parent's Injury

Infants/Toddlers (under age 3)

- Crying, clinging
- Searching for parents/caregivers
- Change in sleep and eating habits
- Regression to earlier behavior (e.g. bedwetting, thumb sucking)
- Repetitive play or talk

Preschoolers/Young Children (3–5 years)

- Separation fears, clinging
- Fighting, crying, tantrums, irritable outbursts
- Withdrawal, regression to earlier behaviors
- Sleep difficulty
- Acting/talking as if the person is not injured
- Increased usual fears (the dark, monsters)

Early School-Age Children (6–9 years)

- Anger, fighting, bullying
- Denial, irritability, self-blame
- Fluctuating moods, withdrawal
- Regression to earlier behavior
- Fear of separation and being alone
- Physical complaints (stomach/headaches)
- School problems (avoidance, academic difficulty, difficulty concentrating)

Middle School–Age Children (9–12 years)

- Crying, sadness, isolation, withdrawal
- Aggression, irritability, bullying
- Resentment, fears, anxiety, panic
- Suppressed emotions, denial, avoidance
- Self-blame, guilt, sleep disturbance
- Physical health symptoms and complaints
- Academic problems or decline, school refusal, memory problems
- Repetitive thoughts or talks with peers
- "Hysterical" expressions of concern and need for help   *(continued)*

Early Teens/Adolescents (13–18 years)

- Numbing, avoidance of feelings
- Resentment, loss of trust, guilt, shame
- Depression, suicidal thoughts
- Distancing, withdrawal, panic, anxiety
- Mood swings, irritability, anger
- Acting out (engaging in risky, antisocial, or illegal behavior), substance abuse
- Appetite and/or sleep changes
- Physical complaints or changes
- Academic decline, school refusal
- Fear or similar events/illness/death/future

When to Talk to Your Child

- The sooner, the better.
- When the panic subsides and you can talk about it more calmly.
- When you know more about the nature and the extent of the injury.
- When you can deliver the news rather than someone else.

Internet Resources

American Academy of Child & Adolescent Psychiatry: www.aacap.org
American Academy of Pediatrics: www.aap.org/terrorism/index.html
National Child Care Information Center: www.nccic.acf.hhs.gov
NYU Child Study Center: www.aboutourkids.org
Parent's Guide to the Military Child During Deployment and Reunion: www.k12.wa.us/operationmilitarykids/resources.aspx

disabled service members and their families with a holistic system of advocacy and follow-up with personal support and liaison to resources, to assist them in their transition from military service to civilian life. AW2 links the Army and other organizations that stand ready to assist these service members and families, such as the Department of Veterans' Affairs and the many eterans' service organizations, to the service member. One key goal of AW2 is to provide a network of resources to severely disabled service members, no matter where they relocate and regardless of their component: active, Reserve or National Guard. The goal is to ensure service members, families, and communities receive responsive support services that meet their needs. The AW2 toll free number is: 800-833-6622.

Navy Safe Harbor Program: The Navy Safe Harbor Program has a coordinated and tailored response for its men and women returning from Iraq, Afghanistan and other areas of conflict with severe debilitating injuries. For immediate, 24-hour response, the Military Severely Injured Center can direct you to a POC and can be reached toll free at 888-774-1361, or you can e-mail severelyinjured@militaryonesource.com.

Marine for Life Injured Support Program (M4L): The Marine for Life Injured Support program provides information, advocacy and assistance from the time of injury through return to full duty or transition to the Veterans Administration, up to one year after separation. The program is currently being introduced by Marine for Life staffers to marines, sailors, and their families at Walter Reed National Military Medical Center with a plan to expand to all major naval hospitals as soon as possible.

Marines who have already been medically discharged are being contacted by phone. Injured marines, sailors or family members needing assistance can call toll-free: 866-645-8762 or e-mail: injuredsupport@M4L.usmc.mil. For more information about the Marine for Life Injured Support Program, go to: www.marines.mil.

Military Severely Injured Center (MSIC): The center is a central Department of Defense (DoD) resource available to offer support services to seriously injured service members and their families. The center works with and complements existing service programs such as the U.S. Army's Wounded Warrior (AW2) Program.

Marine for Life Injured Support System and **Military OneSource:** Support services are provided as long as seriously injured service members and their families require quality of life support. Services are tailored to meet individual's unique needs during recovery and rehabilitation. The center offers counseling and resource referral in such areas as financial support, education, and employment assistance, information on VA benefits, family counseling, resources in local communities, and child care support. For immediate, 24-hour response, the Military Severely Injured Center can be reached toll free at 888-774-1361, or you can contact severelyinjured@militaryonesource.com.

Additionally, families can read up to date information on the DoD Military Homefront website. Go to www.militaryhomefront.dod.mil, and click on the Troops and Families link.

Deployment Health Support Directorate: The DoD established the Deployment Health Support Directorate to see that the medical lessons learned from previous conflicts and deployments are integrated into current policy, doctrine and practice. The Directorate addresses deployment-related health threats to service members. Part of the Deployment Health focus is on outreach. Current information on deployment-related health issues is published on an interactive website, Deployment link: http://deploymentlink.osd.mil. The directorate operates a toll-free, direct hotline number where staff members assist callers in finding the answers they seek in relation to current and past deployments, helping them locate lost medical records, and providing contact information in the Department of Veteran Affairs. That number is 800-497-6261.

THE DISABILITY EVALUATION SYSTEM

The Disability Evaluation System (DES) was created by the Department of Defense (DoD) to provide a uniform procedure for the evaluation of a service member's medical condition and the member's ability to continue his or her military service.

The DES has two stages: the Medical Evaluation Board (MEB) and the Physical Evaluation Board (PEB). In the first stage, the MEB evaluates the service member's injury and ongoing treatment in order to determine whether he or she can continue service in his or her military occupational specialty (MOS) following medical treatment.

In the second stage, the PEB evaluates a service member's physical ability to continue in the military service and provides the service member with a DoD disability rating if the PEB results in separation from the military.

Note: The term MOS is used by the Army and Marine Corps. The Air Force uses Air Force Specialty Code (AFSC), and the Navy uses Navy Enlisted Classification (NEC).

Depending on the nature of the service member's injuries, the MEB may place the service member on temporary limited duty (TLD) or refer the individual to a PEB, which evaluates the service member's ability to continue his or her military service. If the PEB determines that the severity of an injury or illness requires separation, the PEB will order the medical retirement of the service member and assign a disability rating. The disability rating often determines the availability and type of benefits that may be available after separation. In addition, if the PEB believes that the service member may recover from his or her disability over time, the PEB may recommend placing the service member on the Temporary Disability Retirement List (TDRL) until he or she is fit to return to active duty or found unfit and separated from service with appropriate benefits.

The process is complicated, takes time, and can be appealed. The decisions of these boards will affect both the service member and the family. It is a good idea for you as a family member to gain an overall understanding of what these boards do and what the possible outcomes of these boards are.

INTEGRATED DISABILITY EVALUATION SYSTEM (IDES)

The Integrated Disability Evaluation System (IDES) takes the DES to the next level. It is a seamless, transparent disability evaluation system administered jointly by the Departments of Defense (DoD) and Veterans Affairs (VA) to make disability evaluations for wounded, ill or injured service members and veterans simple, seamless, fast and fair. The IDES integrates evaluation processes the DoD and VA each performed separately, to help DoD determine whether a wounded, ill or injured service member is able to continue to serve and quickly returns those who are to duty status. For service members unable to continue service, the IDES determines the disability rating the member will receive through the VA. The advantage of IDES is that it is an evaluation system for both medical separation as well as caregiver and respite benefits. Each branch of the military operates IDES.

The transformation from two separate evaluation and disability systems to the streamlined IDES, will help all current and future service members by delivering:

1. Enhanced Case Management
2. A Single Comprehensive Disability Examination
3. A Single-Sourced Disability Rating
4. Increased Transparency
5. Faster Disability Processing
6. Faster Benefits Delivery

While going through the board process, it is important to keep the service member on track with the various appointments necessary to provide the most complete and up to date picture of health status. The case manager will assist with this as will the PEBLO (Physical Evaluation Board Liaison Officer). There are various points throughout this process that allow the service member to appeal. The service member SHOULD NOT sign anything without a complete understanding of what it is that they are signing and what the ramifications are. If the service member does not understand, seek further clarification from the PEBLO or legal resources.

The Medical Evaluation Board (MEB)

A Medical Evaluation Board (MEB) is the first step in the military's disability evaluation process for determining whether an injured service member is fit to return to active duty.

Integrated Disability Evaluation System (IDES) Timeline

Treatment

- Service member becomes wounded, ill or injured
- Physician assesses and treats Service member

Service members are referred within 1 year of being diagnosed with a medical condition that does not appear to meet medical retention standards.

Medical Evaluation Board Phase (MEB)

- Referral
  - AC 10 days
  - RC 30 days
- Claim Development
  - AC 10 days
  - RC 30 days
- Medical Evaluation
  - AC 45 days
  - RC 45 days
- MEB Stage
  - AC 35 days
  - RC 35 days
- Service member can appeal MEB decision

Physical Evaluation Board Phase (PEB)

DoD

- Informal Physical Evaluation Board (IPEB) 15 days
- Service member can rebut IPEB decision
- Formal Physical Evaluation Board (FPEB) 30 days
- Service member can rebut FPEB decision
- FPEB Appeal 30 days

Unfit

VA

- Preliminary Rating Board 15 days
- Service member can request rating reconsideration
- Rating Reconsideration 15 days

Administrative and record transit 15 days

Transition Phase

- Finalize DES Disposition
- Assign to unit or process for separation

The 45 day goal may be exceeded to allow the Service member to take authorized leave and permissive temporary duty (TDY)

Reintegration Phase

- **Return to Duty**

OR

- **Separate** — *VA benefits letter one month following separation*
- Veteran can appeal VA benefits
- VA Appeals

	Medical Evaluation Board Phase (MEB)	Physical Evaluation Board Phase (PEB)	Transition Phase	Reintegration Phase
Active Component (AC)	100 calendar days	120 calendar days	45 calendar days	30 calendar days = 295 calendar days
Reserve Component (RC)[1]	140 calendar days	120 calendar days	45 calendar days = 305 calendar days	

■ Service Member Decision Points   ☐ IDES Stages

[1] Reserve component member entitlement to VA disability begins upon release from active duty or separation

An MEB typically includes two or three physicians, one of whom is the service member's treating physician. The purpose of an MEB is to determine whether the service member has an injury or illness that is severe enough to compromise his or her ability to return to full duty based on his or her MOS.

The MEB is not a formal hearing, and the service member should not expect to appear before a panel at this stage of the process. Rather, the service member will be evaluated through a series of examinations, and the board will base its findings on a review of the service member's case file. The service member will have the opportunity to review the MEB's report and either agree with or oppose the findings.

While the MEB can determine that a service member is fit for duty, it cannot make a final determination that the service member is unfit for duty, which is required before a service member can be separated because of an injury or medical condition. That determination is left solely to the Physical Evaluation Board (PEB)—see below.

Service members may also seek outside assistance in preparing for the disability evaluation process. Disabled American Veterans, a charitable organization not affiliated with the military, provides numerous advocacy, counseling and outreach services to assist veterans in obtaining benefits and services earned as a result of their military service. Through its National Service Program, the DAV employs national service officers (NSOs) who, upon request, counsel and advocate on behalf of service members.

The service member has the right to see everything considered by the MEB.

If, upon examination, the service member meets retention standards, i.e., the service member's condition allows him or her to return to active duty, then the MEB will clear the service member for return to active duty. If the MEB believes that the service member can return to active duty within a reasonable period of time, it may recommend placing the service member on **Temporary Limited Duty (TLD).** TLD is a specified period of limited duty. The TLD period is normally eight months and generally will not exceed a total of 16 cumulative months. The service member is expected to return to full duty after the specified TLD period. If the MEB is unsure of the service member's ability to return to active duty within a reasonable period of time, or if the service member's condition prevents him or her from returning to full active duty even following a TLD period, the MEB refers the service member to the Physical Evaluation Board (PEB).

The service member's servicing medical treatment facility (MTF) convenes an MEBD to document the service member's medical history, current physical status, and recommended duty limitations. The service member's command prepares a memorandum on the commander's position on the service member's physical abilities to perform PMOS/OS duties in the currently assigned duty position. The MEBD's mission is to determine if the physically impaired service member meets retention standards in accordance with AR 40-501, Standards of Medical Fitness. The PEB, however, is the sole determiner of the service member's physical fitness for duty, as measured by duty performance, in accordance with AR 635-40, Physical Evaluation for Retention, Retirement, or Separation.

The MEBD forwards the service member's case to the PEB for review if the MEBD finds that the service member does not meet retention standards, according to PMOS/OS and grade. However, a service member is not automatically unfit because of a failure to meet the retention standards. AR 635-40 precludes the doctors at the MEBD from making a factual determination as to the service member's physical fitness for duty. This fact-finding authority is solely within the purview of the PEB. If the physician violates this prohibition and renders a fitness assessment, it will simply be ignored by the PEB.

The MEBD findings are recorded on DA Form 3947 (Medical Evaluation Board Proceedings). This form documents the physical or mental conditions that preclude the service member's retention. If the service member does not agree with the findings, he may so indicate on DA Form 3947 and attach a written appeal that sets forth the reasons he or she disagrees. If the Medical Treatment Facility's (MTF) approving authority does not make a favorable change in the original MEBD based upon the service member's appeal, a copy of the service member's appeal will be sent to the PEB along with the results of the MEBD.

Physical Evaluation Board Liaison Officer (PEBLO)

An important actor and source of information for service members throughout the PEB process is the PEBLO. The PEBLO collects and prepares the service member's medical packet for presentation to MEBD and PEB. A service member's medical packet consists of medical records, medical narrative summary of present disabling conditions, commander's memorandum and physical profile, along with other related information.

Each MTF should have a designated PEBLO available to provide counseling for service members from the time they are identified as requiring an MEB through the time that they are separated. The PEBLO will work with the service member's legal counsel and PEB to obtain required documentation and other medical information, and will also serve as the point of contact between physicians and board members. The PEBLO is usually located in the Patient Affairs Division.

Important note: It is very important to seek appropriate advice before going before a physical evaluation board. Depending on the severity of the injury, the family may be approached regarding a medical discharge rather than a PEB. This decision has to be taken very carefully. Equally, there are occasions when it might be advisable to delay your decision to go before the PEB. Again, seek advice before you act.

THE PHYSICAL EVALUATION BOARD (PEB)

Informal Boards

Each case forwarded by the MEBD is reviewed first by an informal PEB. An informal board consists of three voting members: a combat arms colonel/06 serving as the President of the Board; a personnel management officer (PMO), usually reserve combat arms Lieutenant Colonel, and; a physician, either a Medical Corps Officer or a Department of the Army civilian physician. The three board members determine by majority vote based upon a preponderance of the evidence the physical fitness/unfitness of the service member based on PMOS/OS specific performance standards. If the Board determines that the service member is physically unfit for duty in his/her present grade, rank, PMOS/OS and current duty position by reason of a physical disability, the PEB then recommends a disability rating percentage based upon the service member's present degree of severity for each medical diagnosis found to be separately unfitting. The service member processing for physical disability separation possesses no legal right to appear or otherwise participate in the informal board proceedings. The PEB records its informal factual findings and the recommended disability rating on DA Form 199 (Election to Formal Physical Evaluation Board Proceedings). Once the PEB has informally adjudicated a service member's disability case, the service member will consult with his or her PEBLO at the MTF for assistance in choosing an election option. The service member is afforded the following election options: a) concur with the PEB's informal findings and recommendations; b) request a formal administrative hearing, either with or without personal appearance, which is a statutory right; or, c) non-concur and submit a written appeal in lieu of proceeding with a formal board. If electing to proceed with a formal hearing, service members have the option to request minority representation based on race or the female gender. The board typically grants the service member's request if substitute officers are reasonably available.

The membership of the formal board will generally be the same as those members who sat on the informal board. If the informal board members are not available, then a qualified substitute officer will sit on the formal board. All board members are required to familiarize themselves with the case prior to the actual hearing. Once the service member demands a formal hearing, he or she is entitled to regularly appointed military counsel. The service member appearing before a formal hearing may elect to be represented by a private civilian lawyer at no expense to the government.

The Formal Physical Evaluation Board

The formal Physical Evaluation Board is an administrative, fact-finding de novo hearing. The hearing is non-adversarial in nature, that is to say it is a "friendly hearing." In this regard, there is no government representative to oppose or counter the service member's position at hearing. Generally, the formal board is not bound by the military rules of evidence except insofar as the evidence adduced at hearing must be relevant and material to the service member's case. Although termed a formal hearing, the actual proceedings are somewhat relaxed to provide the service member a fair hearing within a friendly atmosphere. Service members usually request a formal hearing to argue for a higher disability rating, believing that the recommended disability made informally did not accurately reflect their current level of severity. Some service members, who were found unfit by the Informal Board, request a formal hearing to argue that they are fit for duty based on uninterrupted and undiminished duty performance. This serves to underscore the fact that PEB proceedings, unlike those of the MEBD, are performance based. It should be noted that service members who are found fit for duty at an informal Board, have no legal right to request a formal hearing. The President of the Board, however, has the discretion to direct a formal hearing when one board member strongly feels that the service member is unfit. A service member may otherwise waive his/her right to a formal hearing should they concur in the finding and recommendation of the informal board.

The mission of the formal PEB is twofold: 1) to determine whether the service member can reasonably perform the duties of his or her primary MOS/OS and grade; and if not, 2) to determine the present severity of the service member's physical or mental disability and rate it accordingly. The three members of the Board—the President, the Personnel Management Officer (PMO) and the medical doctor—may be challenged for cause and replaced if the challenge is sustained. The medical member of the Board is a physician (military or civilian) who may be a general medical officer or a practitioner in any specialized field of medicine. It is administratively impractical to have a physician sitting on the board whose medical specialty pertains to the service member's unfitting condition. The two other board members are active component, reserve component or a DA civilian employee who do not need to be from the same branch or career management field as the boarded service member.

The PMO, however, is usually a reserve AGR officer. This is to accommodate Reserve Component service members processing for physical disability separation who are entitled to have a Reserve Component Officer sitting on the Board.

As the formal hearing is de novo, the PEB is not bound to its previous findings and recommendations. All issues are decided anew which means that the service member's disability rating could be raised, remain the same, or be lowered. The focus of the formal hearing is the medical evidence of record primarily contained in the narrative summary written by the MEBD along with any subsequent medical addenda.

Tip: If your service member requests a formal board they should appear in person. Appearing in person is like a promotion board. Your service member must present a good appearance as a service member. They can bring further documentation, new documentation, witnesses on their behalf, and legal counsel. If bringing legal counsel it is a good idea to get in touch with the legal counsel as soon as the service member makes the decision to demand a formal hearing.

The service member may be represented by appointed military counsel free of charge, generally a JAG officer, or the service member may decide to be represented by civilian counsel of his or her own choosing and at the service member's expense. Also, certain organizations accredited by the VA, such as the DAV, can help service members find free or low-cost legal assistance, including non-attorney counselors. A service member has no right to appear personally before an informal PEB. A service member does have the right to appear personally before a formal PEB. Upon appearing before the formal PEB, the service member may present testimony under oath. If the service member presents testimony under oath, the members of the formal PEB may question the service member. However, the service member is not required to present testimony under oath and, even if under oath, may refuse to answer certain questions.

The Formal Board concludes the opening hearing and then deliberates in private.

Following the closed board deliberations, the service member is recalled to the hearing room where he/she is immediately notified of the Board's decision and given up to ten calendar days to make an election to concur or nonconcur with the formal decision. If the service member disagrees with the formal board results, the service member may submit a written rebuttal to the board's findings and recommendations. The Board will consider the written appeal and issue a written decision to the service member either reaffirming or modifying its formal decision.

If the board reaffirms or modifies their decision, AR 635-40 requires the board to forward the entire formal board record to the Physical Disability Agency (PDA) in Washington, DC, for final approval. The formal board proceedings are tape-recorded for final review by the PDA.

Some terms:

TDRL: Temporary Disability Retirement List. Must be rated at 30% or
    greater. Can be re-evaluated at least every 18 months up to a maximum
    of 5 years.
PDRL: Permanent Disability Retirement List
COAD: Continuance of Disabled personnel on Active Duty
COAR: Continuance of Disabled personnel on Active Reserve

THE PHYSICAL DISABILITY AGENCY (PDA)

The PDA reviews all cases prior to final disposition in which the service
member has non-concurred with the decision of the PEB. The PDA may
modify the PEB's findings and recommendations if it concludes that PEB
made an error. Departing from generally accepted medical principles to adjudicate a case would, for instance, constitute error on the part of the PEB. The
PDA reviews, through its staff psychiatrist, all psychiatric cases.

The PDA, moreover, conducts random disability case reviews based either
on selected categories of medical impairments or reviewing every tenth case
received for final disposition. The PDA conducts random reviews to assure
uniformity of result from the three regional PEBs located at Walter Reed
Army Medical Center, Fort Sam Houston, and Fort Lewis. This means that
the final result of a service member's disability case should be the same ir-
respective of which regional PEB adjudicated the case. In reviewing disability cases, the PDA has full authority to accept or modify the findings and
recommendations of a PEB. In modifying a service member's case, the PDA
may reverse the factual finding of unfitness for duty made by a PEB. Therefore the PDA could find a service member fit for duty who had been previously found unfit by a PEB. With respect to the PEB's recommended disability
rating, the PDA can raise, affirm or lower the disability rating to reflect accurately the service member's present level of physical impairment caused by
the unfitting condition. When the PDA makes a modification after reviewing
a particular case, it gives the affected service member written notice of such,
and provides a sufficient period of time to respond in writing prior to finaliza-
tion of the case.

Rating Disabilities Found to Be Unfitting

Only those service-connected physical impairments which render the service member unfit are ratable under the Physical Disability System. As stated

before, "unfitting" is interpreted to mean service or career interruption. For service members with multiple diagnosed physical impairments, each is potentially ratable provided that the PEB finds each physical impairment to be separately unfitting. The Department of Veterans Affairs (VA), on the other hand, will rate any and all service-connected conditions. Many people mistakenly believe that the military follows the same rules as the VA. This is not the case. The military rates an unfitting condition for present level of severity whereas the VA rates for future progression, which is the prognosis of the illness or injury, and for adverse impact on employability within the civilian job sector.

When a PEB determines that a service member is unfit for continued military service by reason of a physical disability, the disabling condition is rated in accordance with the Veterans Administration Schedule for Rating Disabilities (VASRD) as modified in AR 635-40, Appendix B, and DOD Directives 1332.38 and 1332.39. The mere fact that a service member has an impairment that appears in the VASRD does not automatically result in entitlement to disability rating. As will be remembered, the PEB must first determine that the impairment renders the service member unfit for duty. Contrariwise, when the VA rates a service-connected physical impairment or disease, there is no consideration of performance-based factors.

The VASRD specifies diagnostic codes for a wide spectrum of diseases and physical impairments covering all major body systems. By way of example, there are injuries/diseases of the cardiovascular, respiratory and musculoskeletal systems. Each specific diagnostic code specifies disability ratings percentages in increments of ten, beginning with 0% and continuing to 100%, if so indicated. The specific disability rating expressed as a percentage indicated the degree to which the rated condition has impaired the whole person. Again it must be remembered that the military and VA rate for different purposes. A particular VASRD diagnostic code may have a rating ceiling of 30%. The military cannot exceed the specified upper limit, but the VA can award a 100% disability rating for that condition if it were to find that the severity of this condition rises to the level of rendering the service member incapable of being trained for any type of gainful civilian sector employment. If an impairment is so mild that it fails to meet the minimum criteria listed for an assigned rating under the VASRD, AR 635-40 and DOD directives, the PEB may recommend a zero percent disability rating even if not indicated on the applicable diagnostic code. A zero percent rating is a minimum rating and, as such, is a compensable rating and carries the same military benefits, to include severance pay, as a 10 or 20 percent rating. Zero percent ratings will not be awarded if a mandatory minimum rating is specified. Convalescent ratings contained in the VASRD are for VA use only and do not apply to the military.

Physical Evaluation Board Recommendations

Existed Prior to Service (EPTS)

A service member will not receive a rating for a disability that preexisted entry into military service if the PEB finds that the unfitting condition has not been permanently aggravated by military service. This creates a very difficult standard of proof, especially for reserve component members who must establish a nexus between their unfitting condition and military service. Service aggravation has a narrow definition in AR 635-40, Chapter 5-2, that requires a permanent aggravation of the service member's condition beyond what would have occurred as result of "natural progression." The PDA will conclude that a chronic illness existed prior to service (EPTS) if it manifests itself within a very short period of time, usually 90 days, after entry into active duty. The Army uses accepted medical principles to determine the natural progression or onset of an impairment. For example, it is not unusual for a small number of service members to display bizarre behavior sometime during basic training, AIT or during the first few months of their first overseas assignment. Subsequently, these service members in question are often diagnosed as being schizophrenic. In such cases, the onset of the developmental or prodromal period is dated 90 days prior to the first display of bizarre symptoms. This typically makes this form of mental illness EPTS without permanent aggravation. Therefore, the PEB will find the service member unfit and recommend separation without entitlement to disability benefits.

As in the above example, if the PEB considers a service member's impairment EPTS without permanent service aggravation, the service member will not receive a disability rating. The PEB will recommend separation without disability benefits (i.e., without entitlement to lump sum severance pay) and the service member is medically discharged. By way of further example, the condition of flat feet is a common EPTS condition which often becomes symptomatic for pain as a function of physical activity. The Army's physical training requirements of running, rucksack marches and other equally demanding physical activities, function to increase the intensity of pain for service members whose flat feet have become symptomatic for pain. While these physical activities temporarily aggravate the pain experienced in flat feet, it cannot serve as the basis for "permanent service aggravation" of a congenital condition. The cited condition would be seen merely as natural progression of an EPTS condition. To succeed in gaining a disability rating for an unfitting case of flat feet, the service member would need to show a specific trauma or surgical mishap that has permanently aggravated his/her flat feet. Permanent service aggravation equates to a level of severity caused by military service that is far above a level of severity that can be attributed to natural progression and for which there will be no significant improvement following cessation of physical activity known to aggravate temporarily the unfitting condition. An acceleration of natural progression attributed to military service would also constitute permanent service aggravation.

Fit by Presumption

The presumption of fitness applies whenever a service member's military service is terminated for reasons other than the service member's diagnosed physical impairment. Examples include bars to reenlistment, voluntary or involuntary retirement, Qualitative Management Program (QMP), administrative separations under the provisions of AR 635-200, and the like. The presumption will apply whenever the approval date or imposition date of the cause of termination precedes the dictation date of the MEBD narrative summary. A ruling that the presumption of fitness applies does not necessarily mean that a service member is fit for duty. It merely means that the service member's impairment is not the cause for separation from the service.

A service member can overcome the presumption if he or she shows, by objective medical evidence, that his/her military service was effectively interrupted by reason of a physical impairment. Evidence of prior unfitness may be found in counseling statements for unsatisfactory performance caused by the service member's physical impairment. Comments on OERs/NCOERs pertaining to the service member's/officer's diminished duty performance by reason of a physical impairment are effective in rebutting the presumption of fitness.

The PEB presumes that service members who become retirement eligible or who are within one year of their retention control point (RCP) are fit for duty. If a service member has been able to perform at a minimum level of competence the duties of his/her PMOS up to the point of becoming retirement eligible or reaching the retention control point, he/she cannot convincingly argue sudden unfitness for duty by reason of a physical disability. If there were either an abrupt onset of a disease process or if there were a sudden acute change in a long-standing diagnosed condition (with either event resulting in diminished duty performance falling below a minimum level of competence), the affected service member might well succeed in rebutting the presumption of fitness and thereby gain a disability rating.

Separation with Severance Pay

A service member separated from the service with less than a 30% disability rating will receive severance pay as financial compensation from the military. Severance pay is calculated by doubling the service member's monthly base pay multiplied by the number of active federal service years, not to exceed 12 years. This is a one-time lump-sum payment, and may affect any monetary

VA benefits for which the service member may qualify. Unlike the VA monthly stipend, severance pay from the Army may be taxable income for the service member. Severance pay is not taxable for those service members who were in the Armed Forces on September 24, 1975 or if the disability is due to a combat-related injury or from an instrumentality of war (such as a parachute-related injury). If the VA rates the service member for the same condition which the PEB found unfitting and awarded a disability rating, the severance will then become nontaxable income to the separated service member. Once the calendar year has passed, the military has already transferred the sever-ance pay tax withholdings to the Internal Revenue Service. A service member must then request a refund with the IRS by filing a 1040X form along with his/her tax return. The service member must also attach a copy of her DD 214, DA Form 199, and a letter from the VA documenting the service member's disability percentage. The IRS will review and consider the service mem-ber's filed tax return on a case by case basis.

Permanent Disability Retirement

A service member with less than 20 years of active federal service qualifies for disability/medical retirement if his/her disability rating is 30 percent or higher. Disabled service members with a medical retirement rated at 30% will draw for a lifetime 30% of their base pay calculated at their retirement date. Active component service members with vested retirement based on 20 or more years of active federal service, who are found unfit and awarded a dis-ability rating of 30% or higher, being eligible for both a longevity and medi-cal retirement, will always draw a retirement based on the higher amount. If, for instance, a service member's disability rating percentage exceeds that percentage of retired pay based on years of service, he/she will receive as retired pay the higher amount based on the disability rating percentage.

Contrariwise, if the percentage of retired pay based on years of service is higher than the disability rating percentage, the retired pay based on years of service will take precedence over the disability rating percentage. By way of a specific example, an unfit service member with 22 years of service is enti-tled to receive 55% of his/her base pay as regular retirement pay.

But if the PEB were to rate the unfitting condition at a 60% disability, that service member would receive a monthly pension equal to 60% of his/her base pay. Additionally, the service member's retired pay will be classified as disability retired pay. There is, however, no "double dipping"; the 60% disability amount will not be added to the service member's 55% retirement amount. If that same service member received a disability rating of 40%, and qualified for 55% of his/her current base pay, the service member will receive

40% of base pay for disability retirement, and 15% of base pay for standard longevity retirement.

This distinction is significant for two reasons: (1) it can figure in reducing tax liability, and (2) disability retirement pay is not subject to division under the Former Spouses' Protection Act. Note that by law a retired service member is prohibited to receive more than 75% of his/her military base pay, whether retired medically or retired for years of service. A disability rating less than 75% will result in pensions equal to that amount of base pay (e.g., a service member with 24 years' service who is rated at a 40% disability rating, disability retired pay will be 40% of base pay with an additional 20% in ordinary retired pay). Permanent disability ratings in excess of 75% will result in compensation limited to 75% of the service member's base pay. Service members placed on the Temporary Disability Retirement List by regulation will receive no less than 50% of their current base pay, even if their disability rating is 30%.

Reserve component members found unfit at a disability rating of less than 30%, but who have a vested reserve retirement as evidenced by a twenty year retirement letter, have the election of choosing between immediate receipt of disability severance pay or delayed receipt of the vested reserve retirement at age 60. The reserve component member will not be able to receive both benefits and should base an election upon factors such as age, immediate financial needs, life expectancy, and other relevant factors. It is usually to the financial benefit of the reservist to retain the retirement based on years of service.

Temporary Disability Retirement List (TDRL)

Service members rated at 30% or more and whose impairments are considered to be unstable for rating purposes are placed on the TDRL and required to be re-examined in 12 or 18 months. This is a "wait and see" approach for medical conditions that are likely to either improve or deteriorate within the next 18 months. Such conditions are not considered stable for rating purposes inasmuch as the PEB rates solely for present severity and not for future progression. The service member can be retained on the TDRL for a maximum of five years if the service member's condition remains unstable and continues to meet the minimum criteria for a rating of 30% or more. If a service member's impairment stabilizes within the five-year period, the PEB will recommend a permanent disability rating and remove the service member from the TDRL. All of the initial options (fit for duty, separation with severance pay, separation without benefits, and permanent disability retirement) are available to the PEB when making a final adjudication of the case. Should the service member disagree with PEB's final findings and recommendations, he/she has a right to demand a formal hearing.

If a service member's unfitting condition has not stabilized within the five-year period, the PEB will proceed to rate the service member for the level of severity attained at the end of the five-year period.

Line of Duty Determinations (LOD)

Injuries or diseases contracted in the line of duty entitle the unfit service member to disability compensation in the form of severance pay or a medical retirement. An unfavorable LOD determination disqualifies a service member from receiving disability compensation. If, for example, the PEB receives a negative line of duty determination after it has adjudicated a disability case, it will revise its findings and recommendations, reversing any award of benefits. Usually, if an active duty service member is pending an LOD, the PEB will conditionally adjudicate (noted on DA Form 199 as such) the case pending final outcome of the LOD. In the case of reservists, the PEB will not recommend a disability rating without first having received an LOD determination for the unfitting disability. Although the PEB cannot modify the LOD determination, it can return the case to the casualty branch. The casualty branch determines if there are LOD issues which require further examination.

Eligibility for Processing

Service members who are under investigation or pending charges which could result in dismissal, punitive discharge, or an administrative separation under other than honorable (OTH) conditions, are not eligible for processing for physical disability separation. The PEB will return the service member's case file to the MTF awaiting resolution of the charges before the PEB will take additional action. If the action is favorably resolved for the service member and the possibility of an adverse discharge or separation no longer exists, processing will then continue. Additionally, cadets, AWOL service members, and service members confined for civil offenses are not eligible for processing through the physical disability system.

THE TRANSITION PROCESS

The shift of a service member to medical retirement, transit on to the Department of Veterans Affairs, or separation from the military is known as Transition. The DoD has a mandatory Transition Assistance Program (TAP) for all transitioning and/or separating service members. You can read more about transition at www.turbotap.org.

DIFFERENCES BETWEEN MILITARY AND VA DISABILITY RATINGS

The VASRD is the standard used by both the VA and the military to quantify a service member's disability. PEBs use the VASRD to assign a disability rating when the PEB finds a service member unfit. The military's disability rating is used to determine eligibility for certain military benefits such as separation pay and medical retirement. The VA uses the VASRD to assign a disability rating when determining a veteran's eligibility for VA benefits.

Not all general policy provisions in the VASRD are applicable to the military departments, and, consequently, a service member may receive a disability rating from the VA that differs from the rating assigned by the military. More specifically, the military will only consider the service member's physical conditions that make him or her unfit for continued service. In contrast, the VA will consider all service-connected disabilities when assigning a disability rating. In addition, the VA process permits re-evaluation of service-connected disabilities if a condition worsens over time, if medical science permits an improved evaluation or if there is a change in the law governing the assignment of disability ratings. As a consequence, a VA disability rating generally is expected to be equal if not higher than the military disability rating, and it may increase after the service member's separation from the military.

Separation with severance pay

- Disability permanent, **and**
- Disability rating of less than 30% **and**
- Less than 20 years on active duty.

Permanent retirement

- Disability permanent, **and**
- Disability rating of 30% or higher, **or**
- 20 or more years of active service.

Retention on the temporary disability retirement list

- Disability unstable, with potential for recovery, **and**
- Disability rating of at least 30%.

Transitional Health Care for You and Your Family

The Transitional Assistance Management Program (TAMP) offers transitional TRICARE coverage to certain separating active duty members and their eligible family members. Care is available for a limited time. TRICARE

PEB LOCATIONS

U.S. Air Force
Lackland Air Force Base
San Antonio, TX
www.lackland.af.mil

U.S. Army
Fort Lewis
Tacoma, WA
www.lewis.army.mil

Fort Sam Houston
San Antonio, TX
www.samhouston.army.mil

Walter Reed National Military Medical Center
Bethesda, MD
www.wramc.amedd.army.mil

U.S. Navy and U.S. Marine Corps
National Naval Medical Center
Bethesda, MD
www.bethesda.med.navy.mil

eligibility under the TAMP has been permanently extended to 180 days. There are four categories of eligibility for TAMP:

- Members involuntarily separated from active duty and their eligible family members.
- National Guard and Reserve members, collectively known as the Reserve Component (RC), separated from active duty after being called up or ordered in support of a contingency operation for an active duty period of more than 30 days and their family members.
- Members separated from active duty after being involuntarily retained in support of a contingency operation and their family members; and
- Members separated from active duty following a voluntary agreement to stay on active duty for less than one year in support of a contingency mission and their family members.

Active duty sponsors and family members enrolled in TRICARE Prime who desire to continue their enrollment upon the sponsor's separation from active duty status are required to reenroll. To reenroll, the sponsor or family member must complete and submit a TRICARE Prime enrollment application. Contact your servicing personnel center prior to separating to see if you are TAMP eligible. Under TAMP, former active duty sponsors, former activated reservists, and family members of both are not eligible to enroll or reenroll in TRICARE Prime Remote or in TRICARE Prime Remote for Active Duty Family Members because both programs require the sponsor to be on active duty. Under the TAMP, the sponsor is no longer on active duty and is treated as an active duty family member for benefits and cost-sharing purposes.

Health Insurance

Health Care Insurance Planning Is Critical

TRICARE

Referral: The act or instance of referring a beneficiary to another authorized provider for necessary medical or behavioral health care treatment.

Prior Authorization: A decision issued electronically or in writing stating that TRICARE will cover services that have not yet been received. Failure to obtain a prior authorization when required may result in a denial of payment for those services.

Active Duty Service Members: Active duty service members (ADSMs) should always seek care first at an MTF, when available. ADSMs must have a referral from their primary care manager (PCM) and have prior authorization from their regional contractor before seeking any behavioral health care services outside the MTF. If enrolled in TRICARE Prime Remote, you may receive authorization from your service point of contact (SPOC) for civilian behavioral health care.

TRICARE Prime Beneficiaries (Other than Active Duty Service Members): If you are enrolled in TRICARE Prime, you may receive the first eight behavioral health care outpatient visits per fiscal year (October 1–September 30) from a TRICARE network provider without a referral from your PCM or prior authorization from your regional contractor. If you obtain services from a non-network provider, the office visit will be covered under the point of service (POS) option, resulting in higher out of pocket costs.

After the first eight visits (starting with the ninth visit), your behavioral health care provider must receive prior authorization from your regional contractor, however PCM referrals are not required if you are non-active-duty status.

Additional prior authorization requirements apply for inpatient services, outpatient treatment programs, residential treatment center services, and other services. Refer to your regional contractor's website for details.

Note: These rules also apply to you if you are enrolled in TRICARE Prime Remote for Active Duty Family Members (TPRADFM) and the US Family Health Plan.

Beneficiaries Using TRICARE Standard or TRICARE Extra: Under TRICARE Standard and TRICARE Extra, referrals are never required. You may receive your first eight behavioral health outpatient visits per fiscal year without prior authorization. After the first eight visits, your behavioral health care provider must receive prior authorization from your regional contractor (see below). Additional prior authorization requirements apply for inpatient services, outpatient treatment programs, residential treatment center services, and other services.

Refer to your regional contractor's website for details. Regional contractors:

TRICARE North Region: Health Net Federal Services, Inc.
TRICARE South Region: Humana Military Healthcare Services, Inc.
TRICARE West Region: TriWest Healthcare Alliance Corp.

Remember to obtain care only from TRICARE network providers or TRICARE authorized non-network providers. Obtaining care from a TRICARE network provider will reduce your out-of-pocket expenses.

Dual-Eligible Beneficiaries: If you are using Medicare as your primary payer and TRICARE as secondary payer, you are not required to obtain referrals or prior authorization from TRICARE for inpatient behavioral health care services. However, when your behavioral health care benefits are exhausted under Medicare and TRICARE becomes the primary payer, TRICARE referral and authorization requirements apply. Refer to your regional contractor's website for details.

Note: Additional prior authorization requirements are listed in the Covered Behavioral Health Care Services section.

Behavioral Health Care Providers

The following types of behavioral health care providers may be authorized providers under TRICARE:

- Psychiatrists
- Clinical psychologists
- Certified psychiatric nurse specialists
- Clinical social workers
- Certified marriage and family therapists with a TRICARE participation agreement
- Pastoral counselors—with physician referral and supervision

- Mental health counselors—with physician referral and supervision
- Licensed professional counselors—with physician referral and supervision

If you are unsure which type of provider would best meet your needs, you can contact your regional contractor for assistance. To ensure that your behavioral health care is covered, remember the following:

- If you are taking prescription medications for a behavioral health care condition, you must be under the care of a provider authorized to prescribe those medications. While this can be a primary care provider, it is often preferable to receive psychiatric medication management services from a psychiatrist who is an expert in this area.
- Nonphysician behavioral health care providers (e.g., clinical psychologists, clinical social workers, psychiatric nurse specialists, and marriage/family therapists) may deliver covered services without a physician referral and supervision. Other behavioral health care providers require a referral from an M.D. or D.O., and ongoing supervision. These providers are pastoral counselors, mental health counselors, and licensed professional counselors.
- Your behavioral health care provider is expected to consult with (or refer you to) a physician for evaluation and treatment of physical conditions that may co-exist with or contribute to a behavioral health care condition.

Costs and Fees

Your financial responsibility for behavioral health care services depends on which TRICARE option (TRICARE Prime, TRICARE Standard, etc.) you use. For specific cost information, visit www.tricare.mil/tricarecost or see the *TRICARE: Summary of Beneficiary Costs* brochure. The brochure is available from your regional contractor or local TRICARE Service Center (TSC), or it can be found online at www.tricare.mil/tricaresmart.

Covered Behavioral Health Care Services

TRICARE offers a wide range of coverage for behavioral health care services.

Psychotherapy

TRICARE covers both outpatient and inpatient psychotherapy. Outpatient psychotherapy is limited to a maximum of two sessions per week in any combination of individual, family, collateral, or group sessions, and is not covered if you are an inpatient in an institution. Inpatient psychotherapy is limited to five sessions per week in any combination of individual, family, collateral, or group sessions. The duration and frequency of care is dependent upon medical necessity.

Covered psychotherapy includes:

Family Therapy—Family therapy is directed toward the family as a unit and is based on the assumption that the mental or emotional illness of the patient is related to family interactions. Family therapy could include part of or the entire family and would normally involve the same therapist or treatment team.

Collateral Visits—A collateral visit is not a therapy session or a treatment planning session. It is used to gather information and implement treatment goals. Collateral visits are included as an individual psychotherapy visit and can last up to one hour. They may be combined with another individual or group psychotherapy visit.

Play Therapy—Play therapy is a form of individual psychotherapy used to diagnose and treat children with psychiatric disorders and is covered as an individual psychotherapy session.

Psychoanalysis—Psychoanalysis is covered when provided by a graduate or candidate of a psychoanalytic training institution and requires prior authorization from your regional contractor.

Psychological Testing—Psychological testing and assessment is covered when provided in conjunction with otherwise covered psychotherapy and is generally limited to six hours per fiscal year.* Psychological testing is not covered under the following circumstances:

- Academic placement
- Job placement
- Child custody disputes
- General screening in the absence of specific symptoms
- Teacher or parental referrals
- Diagnosed specific learning disorders or learning disabilities

Acute Inpatient Psychiatric Care

Acute inpatient psychiatric care may be covered on an emergency or non-emergency basis.

- All non-emergency inpatient admissions require prior authorization from your regional contractor.
- Emergency behavioral health care inpatient admissions should be reported to your regional contractor within 24–72 hours.

---

* Fiscal year is October 1–September 30.

- Ongoing authorization is based upon medical necessity reviews.
- Patients ages 19 and older are limited to 30 days per fiscal year.
- Patients ages 18 and under are limited to 45 days per fiscal year.
- Inpatient admissions for substance use disorder detoxification and rehabilitation count toward the 30 or 45 day limit.

Partial Hospitalization

Partial hospitalization provides interdisciplinary therapeutic services at least three hours per day, five days per week in any combination of day, evening, night, and weekend treatment programs.

- Requires prior authorization from your regional contractor.
- Facility must be TRICARE-authorized and must agree to participate in TRICARE.
- Limited to 60 treatment days (whether a full or partial day treatment) in a fiscal year. These 60 days are not offset or counted toward the 30 or 45 day inpatient limit.

Residential Treatment Center Care

Residential treatment center care provides extended care for children and adolescents with psychological disorders that require continued treatment in a therapeutic environment.

- Requires prior authorization from your regional contractor.
- Care must be recommended and directed by a psychiatrist or clinical psychologist.
- Facility must be TRICARE authorized.
- Care is considered elective and will not be covered for emergencies.
- Admission primarily for substance use rehabilitation is not authorized.
- Limited to 150 days per fiscal year, based upon medical necessity reviews.
- Not available in all overseas locations.

Substance Use Disorders

A substance use disorder includes alcohol, drug abuse, or dependence. TRICARE may cover services for the treatment of substance use disorders, including detoxification, rehabilitation, and outpatient group and family therapy.

   Note: All treatment for substance use disorders requires prior authorization from your regional contractor.

Detoxification. Covered if the medical necessity is documented. In a diagnosis-related group (DRG) exempt facility, detoxification services are limited to seven days per year, unless the limit is waived.

Rehabilitation. Limited to one inpatient stay, up to 21 days per benefit period, in a DRG-based reimbursement system. Rehabilitation may consist of a combination of inpatient days and partial hospitalization days.

Benefit Period. A substance use disorder treatment benefit period begins with the first date of covered treatment and ends 365 days later. You are allowed three benefit periods in your lifetime.

Outpatient Care. Must be provided by an approved substance use disorder facility in a group setting only. Up to 60 visits per benefit period are covered.

Family Therapy. Outpatient family therapy is covered beginning with the completion of rehabilitative care. You are covered for up to 15 visits per benefit period.

Medication Management

If you are taking prescription medications for a behavioral health care condition, you must be under the care of a provider who is authorized to prescribe those medications. Your provider will manage the dosage and duration of your prescription to ensure you are receiving the best care possible.

For additional information about covered and noncovered behavioral health care services, consult the handbook for your TRICARE program option or contact your regional contractor.

For Information and Assistance

TRICARE North Regional Contractor
Health Net Federal Services, Inc.
877-TRICARE (877-874-2273) www.healthnetfederalservices.com

TRICARE South Regional Contractor
Humana Military Healthcare Services, Inc. 800-444-5445
www.humana-military.com
ValueOptions 800-700-8646

TRICARE West Regional Contractor
TriWest Healthcare Alliance Corp. 888-TRIWEST (888-874-9378)
www.triwest.com

TRICARE Overseas
(TRICARE Europe, TRICARE Latin America and Canada, and TRICARE Pacific)
888-777-8343

TRICARE Prime Remote
Service Point of Contact (SPOC)
DoD: 888-647-6676
Coast Guard: 888-647-6676 or 800-942-2422
NOAA: 800-662-2267
USPHS: 800-368-2777, option 2

US Family Health Plan
A TRICARE Prime Option 800-74-USFHP (800-748-7347)
www.usfamilyhealthplan.org

DEERS—Verify and Update Information
800-538-9552
www.tricare.mil/DEERS

Echo: Extended Health Care Option
Companion coverage to TRICARE providing medical equipment that TRI-
CARE doesn't cover with its basic coverage. Apply through your TRICARE
Regional Contractor—see above.

4

Support

OUR PLEDGE TO THE WOUNDED AND SICK
OF OUR ARMED FORCES

We pledge on our honor
To remember and assist the wounded
And ill of our Armed Forces
From ALL wars to the best of our ability.

We pledge that we will never forget
That we will always remember
The sacrifices you have made.
The blood sweat and tears that you shed

Will remain on our minds and in our hearts
And we will forever be grateful
We pledge that we will remind others

So that all remember
That you gave up so much
So that this Nation would not perish from the face of the earth.
God bless the United States of America

This is the pledge of Silver Star Families of America, which designated May 1 as Silver Star Day—an annual celebration to honor our wounded. Over 2,907 cities and counties, 49 states and the District of Columbia celebrated Silver Star Day in 2010.

Replacing Military Records

If discharge or separation documents are lost, veterans or the next of kin of deceased veterans may obtain duplicate copies by completing forms found on the Internet at www.archives.gov/research/index.html and mailing or faxing them to the NPRC.

Alternatively, write the National Personnel Records Center, Military Personnel Records, 9700 Page Ave., St. Louis, MO 63132-5100. Specify that a duplicate separation document is needed. The veteran's full name should be printed or typed so that it can be read clearly, but the request must also contain the signature of the veteran or the signature of the next of kin, if the veteran is deceased. Include the veteran's branch of service, service number or Social Security number and exact or approximate dates and years of service. Use Standard Form 180, "Request Pertaining to Military Records." It is not necessary to request a duplicate copy of a veteran's discharge or separation papers solely for the purpose of filing a claim for VA benefits. If complete information about the veteran's service is furnished on the application, VA will obtain verification of service.

Correction of Military Records

The secretary of a military department, acting through a Board for Correction of Military Records, has authority to change any military record when necessary to correct an error or remove an injustice.

Note: With the transcription of paper to electronic records, errors can occur. Medical records should be reviewed periodically for accuracy so that errors do not translate into risks or misinterpretations.

The veteran, survivor or legal representative must file a request for correction within three years after discovering an alleged error or injustice. Applications should include all evidence, such as signed statements of witnesses or a brief of arguments supporting the correction. Application is made with DD Form 149, available at VA offices, veterans organizations or www.dtic.mil/whs/directives/infomgt/forms/eforms/dd0149.pdf.

Replacing Military Medals

Medals awarded while in active service are issued by the individual military services if requested by veterans or their next of kin. Requests for replacement medals, decorations, and awards should be directed to the branch of the military in which the veteran served.

However, for Air Force (including Army Air Corps) and Army veterans, the National Personnel Records Center (NPRC) verifies awards and forwards requests and verification to appropriate services. Requests for replacement medals should be submitted on Standard Form 180, "Request Pertaining to Military Records," which may be obtained at VA offices or the Internet at www.archives.gov/research/order/standard-form-180.pdf. Forms, addresses, and other information on requesting medals can be found on the Military Personnel Records section of NPRC's website at www.archives.gov/st-louis/military-personnel/index.html. For questions, call Military Personnel Records at 314-801-0800 or e-mail questions to: MPR.center@nara.gov.

When requesting medals, type or clearly print the veteran's full name, include the veteran's branch of service, service number or Social Security number and provide the veteran's exact or approximate dates of military service. The request must contain the signature of the veteran or next of kin if the veteran is deceased. If available, include a copy of the discharge or separation document, WDAGO Form 53-55 or DD Form 214.

Applying for Review of Discharge

Each of the military services maintains a discharge review board with authority to change, correct or modify discharges or dismissals not issued by a sentence of a general courts-martial. The board has no authority to address medical discharges.

VA DISABILITY BENEFITS

The VA pays disability compensation to veterans who become disabled while serving in the armed forces or whose pre-service ailments are made worse by such service. As is often the case, the same disability that entitles the service member to monthly disability retirement payments or a lump-sum severance payment from the DoD also entitles service members to monthly VA disability compensation.

The VA's disability compensation is paid monthly and is calculated on the basis of the service member's VA disability rating—rank and years of service do not factor into the VA disability compensation calculation. VA disability payments do vary, however, based on the degree of a service member's disability and the number of dependents he or she has. For more information see chapter 7.

The VA's disability rating is entirely separate from the DoD's. While the PEB and MEB (see chapter 3) make a determination on the service member's medical condition and ability to continue to serve based on a service member's particular injury, the VA disability rating takes into account all the service member's disabilities and medical conditions to arrive at a combined disability rating. Service members with at least a 10% combined disability rating are eligible to receive VA disability compensation payments.

SEVERANCE PAY AND DISABILITY RETIREMENT PAY

As a preliminary matter, a service member will be eligible for DoD disability compensation—severance pay or disability retirement pay—only following a determination that the service member is unfit for duty and assigned a disability rating by a PEB. On occasion, a service member may have a scheduled separation date (e.g., end-of-service contract, administrative separation, voluntary retirement) that occurs prior to a fitness-for-duty determination by a PEB. (Service members generally will not be separated while awaiting an MEB/PEB.) In such a situation, the service member's separation will be subject to a "presumption of fitness," which means that the separation is presumed to occur not as a result of a medical condition, even though the service member may actually be separated after an "unfit for duty" determination by a PEB. This presumption of fitness is not the same as a finding of fitness, but it does mean that the service member would not be entitled to DoD disability compensation unless the service member can show that that military service was in fact interrupted because of the medical condition.

Disabled service members separated from the military as a result of their disability are entitled to either severance pay or disability retirement pay, depending on factors such as the disability rating assigned by the PEB and the number of years of qualifying military service the individual has as of the date of separation.

Severance pay is a lump-sum, one-time payment that is calculated on the basis of the service member's base pay and number of years of service. A service member who is found unfit to continue in the military, but who has a disability rating of less than 30% and less than 20 years of military service, is entitled to severance pay (but no disability retirement pay).

Disability retirement pay is the monthly compensation paid under certain circumstances by the DoD to a service member following separation. A service member will be entitled to disability retirement pay when he or she is separated from military service and placed on either the Permanent Disability Retirement List (PDRL) or Temporary Disability Retirement List (TDRL). Whether a service member is placed on the PDRL or TDRL will determine the amount of disability retirement pay he or she receives. Service members placed on the PDRL will receive disability retirement pay for life. However, there are no spouse or survivor benefits upon the service member's death unless the service member elects to participate in the Survivor Benefit Plan.

Generally, the service member's retired base pay is his or her highest basic pay received at the time of separation.

SPECIAL COMPENSATION

Depending on the severity of a service member's injury and number of dependents, he or she may be entitled to Special Monthly Compensation, additional compensation for dependents and payments to overcome a lack of employability.

Special Monthly Compensation (SMC). Service members who sustain particularly severe injuries, such as amputations, blindness, and other severe traumas, are eligible to receive additional monthly payments above and beyond the basic VA disability compensation. SMC rates take into account attendant care or other special needs resulting from severe injuries.

Dependents. Veterans receiving VA disability compensation and assigned a disability rating of at least 30%are eligible for adjustments to their VA disability payments according to the number and, in the case of children, the ages of their dependents. Additional adjustments are made for each additional child and certain further adjustments are made for children who enrolled in school after age 18.

Individual Unemployability (IU). The VA provides additional benefits to veteran service members who are unemployable because of their service-connected disabilities. Under the program, the VA can grant total disability compensation (as if the service member had a 100% disability rating) to service members with disabilities rated 60% or higher and who cannot work. In certain cases, service members with disabilities rated less than 60% may be given Individual Unemployability benefits. Thus, under certain circumstances, a service member who is not employable due to his or her disability can still receive total disability compensation, despite not being rated 100% disabled by the VA.

Generally, the DoD retirement benefit is offset dollar-for-dollar by the amount of the VA compensation benefit.

Concurrent Receipt Payments

The Combat-Related Special Compensation (CRSC) programs and Concurrent Retirement & Disability Payments (CRDP) programs are DoD programs that provide extra payments to qualifying veterans whose DoD disability retirement benefit payments are offset by VA disability compensation. Veterans who are eligible for both programs may only receive one benefit at a time, either the CRSC or the CRDP, but they may switch programs on a yearly basis. Qualifying veterans are automatically enrolled in the CDRP; no separate application is necessary to enroll in the CRDP.

Traumatic Injury Protection Insurance (TSGLI)

Service members who suffer a qualifying loss due to a traumatic injury incurred on or after October 7, 2001 through and including November 30, 2005, in Operation Enduring Freedom (OEF) or Operation Iraqi Freedom are eligible as are service members covered under SGLI who suffer a qualifying loss due to a traumatic injury on or after December 1, 2005. Effective October 1, 2011, TSGLI will be payable for all qualifying injuries incurred during the period of October 7, 2001, to November 30, 2005, regardless of where they occurred and regardless of whether the member had SGLI coverage at the time of the injury (see also chapter 1).

Injuries Covered

- Total and permanent loss of sight in one or both eyes;
- Loss of hand or foot by severance at or above the wrist or ankle;
- Total and permanent loss of hearing in one or both ears;
- Loss of thumb and index finger of the same hand by severance at or above the metacarpophalangeal joints;
- Quadriplegia, paraplegia, or hemiplegia;
- 3rd degree or worse burns covering 30 percent of the body or 30 percent of the face.
- Coma or the inability to carry out two of the six activities of daily living.

For the complete schedule of losses, go to www.insurance.va.gov/sgliSite/TSGLI/TSGLI.htm.

Benefits

TSGLI coverage pays a benefit of between $25,000 and $100,000 depending on the qualifying loss incurred. The amount paid for each qualifying loss is listed on a schedule available at the following website: www.insurance.va.gov/sgliSite/TSGLI/TSGLI.htm.

How to Claim

In order to make a claim for the TSGLI benefit, the member (or someone acting on his or her behalf) should:

1. Download the TSGLI Certification Form GL.2005.261 at www.insurance.va.gov/sgliSite/TSGLI/TSGLI.htm. You can also obtain this form from

your service department point of contact or from the Office of Service members' Group Life Insurance by toll-free phone at 800-419-1473 or by email at osgli.claims@prudential.com.

2. Contact your service department point of contact to begin the certification process. The certification form has three parts:
   - Part A is to be completed by the service member or, if incapacitated, by the member's guardian, or the member's attorney-in-fact.
   - Part B is to be completed by the attending medical professional.
   - Part C is to be completed by the branch of service prior to submission of the claim form to OSGLI.

TRICARE FOR LIFE

If a member or family member becomes entitled to Medicare Part A, whether due to a disability or when they turn 65, they are eligible for TRICARE for Life (TFL). There are no TFL enrollment fees, but you are required to pay Medicare Part B premiums (unless the sponsor is on active duty). When using TFL, TRICARE is the second payer after Medicare in most cases. For more information about TFL visit www.tricare.mil/tfl or search on "TRICARE for Life"; you may also call Wisconsin Physicians Service-TFL at 866-773-0404 (866-773-0405 TTY/TDD for the hearing impaired).

Survivors

Family members are entitled to TRICARE benefits as transitional survivors or survivors if their active duty service sponsor died while serving on active duty for a period of more than 30 days. TRICARE pays transitional survivor claims at the active duty family member payment rate and pays survivor claims at the retiree payment rate for surviving spouses while eligible children claims process at the active duty family member rate. Transitional survivors pay no enrollment fees or co-payments when they use TRICARE Prime. They will, however, pay cost shares and deductibles at the active duty family member rate to use TRICARE Standard or TRICARE Extra. Contact your regional contractor or visit www.tricare.mil.

CONTINUED HEALTH CARE BENEFIT PROGRAM

Your Option to Purchase Temporary Medical Coverage

Following the loss of eligibility to military medical benefits, you or a family member may apply for temporary, transitional medical coverage under the

Continued Health Care Benefit Program (CHCBP). CHCBP is a premium-based health care program providing medical coverage to a select group of former military beneficiaries. CHCBP is similar to, but not part of, TRI-CARE. The CHCBP program extends health care coverage to the following individuals when they lose military benefits:

- The service member (who can also enroll his or her family members)
- Certain former spouses who have not remarried
- Certain children who lose military coverage

Enrollment and Coverage

Eligible beneficiaries must enroll in CHCBP within 60 days following the loss of entitlement to the Military Health System. To enroll, you will be required to submit:

- A completed DD Form 2837, "Continued Health Care Benefit Program (CHCBP) Application."
- Documentation as requested on the enrollment form, e.g., DD Form 214, "Certificate of Release or Discharge from Active Duty"; final divorce decree; DD Form 1173, "Uniformed Services Identification and Privilege Card." Additional information and documentation may be required to confirm an applicant's eligibility for CHCBP.
- A premium payment for the first 90 days of health coverage. For enrollments with an effective date of September 30, 2010, or before, the premium rates are approximately $933 per quarter for individuals and $1,996 per quarter for families. For enrollments with an effective date of October 1, 2010, or after, and quarterly payments to pay for periods beginning October 1, 2010, and after, the rate is $988 per quarter for individuals and $2,213 per quarter for families.
- Humana Military Healthcare Services, Inc., will bill you for subsequent quarterly premiums through your period of eligibility once you are enrolled.
- The program uses existing TRICARE providers and follows most of the rules and procedures of the TRICARE Standard program. Depending on your beneficiary category, CHCBP coverage is limited to either 18 or 36 months as follows:
- 18 months for separating service members and their families
- 36 months for others who are eligible (in some cases, former spouses who have not remarried may continue coverage beyond 36 months if they meet certain criteria)

You may not select the effective date of coverage under CHCBP. For all enrollees, CHCBP coverage must be effective on the day after you lose military benefits.

All Others

If you separate voluntarily, you and your family are not eligible to use military treatment facilities or TRICARE. However, you may purchase extended transitional health care coverage (CHCBP) for up to 18 months of coverage. You have 60 days after separation to enroll in CHCBP. Your coverage will start the day after your separation.

DoD contracted with Humana Military Healthcare Services, Inc., to administer CHCBP. You may contact Humana Military Healthcare Services, Inc., in writing or by phone for information:

Humana Military Healthcare Services, Inc.
Attn: CHCBP
P.O. Box 740072
Louisville, KY 40201
800-444-5445

A copy of the CHCBP enrollment application can also be found at www
.tricare.mil and www.humana-military.com.

5

Recovery and Transition

RECOVERY

Returning to Duty after Injury

Service members wanting to return to active duty often undergo extensive periods of rehabilitation to ensure they reach their maximum fitness and performance levels. During this time they are constantly evaluated by their medical team, which produces a functional assessment report. In order to remain on active duty, the report must find that the service member meets retention standards for each of his or her medical conditions.

This report is one of many documents compiled by medical and civilian personnel who determine the service member's fitness for duty. These documents are presented to an informal Physical Evaluation Board (PEB) along with the service member's personnel records and performance requirements for their primary Military Occupational Specialty (MOS). The PEB is called informal because the service member does not attend.

The informal PEB deliberations determine whether the service member is fit for duty or not. The inability to be deployed to any geographic location under any condition cannot be used as a sole basis for finding the soldier unfit. Following the findings the service member has 10 days to appeal the decision. If the PEB determines the service member is fit to return to duty, he or she will either be sent back to their unit or assigned for new training.

Until recently the idea of amputees returning to duty was not even considered an option but thanks to modern prosthetics, a growing number of wounded warriors are able to continue in the military and meet the rigorous performance standards required of them. The severity of limb loss and the nature and extent of associated injuries are the main factors taken into consideration when considering suitability for return to active duty. Service members most likely to return to active duty are those with highly valued military skills and strong service records prior to their injuries. Many amputees are assigned to a Medical Holding Company (MHC) while they recover and where they receive treatment and are assessed. Service members who want to remain in the military often spend many more weeks of rehabilitation at the MHC than those seeking to transition. The service members' medical team will prepare a detailed profile which will be presented to the Physical Evaluation Board and the Medical Evacuation Board. If the service member is considered fit for duty, he or she will be sent back to their unit or assigned to new training.

LEAVING THE MILITARY

Mentoring

The VetConnect program is designed to "provide wounded warriors with a critical link to resources . . . and to engage local community and business leaders in the reorientation of disabled veterans to their communities," Scott Heintz, the program's director, said. The program is run by "Enable America," a non-profit group dedicated to increasing employment opportunities for Americans with disabilities.

VetConnect also offers early intervention support by matching wounded warriors with casualty mentors and coordinating their participation in wellness activities, he said. This program has been expanded to wounded special operations troops through the Care Coalition Recovery Pilot Program. The program, similar to VetConnect's mentoring program, was developed and implemented with the help of U.S. Special Operations Command.

"The objective of the pilot program is to improve the recovery outcome of special operations forces wounded warriors through the early introduction of casualty mentors and wellness activities designed to boost wounded warriors' confidence and self-esteem," Heintz said.

The mentors, wounded warriors themselves, are matched with a newly wounded warrior and trained to provide support and guidance throughout and beyond the recovery process. The matches are made based on similarity of injures, unit affiliations and family situations.

"Mentors offer valuable insight and counsel from the perspective of someone who has successfully navigated similar physical and emotional challenges," Heintz said. "Spouses and family members of wounded (special operations force members) also serve as mentors and provide guidance to their counterparts."

When service members and their family members are ready to try Enable America's wellness activities, the organization will help them find the right one. All of the activities—camping, skiing, yoga and photography, to name a few—are offered through organizations that are able to accommodate the participant's needs.

"As their recovery progresses, Enable America provides wounded warriors and their families with access to a comprehensive network of community and employment resources," Heintz said. "The final component of the program is that of providing the wounded warrior with an employment resource network that will (offer) them meaningful and challenging work that is commensurate with their unique skill sets."

Enable America recently became a supporter of America Supports You, a Defense Department program connecting citizens and companies with service members and their families serving and home and abroad.

Pre-Separation

Review the Pre-separation Counseling Checklist

Your Transition Counselor or Command Career Counselor will walk you through the Pre-separation Counseling Checklist, which helps ensure that you will receive the necessary assistance and advice to benefit fully from the wide range of services and entitlements available to you. The checklist is required by law to be filed in the official military personnel record of each service member receiving the counseling.

At this meeting, the Transition Assistance Office or Command Career Counselor will:

- **Assist** you in developing an individual needs assessment.
- **Identify** helpful relocation resources.
- **Offer** immediate and long-range career guidance.
- **Provide** benefits counseling.
- **Refer** you to other service providers for any additional assistance you may require.

Draft Your Individual Transition Plan

Information on drafting your Individual Transition Plan (ITP) is available through the Transition Assistance Office. You may choose to use your Pre-separation Counseling Checklist as a guide for developing your own unique ITP. Once you have created your ITP, show it to your Transition Counselor or Command Career Counselor. They will provide you further assistance or refer you to a subject matter expert to assist you. Full participation in this process by you and your spouse is encouraged.

Phases of Individual Transition Planning

All military personnel transitioning out of the service go through the same fundamental stages. These stages can be divided into the following seven different phases: Self-Assessment, Exploration, Skills Development, Intern Programs, Job Search, Job Selection, and Support.

Self-Assessment

Ask yourself: Who am I? What are my talents and experiences? Why would someone want to hire me?

In this phase, document your portfolio of knowledge, experience, skills, talents, and abilities. For starters, create a list using your personal DD Form 2586, "Verification of Military Experience and Training." Your VMET outlines the training and experience you received during your military career. It is designed to help you, but it is not a resume. To get your verification document, go to the VMET website at www.dmdc.osd.mil/vmet. All separating military personnel can electronically download and print their VMET document and personal cover letter from your military service from the VMET website. Simply click the "Request Document" and "Request Cover Letter" tabs and print each of these documents after they are downloaded. You can get your verification document online as long as you have a current DoD Common Access Card (CAC) or have a current Defense Finance, Accounting Service (DFAS) myPay Personal Identification Number (PIN). However, you should retrieve it within 120 days prior to your separation. If you have problems getting your VMET and need assistance, check with your local Transition Counselor. Add anything else you can think of to this list. In essence, you are now creating an "asset bank" from which you can draw later when called upon to write a resume or attend a job interview. If you need help, use the professional guidance available through your local installation Transition Assistance Office or Education Center. Or refer to the self-help section of your local library or bookstore for useful career-planning books.

In addition you can get an official transcript of your education and training credits from your service branch. Each branch has their own system for recording your military (and civilian) education and experience. The following explains how to:

- **Army.** The **Army's AARTS** (Army/American Council on Education Registry Transcript System) automatically captures your military training, your Military Occupational Specialty (MOS) and college-level examinations scores with the college credit recommended. AARTS Home Page: aarts.army.mil.

- Navy and Marines. The **Navy and Marine Corps use the SMART system**. This system automatically captures your training, experience and standardized test scores. SMART website: https://www.navycollege.navy.mil/transcript.html.
- **Air Force.** The **Community College of the Air Force** (CCAF) automatically captures your training, experience and standardized test scores. Transcript information may be viewed at the CCAF website: www.au.af.mil/au/ccaf.
- **Coast Guard.** The **Coast Guard Institute** (CGI) requires each service member to submit documentation of all training (except correspondence course records), along with an enrollment form, to receive a transcript. Transcript information can be found at the Coast Guard Institute website: www .uscg.mil/hr/cgi.

If you are able, the investment you make now in conducting your assessment is crucial. It will bring the "professional you" into clearer focus, and it will have a major impact on your career decisions. The key to a smooth transition is to be prepared well before you separate from the military. Start early. Make connections and build networks that will help you transition into the civilian world.

Exploration
Ask Yourself: What are the current and emerging occupational areas that are attractive to me? Do these jobs coincide with my values and aptitudes? How do I find these jobs?

With your assessment in hand, you probably have some ideas about what you want to do. Now is not the time to limit your opportunities. Expand the list of job titles and career paths that appeal to you. Broaden your geographic horizons to include several places where you might like to pursue your career. Many resources are available to help you explore your expanded set of options.

The Transition Assistance Office can help you focus on jobs that employers need to fill today and will need to fill in the near future. Transition staff can help you identify the geographic areas that have opportunities in your fields of interest.

Your state employment office is another good resource during this phase, offering such services as job interviewing; selection and referral to openings; job development; employment counseling; career evaluation; referral to training or other support services; and testing. Your state office can also lead you to information on related jobs nearby and introduce you to the Department of

Labor database, DoD Job Search, which has listings of thousands of jobs across the nation. And don't forget your local library's reference section. Most of them are full of helpful publications relating to job searches.

Skills Development

Ask Yourself: How do I prepare myself to be an attractive candidate in the occupational areas that I have chosen? Do I need additional education or training?

As you continue through the exploration phase, you may find some interesting opportunities for which you feel only partially qualified. Your local Transition Assistance Office and Education Center can help you determine the academic credentials or vocational training programs you will need and how to get them.

Intern Programs

Ask Yourself: Do I have the aptitude and experience needed to pursue my occupational interests? Are there internships, volunteer jobs, temporary services, or part-time jobs where I might try out the work that interests me?

To learn about intern programs, inquire at your Transition Assistance Office, your local civilian personnel office, or the state employment office. Some government-sponsored programs, such as obtaining teaching credentials, can provide income and training in exchange for guaranteed employment. Check local and base libraries and the education office for books containing intern program information.

Temporary agencies are also a great way to become familiar with a company or industry. Explore internship possibilities with private employers: Many companies have such programs but do not advertise them. Don't necessarily turn down an interesting volunteer position. Volunteering increases your professional skills and can sometimes turn into a paid position.

The Job Search

Ask Yourself: How do I identify job requirements and prospective companies, find networks and placement agencies, and generally increase my knowledge and experience in the job market? How do I write a resume, develop leads, conduct an interview, and complete a job application?

Once you have selected your future career, you must now begin the challenge of finding work. Millions of people are hired all across the country every year. Employee turnover opens up existing positions, and entirely new jobs are created every day. Nevertheless, the job market is competitive. The best way to improve your odds is to play your best hand: Seek the opportunities for which you are best prepared.

Work hard at finding a job. Network! The vast majority of jobs are filled by referrals, not the want ads. Use your network of friends, colleagues, and family, as well as the job listings provided by your installation's Transition Assistance Office, the local personnel office, or even the nearest community college. Take advantage of job-hunting seminars, resume-writing workshops, and interviewing techniques classes too. Attend job fairs and talk to as many company representatives as possible.

Job Selection
Ask Yourself: How do I select the right job?

Although it might be tempting, you don't have to take the first job that comes along. Consider the type of work, location, salary and benefits, climate, and how the opportunity will enhance your future career growth. Even if you take the first job offer, you are not necessarily locked into it. Some experts say employers are biased against hiring the unemployed. A shrewd move might be to look for a job from a job. Take a suitable position—and then quickly move on to a better one.

Support
Ask Yourself: How do I make a smooth transition to a new career?

For your transition to be truly successful, you should manage the personal affairs side of your career change with the same professionalism and care as your job search. Things like out-processing, relocation, financial management, taking care of your family, and coping with the inevitable stress are important too.

Your Transition Assistance Office can offer support as you go through this process. In addition your ITP provides an opportunity to integrate these issues with the career-oriented activities that are the central focus of your transition effort.

TRANSITION

You have been in the military for a number of years, and you are now making the transition back to civilian life. Understanding stress and coping with it, are essential skills you will need to get through this difficult time. The following information and resources will help you prepare for a successful transition. For more detailed information see *Life After the Military* published by GI.

Leaving the Military Challenges Your Identity

You have worked hard to become a captain, sergeant, or petty officer. When asked what you do, you probably replied, "I'm in the Army (Air Force, Navy, Coast Guard, or Marines)." Now you must start over as a civilian. Now you are just another civilian.

Changing careers is a stressful undertaking, perhaps even more so for those leaving military service after many years. A service member may have worked for 30 years to achieve a rank or grade, but upon leaving the Armed Forces, he or she leaves this rank behind—and with it, a large portion of his or her identity.

Coping with Transition-Related Stress

The experiences of thousands of service members who have recently separated suggest that this transition is likely to be stressful for you and your family. Those that have transitioned in the past have found several tactics extremely important in dealing with the stress related to separation from the military:

- **Get going**: It is your transition; no one can do it for you. Work through the transition process and do not procrastinate. Put your situation in perspective and get on with your life. After all, you are not the first person to go through transition, and you will not be the last. You'll do okay too.
- **Sell yourself**: You have a great product—YOU! So sell yourself! Now is not the time to be modest about your accomplishments. No one will come looking for you unless they know you are available. Once you let them know, you will find many people who will help you.
- **Work at it**: Work at planning your transition as if it were a job. However, if you spend every waking hour working on it, you will burn out. Take time for yourself and your family.
- **Lighten up**: This is probably the most important piece of advice. Do not lose your sense of humor. An upbeat disposition will see you through.
- **Keep your family involved**: Your family has a large stake in your transition. They are experiencing many of the same feelings, worries, and uncertainties as you are. Do not keep your plans to yourself; get your family involved in this process. Let them in on your plans and ask for their input throughout the process. It's their life too.
- **Volunteer**: Consider doing volunteer work. Your charitable actions will help others and assist you in getting to know the community beyond the military installations and enhance your networking.
- **Take a change management course**: Consider taking a change management course before stress appears, or at the first signs of stress.

Where to Go for Help

We all deal with stress every day. However, during a major life transition stress can manifest itself in unforeseen and undesirable ways. Fortunately, help is only a phone call away. Various agencies on and off base provide counseling for personal issues, marital issues, parent-child conflicts, stress-related concerns, and alcohol and drug abuse. Remember, while you are on active duty, these services are free on military installations.

For information, assistance, and referrals, contact any of the following:

- Local assistance: family center, chaplain's office, and military mental health care facility: www.nvti.ucdenver.edu/home/infoVeterans.htm
- Military mental health resources: www.samhsa.gov/militaryfamilies
- The Dept. of Veterans Affairs: 800-827-1000, www2.va.gov/directory
- Military OneSource 24/7 Support: 800-342-9647, www.militaryonesource .com
- Marine for Life: www.marineforlife.org
- Military Family Network: www.emilitary.org

Transition Assistance

All separating and retiring service members should make an appointment to see their local Transition Counselor for information on transition services and benefits. Transition Counselors are located in the following offices at local military installations:

- **Army**: Army Career and Alumni Program—The Army Career and Alumni Program (ACAP) is a military personnel function and the centers are found under the Director of Human Resources (DHR) or the Military Personnel Office (MILPO). www.acap.army.mil
- **Air Force**: Airman and Family Readiness Center. You can find the nearest office using the military installation finder at: www.militaryinstallations.dod .mil
- **Navy**: Fleet and Family Support Center. www.cnic.navy.mil
- **Marines**: Career Resource Management Center (CRMC)/Transition & Employment Assistance Program Center. www.usmc-mccs.org/tamp/index .cfm
- **Coast Guard**: Worklife Division—Transition Assistance. Coast Guard Worklife staffs can be found at your nearest Integrated Support Command. www.uscg.mil/worklife/transition_assistance.asp

VA Seamless Transition

VA has stationed personnel at major military hospitals to help seriously in-jured service members returning from OEF and OIF as they transition from military to civilian life. OEF/OIF service members who have questions about VA benefits or need assistance in filing a VA claim or accessing services can contact the nearest VA office or call 800-827-1000.

Transition Assistance Program

The Transition Assistance Program (TAP) consists of comprehensive three-day workshops at military installations designed to help service members as they transition from military to civilian life. The program includes job search, employment and training information, as well as VA benefits information, to service members who are within 12 months of separation or 24 months of retirement. A companion workshop, the Disabled Transition Assistance Program, provides information on VA's Vocational Rehabilitation and Employment Program, as well as other programs for the disabled. Additional information about these programs is available at www.dol.gov/vets/programs/tap/tap_fs.htm.

Military Services Provide Pre-Separation Counseling

Service members may receive pre-separation counseling 24 months prior to retirement or 12 months prior to separation from active duty. These sessions present information on education, training, employment assistance, National Guard and reserve programs, medical benefits and financial assistance.

Verification of Military Experience and Training

The Verification of Military Experience and Training (VMET) Document, DD Form 2586, helps service members verify previous experience and training to potential employers, negotiate credits at schools and obtain certificates or licenses. VMET documents are available only through Army, Navy, Air Force and Marine Corps Transition Support offices and are intended for service members who have at least six months of active service. Service members should obtain VMET documents from their Transition Support office within 12 months of separation or 24 months of retirement.

Transition Bulletin Board

To find business opportunities, a calendar of transition seminars, job fairs, information on veterans associations, transition services, training and education opportunities, as well as other announcements, visit the website at www.dol.gov/vets/programs/tap/tap_fs.htm.

Educational and Vocational Counseling Services

The Vocational Rehabilitation and Employment (VR&E) program provides educational and vocational counseling to service members, veterans, and certain dependents (U.S.C. Title 38, Section 3697).

These counseling services are designed to help an individual choose a vocational direction, determine the course needed to achieve the chosen goal, and evaluate the career possibilities open to them. Assistance may include interest and aptitude testing, occupational exploration, setting occupational goals, locating the right type of training program, and exploring educational or training facilities which can be utilized to achieve an occupational goal. Counseling services include, but are not limited to, educational and vocational counseling and guidance; testing; analysis of and recommendations to improve job marketing skills; identification of employment, training, and financial aid resources; and referrals to other agencies providing these services.

Eligibility for this service is based on having eligibility for a VA program such as Chapter 30 (Montgomery GI Bill); Chapter 31 (Vocational Rehabilitation and Employment); Chapter 32 (Veterans Education Assistance Program—VEAP); Chapter 35 (Dependents Education Assistance Program) for certain spouses and dependent children; Chapter 18 (Spina Bifida Program) for certain dependent children; and Chapters 106 and 107 of Title 10.

Educational and vocational counseling is available during the period the individual is on active duty with the armed forces and is within 180 days of the estimated date of his or her discharge or release from active duty. The projected discharge must be under conditions other than dishonorable. Service members are eligible even if they are only considering whether or not they will continue as members of the armed forces. Veterans are eligible if not more than one year has elapsed since the date the individual was last discharged or released from active duty.

Veterans and service members may apply for the counseling services using VA Form 28-8832, Application for Counseling. Veterans and service members may also write a letter expressing a desire for counseling services. Upon receipt of either type of request for counseling from an eligible individual, the VR&E Division will schedule an appointment for counseling. Counseling services are provided to eligible persons at no charge.

Veterans' Workforce Investment Program

Recently separated veterans and those with service-connected disabilities, significant barriers to employment or who served on active duty during a period in which a campaign or expedition badge was authorized can contact the nearest state employment office for employment help through the Veterans' Workforce Investment Program.

The program may be conducted through state or local public agencies, community organizations or private, nonprofit organizations.

State Employment Services

Veterans can find employment information, education and training opportunities, job counseling, job search workshops, and resume preparation assistance at state Workforce Career or One-Stop Centers. These offices also have specialists to help disabled veterans find employment.

Unemployment Compensation

Veterans who do not begin civilian employment immediately after leaving military service may receive weekly unemployment compensation for a limited time. The amount and duration of payments are determined by individual states. Apply by contacting the nearest state employment office listed in your local telephone directory.

Veterans Preference for Federal Jobs

Since the time of the Civil War, veterans of the U.S. armed forces have been given some degree of preference in appointments to federal jobs. Veterans' preference in its present form comes from the Veterans' Preference Act of 1944, as amended, and now codified in Title 5, United States Code. By law, veterans who are disabled or who served on active duty in the U.S. armed forces during certain specified time periods or in military campaigns are entitled to preference over others when hiring from competitive lists of eligible candidates, and also in retention during a reduction in force (RIF).

To receive preference, a veteran must have been discharged or released from active duty in the U.S. armed forces under honorable conditions (honorable or general discharge). Preference is also provided for certain widows and widowers of deceased veterans who died in service; spouses of service-connected disabled veterans; and mothers of veterans who died under honorable conditions on active duty or have permanent and total service-connected disabilities. For each of these preferences, there are specific criteria that must be met in order to be eligible to receive the veterans' preference. Recent changes in Title 5 clarify veterans' preference eligibility criteria for National Guard and Reserve service members. Veterans eligible for preference include National Guard and Reserve service members who served on active duty as defined by Title 38 at any time in the armed forces for a period of more than

180 consecutive days, any part of which occurred during the period beginning on September 11, 2001, and ending on the date prescribed by presidential proclamation or by law as the last date of OIF. The National Guard and Reserve service members must have been discharged or released from active duty in the armed forces under honorable conditions.

Another recent change involves veterans who earned the Global War on Terrorism Expeditionary Medal for service in OEF. Under Title 5, service on active duty in the armed forces during a war or in a campaign or expedition for which a campaign badge has been authorized also qualifies for veterans' preference. Any Armed Forces Expeditionary medal or campaign badge qualifies for preference. Medal holders must have served continuously for 24 months or the full period called or ordered to active duty. As of December 2005, veterans who received the Global War on Terrorism Expeditionary Medal are entitled to veterans' preference if otherwise eligible. For additional information, visit the Office of Personnel Management (OPM) website at www.opm.gov/veterans/html/vetguide.asp#2.

Veterans' preference does not require an agency to use any particular appointment process. Agencies can pick candidates from a number of different special hiring authorities or through a variety of different sources. For example, the agency can reinstate a former federal employee, transfer someone from another agency, reassign someone from within the agency, make a selection under merit promotion procedures or through open, competitive exams, or appoint someone noncompetitively under special authority such as a Veterans Readjustment Appointment or special authority for 30 percent or more disabled veterans. The decision on which hiring authority the agency desires to use rests solely with the agency.

When applying for federal jobs, eligible veterans should claim preference on their application or resume. Veterans should apply for a federal job by contacting the personnel office at the agency in which they wish to work. For more information, visit www.usajobs.gov for job openings or help creating a federal resume.

Veterans' Employment Opportunities Act. When an agency accepts applications from outside its own workforce, the Veterans' Employment Opportunities Act of 1998 allows preference eligible candidates or veterans to compete for these vacancies under merit promotion procedures. Veterans who are selected are given career or career-conditional appointments. Veterans are those who have been separated under honorable conditions from the U.S. armed forces with three or more years of continuous active service. For information, visit www.usajobs.gov.

Veterans' Recruitment Appointment. Allows federal agencies to appoint eligible veterans to jobs without competition. These appointments can be converted to career or career-conditional positions after two years of satisfactory work. Veterans should apply directly to the agency where they wish to work. For information, visit www.usajobs.gov.

REINTEGRATION CHALLENGES

The changing nature and complexity of the Iraq war has contributed to reintegration stresses experienced by service members, their spouses and families.

The biggest task for the returning service member is to transform a sense of purpose created by the intensity of war into the routines and safety of everyday life. Similarly, the service member's family has established a sense of purpose sustaining the home and its routines in the absence of the spouse. Helping couples respect each other's perspective and reestablish a shared sense of purpose is a constructive paradigm that addresses standard concepts such as emotional changes, expectations and adjustments, and reframes them into an action-oriented, positive approach for moving couples forward.

The four steps to achieving a shared sense of purpose are:

1. Understand common factors that have shaped the service member's and spouse's sense of purpose during separation;
2. Recognize common concerns shared by service member and spouse resulting from the separation;
3. Be aware of relationship breakers: common, sensitive issues that can distance couples;
4. Focus on relationship makers: ways to build shared experiences, shared sense of purpose and closeness.

Civilian Transition

For those exiting military service, there are many resources to ease the transition. For the family, there are many considerations to reflect on as actual homecoming approaches.

While at the MTF, you have been surrounded by other families and service members who have experienced journeys similar to your own. There is a shared sense of "being in the trenches" with others living at the post lodging. The focus has been on healing and rehabilitation. The medical and support services at the MTF are superb. There are agencies available to help with just about any need that the service member or family has had while at the MTF. All this is about to change.

Though you may have been home with your warrior already during periods of convalescent leave, there is a difference when it is time to go home to stay.

A new normal will have to be established, and like any change, this will take some getting used to. Even if your service member has healed to the point of returning to active duty/active reserve, you have been changed by the experiences endured. The entire family has been through a tremendous ordeal, and the full extent of how your lives have been changed will become even more evident once beginning your new routines.

Some changes you may be facing are:

- Adapting your home to be accessible to your service member
- Resuming/redefining parenting roles, especially if your children were not with you at the MTF
- Getting back to household chores, i.e., cooking and cleaning
- Going back to work or having to find a job
- Reunion with friends and family
- Being the only family of a seriously wounded service member in your community
- Becoming your spouse's or adult child's caregiver away from the MTF
- Relinquishing your role as the caregiver as your service member regains health
- Sharing your role as head of household after separation
- Relocating and all that entails
- Using a new medical facility and establishing relationships with new health care staff
- As a parent of a seriously wounded service member, allowing the adult child to resume control of their lives
- Dealing with a change in status from Army family to civilian family
- Redefining life goals
- Sending your service member back to duty or even returning to theater

These are just a few of the changes and challenges that could be looming ahead. While the medical team has been busy from day one with discharge planning for your service member, it is critical that the family do some family "discharge planning." Make a conscious effort to devise an action plan for your transition home. Begin constructing your support network and thinking of local resources to tap into. Develop an action plan for the transition home.

Develop your plan with your service member. Communicate your thoughts, feelings, and ideas so that you both develop realistic expectations about this final homecoming. Listen to your service member's concerns, thoughts and feelings. Problem solve together to help forge a strong family team. The transition home could bring about more reunion-related issues. Keep in mind that this is normal and to be expected. Getting help is not an admission of failure, it is an admission of caring.

There are professionals at many of the organizations supporting wounded warriors and their families who can help you through this time of transition and beyond. This is not a journey that you have to make alone.

Get in touch with the VA and begin working to determine how to best navigate their system. There are organizations listed in the resource section of this handbook that can assist you with obtaining VA benefits. There is a time limit for signing up for VA benefits so make an appointment with the VA representatives at the MTF to begin the process.

Readjustment counseling

Readjustment counseling assists combat veterans in their transition from military to civilian life. Readjustment counseling includes the following services:

- Individual counseling;
- Group counseling;
- Marital and family counseling;
- Bereavement counseling;
- Medical referrals;
- Assistance in applying for VA benefits;
- Employment counseling;
- Substance abuse assessment and referral; and
- Military sexual trauma counseling.

Readjustment counseling is provided at community Vet Centers in all 50 states and most U.S. territories and possessions. All discharged service members who served in any combat zone and received a military campaign ribbon are eligible for free readjustment counseling. Family members of combat veterans are also eligible for readjustment counseling for military-related issues.

Resources

Transition Assistance

VA Seamless Transition. VA has stationed personnel at major military hospitals to help seriously injured service members returning from OEF and OIF as they transition from military to civilian life. OEF/OIF service members who have questions about VA benefits or need assistance in filing a VA claim or accessing services can contact the nearest VA office or call 800-827-1000.

Transition Assistance Program. The Transition Assistance Program (TAP) consists of comprehensive three-day workshops at military installations designed to help service members as they transition from military to civilian life. The program includes job search, employment and training information, as well as VA benefits information, to service members who are within 12 months of separation or 24 months of retirement. The program is geared to soldiers separating from the service. Pre-separation counseling, veterans' benefits briefings, and pre-discharge program are offered.

A companion workshop, the Disabled Transition Assistance Program, provides information on VA's Vocational Rehabilitation and Employment Program, as well as other programs for the disabled.

Additional information about these programs is available at www.dol.gov/vets/programs/tap/tap_fs.htm.

Transition Resources

Recovery and Employment Lifelines: www.dol.gov/vets/programs/Real-life/main.htm, 888-774-1361. The program seeks to support the economic recovery and reemployment of transitioning wounded and injured service members and their families by identifying barriers to employment or reemployment and addressing those needs. The program facilitates collaboration of federal and state programs and services with follow-up and technical assistance to assure success of wounded and injured service members.

E-VETS Resource Advisor: www.dol.gov/elaws/evets.htm. The e-VETS Resource Advisor assists veterans preparing to enter the job market. It includes information on a broad range of topics, such as job search tools and tips, employment openings, career assessment, education and training, and benefits and special services available to veterans.

The e-VETS Resource Advisor was created to help veterans and their family members sort through the vast amount of information available on the Internet. Based on your personal profile and/or the various services you select, the e-VETS Resource Advisor will provide a list of website links most relevant to your specific needs and interests. The e-VETS Resource Advisor is one of several elaws Advisors developed by the US Department of Labor to help employees and employers understand their rights and responsibilities under numerous federal employment laws. The e-VETS Resource Advisor has two sections: General Services and Personal Profile. You are encouraged to use both sections to achieve the best results.

Army Community Service Employment Readiness Program: The goal and focus of this program is to help the military spouse find employment. The program provides education, employment, and volunteer information as well as career counseling and coaching. Job search assistance is provided.

Heroes to Hometowns: Helping severely injured service members and their families connect with their hometowns or new communities. The recuperation time after hospitalization and rehabilitation is crucial to an individual's recovery. Knowing that they are welcome in their new community and that there is a new life ahead can be the most significant part of this process. The purpose of the Heroes to Hometowns Program is to help communities:

• Recognize the severely injured and embrace them as part of the community
• Assist them in making a seamless transition into their new hometown
• Provide a support network they can access when needed

This program will promote community growth and:

• Bring in a "champion" to support your community, or reach out to assist another community in need.
• Rally the community to provide what is needed.
• Connect the community with nation-wide efforts and nationally accessible resources.
• Keep the community informed of severely injured service members interested in becoming a member of the community.
• Comfort all active duty and reserve military and their families by knowing that their communities support them.

Call the Military Severely Injured Center at 888-774-1361 for more information or Pentagon Severely Injured Center at 703-692-2052.

Seamless Transition Assistance Program for all veterans: www.oefoif.va.gov

Seamless Transition Benefits:

• Compensation and Pension: VA website hosting benefits information for veterans with disabilities.
• Education: Information on VA education benefits available for veterans.
• Home Loan Guaranty: VA's Home Loan Guaranty eligibility website.
• Vocational Rehabilitation and Employment: Rehabilitation counseling and employment advice for veterans who are disabled and in need of help readjusting.
• Insurance: VA life insurance program for disabled veterans.
• Burial: Information on burial benefits for certain qualified veterans.
• Women Veteran Benefits and the Center for Women Veterans: Two separate websites where you will find benefits issues and other programs unique to women veterans.
• Health and Medical Services: VA website for complete health and medical services information.

- Medical Care for Combat Theater Veterans: VA website with specific information for veterans of combat theater of operations.
- Special Health Benefits Programs for Veterans of Operations Enduring Freedom/Iraqi Freedom: VA health information website for OEF/OIF veterans specific to environmental agents issues.
- HealtheVet Web Portal: VA's health portal has been developed for the veteran and family: to provide information and tools to enable one to achieve *the* best health.
- CHAMPVA (Civilian Health and Medical Program of the Department of Veterans Affairs): CHAMPVA is a federal health benefits program administered by the Department of Veterans Affairs. CHAMPVA is a Fee for Service (indemnity plan) program. CHAMPVA provides reimbursement for most medical expenses: inpatient, outpatient, mental health, prescription medication, skilled nursing care, and durable medical equipment (DME). There is a very limited adjunct dental benefit that requires pre-authorization. CHAMPVA is available to certain veterans' family members who are not eligible for TRICARE.
- Transitioning from War to Home: Go to the VA website of the Vet Center Readjustment Counseling Service. Provides war veterans and their family members quality readjustment services in a caring manner, assisting them toward a successful post-war adjustment in or near their respective communities.
- State Benefits: Many states offer benefits for veterans. You should contact the VA regional office that serves your area to find out what your state may offer. You will find the area(s) served in the right hand column of the web page at the other end of the link.

Transportation to Your New Home

Once you have chosen your new hometown, you should arrange for transportation counseling. Schedule an appointment with your installation's Transportation Office as soon as you have your orders. This is extremely important, because the availability of movers is limited. The reimbursement amount is determined by the regulations pertaining to your particular entitlement. Entitlements vary with individual situations. Your exact entitlement and the time limits for its use will be explained to you during your appointment.

For example: If you are overseas, you may be authorized to ship an automobile to the United States. Motorcycles may be shipped as part of your personal property. **Note:** Airline tickets must be purchased from the Commercial Travel Office (CTO) under contract to your respective organization.

For more information, please go to: www.defensetravel.dod.mil/site/perdiem Calc.cfm.

RELOCATION ASSISTANCE

Planning your final move is a critical part of your transition from the military. Knowing about the basic procedures and your rights is essential to helping you make informed decisions and ensures your last move will be a smooth one.

Choosing Where to Live

Think about where you'd like to live and then consider the realities. For example, if you were a ship navigator during your military career, you could have a difficult time finding a similar job in Idaho. On the other hand, if you were an Army nurse, you may find several excellent opportunities in Idaho's many fine hospitals.

Most career placement specialists recommend that job applicants choose the type of job they want first, then go where the jobs are. In making a decision to relocate, you might prioritize as follows:

1. Job potential: Which community is most likely to offer job opportunities that match your skills, experience, and career goals?
2. Affordability: Consider the not so obvious expenses in addition to the cost of living. Compare local, state income, property, and sales taxes. Does the state tax your military retirement pay? Does the location have income and career potential?
3. Community: Do you have family or friends there? Can you count on them to help make your transition easier? Do you need to be close to your aging parents for economic or medical reasons? Are you seeking upward mobility with the potential to move, or are you looking for a community to settle for the long term?
4. Environment: Would you be happiest living in a city, the suburbs, a small town, or a rural area? Does the climate suit you?

Moving Out of the Area

Before moving consult your nearest Family Center, the best source of relocation information and planning assistance. Other useful resources include local chambers of commerce, libraries, bookstores, and the Internet. Use them to find out what you need in order to make informed moving decisions.

Family Centers

Family Centers can refer you to offices, programs, and services that may be of assistance as you prepare to leave the military. Examples include the Relocation Assistance Program (RAP), the Personal Financial Management

Program, Information and Referral, Spouse Employment Assistance Program, and the Exceptional Family Member Program (EFMP). The term "Family Centers" is used here to refer to the following service-specific entities:

- **Army:** Army Community Service Center
- **Air Force:** Airman & Family Readiness Center
- **Navy:** Fleet and Family Support Center
- **Marine Corps:** Marine and Family Services

Take advantage of the information and referrals available through the Relocation Assistance Program.

Chambers of Commerce

Many communities across America have chambers of commerce. Each chamber of commerce promotes its community and is a good source of information about the surrounding area: the local job market, housing costs, local realtors, cost of living, local taxes, climate, schools and availability of recreation or child care. Ask for the chamber's booklet—much like the relocation packet you received about a new installation when you changed stations. You can find any chamber of commerce office in the nation at www.chamberofcommerce.com.

Libraries and Bookstores

Each of the Service Library Programs provides electronic content through their respective portals (https://wwwa.nko.navy.mil/portal/home; www.army.mil/ako; www.my.af.mil). The electronic content provides information on relocating, career opportunities, and educational opportunities. The reference section of your nearest installation library, public library or bookstore may offer atlases, maps, and geographical information that provide useful information. Tour books and guides in the travel section may provide insights into the community you may someday call home. Military libraries and public libraries also have many other free resources. Libraries also offer computers which can help you keep up to date on the latest news in your new community, apply for a job, check your e-mail, or just chat with friends.

Some Helpful Websites

Relocation:
www.rileyguide.com
www.relo.usa.com
www.militaryonesource.com

(*continued*)

Education:
www.voled.doded.mil
www.collegeboard.com
education.military.com

Jobs:
www.ajb.dni.us
www.acinet.org/acinet
www.careersingovernment.com
www.khake.com
www.military.com/spouse

Housing

The following is important guidance about making the transition from your old housing to your new.

If you live in government quarters: You must arrange a time for a member of the Housing staff to come to your home to perform a pre-inspection and explain the requirements for cleaning and vacating quarters, as well as options available for you to accomplish them. If you live in government housing, you must make an appointment with the Housing Office as soon as your departure date is established.

If you are moving from a rental property: Notify your landlord as soon as possible. The Housing Office can assist you with any landlord problems you may have in conjunction with your separation—e.g., breaking a lease or early termination of a lease.

Shipment and Storage of Household Goods

The following guidance applies to the shipment and storage of household goods:

- Eligibility Involuntary Separatees and Retirees: You are authorized storage and shipment of household goods for up to one full year. Your items may be shipped to:
  - Any destination within the United States
  - Your home of record outside the United States—Your home of record is the place you lived when you entered the military.
  - The place from which you were initially called to active duty
- All Others: You are authorized storage and shipment of household goods up to six months. Your items may be shipped to whichever of the following points for which you collected separation travel pay:

- Your home of record—Your home of record is the place you lived when you entered the military.
- The place from which you were initially called to active duty.

Special-Needs Family Members

Families with special needs members can find information on the services available in your new hometown through the Family Center, the United Way/Community Chest, the community social services office listed in the local telephone directory, or the closest veterans' hospital. Information is also available through the "Special Needs" website at www.militaryhomefront.dod.mil or National Organization on Disability Collaboration: www.aapd-dc.org/employment/positions/nod.doc. For more detailed information see *Special Needs Families in the Military* published by GI.

HEALTH CARE COVERAGE

Programs for Service Members

The VA provides medical care for service members who are discharged from the military (including discharged reservists and members of the National Guard who were activated for federal service) and meet certain eligibility requirements.

For example, discharged service members who served in combat are entitled to free VA medical care for certain medical conditions during a 2-year period following separation from the military. The VA generally determines eligibility on the basis of any disabilities, whether such disabilities were incurred in the line of duty and the financial resources of the individual. Generally, all discharged service members who were disabled by an injury or disease that was incurred or aggravated in the line of duty during active military service are eligible for VA medical care, including care for illnesses or injuries unrelated to the military service.

Medicare

Medicare provides health care coverage to persons over 65 years of age, some younger disabled persons, and in limited cases, to other persons under 65.

Medicare (Part A) provides coverage for care in hospitals as an inpatient, critical access hospitals (which are small facilities that give limited outpatient and inpatient services to people in rural areas), skilled nursing facilities, hospice care and some home health care. Persons eligible for Medicare (Part A) do not have to pay any monthly premiums for Medicare (Part A) coverage.

SPECIAL ACCESS TO CARE

Service Disabled Veterans: Veterans who are 50 percent or more disabled from service-connected conditions, unemployable due to service-connected conditions, or receiving care for a service-connected disability receive priority in scheduling of hospital or outpatient medical appointments.

Combat Veterans: Veterans who served in combat locations during active military service after November 11, 1998, are eligible for free health care services for conditions potentially related to combat service for two years following separation from active duty. For additional information call 877-222-VETS (8387).

Medicare (Part B) provides coverage for doctors' services, outpatient hospital care, and some other medical services that Medicare (Part A) does not cover, such as the services of physical and occupational therapists, and some home health care. Medicare (Part B) helps pay for these covered services and supplies when they are medically necessary.

Enrollees pay a monthly premium for Medicare (Part B). Medicare (Part C), also called Medicare Advantage Plans, provides Medicare beneficiaries the option to receive their Medicare benefits through private health insurance plans. Part C is available only to those individuals who qualify for both Part A and Part B and live in certain coverage areas. Medicare (Part D) provides prescription drugs for Medicare Part A or Part B beneficiaries. The beneficiaries must affirmatively enroll in Part D. Enrollees will pay the full cost of their prescriptions until they meet the annual deductible and then they will pay a percentage of the remaining costs. For more information on Medicare, please visit www.medicare.gov.

Generally, individuals over the age of 65 are usually eligible for Part A. Individuals below the age of 65 and receiving Social Security disability benefits for 24 months are eligible for Part B.

Medicaid

Medicaid provides health care coverage to some individuals and families with low incomes and resources. Although the federal government establishes general guidelines for the program, the Medicaid eligibility requirements are established by each state. Therefore, whether or not a person is eligible for Medicaid depends on the state where he or she lives. Medicaid benefits vary by state, but all states must cover certain services, including medical and surgical dental care, hospital care and physicians' services.

Travel to VA Medical Care May Be Reimbursed

Certain veterans may be reimbursed for travel costs to receive VA medical care. Reimbursement is paid per mile. Two exceptions to the deductible are travel for C&P exam and special modes of transportation, such as an ambulance or a specially equipped van.

Eligibility

Payments may be made to the following veterans:

• whose service-connected disabilities are rated 30 percent or more;
• traveling for treatment of a service-connected condition;
• who receive a VA pension;
• traveling for scheduled compensation or pension examinations;
• whose gross household income does not exceed the maximum annual VA pension; and
• whose medical condition requires a special mode of transportation, if they are unable to defray the costs and travel is pre-authorized. Advance authorization is not required in an emergency if a delay would be hazardous to life or health.

INSURANCE

Life Insurance

For complete details on government life insurance, visit the VA Internet site at www.insurance.va.gov or call toll-free 800-669-8477. Specialists are available between the hours of 8:30 a.m. and 6 p.m., Eastern time, to discuss premium payments, insurance dividends, address changes, policy loans, naming beneficiaries and reporting the death of the insured.

If the insurance policy number is not known, send whatever information is available, such as the veteran's VA file number, date of birth, Social Security number, military serial number or military service branch and dates of service to:

Department of Veterans Affairs
Regional Office and Insurance Center
Box 42954
Philadelphia, PA 19101

Service Members' Group Life Insurance (SGLI)

Service Members' Group Life Insurance is low-cost term insurance protection for members of the uniformed services. The following are automatically insured for $400,000 under Service Members' Group Life Insurance (SGLI):

1. Active-duty members of the Army, Navy, Air Force, Marines and Coast Guard.
2. Commissioned members of the National Oceanic and Atmospheric Administration and the Public Health Service.
3. Cadets or midshipmen of the service academies.
4. Members, cadets and midshipmen of the ROTC while engaged in authorized training.
5. Members of the Ready Reserves who are scheduled to perform at least 12 periods of inactive training per year.
6. Members who volunteer for a mobilization category in the Individual Ready Reserve or Inactive National Guard.

Individuals may elect in writing to be covered for a lesser amount or not at all. Part-time coverage may be provided to reservists who do not qualify for full-time coverage. Premiums are automatically deducted from the service member's pay. At the time of separation from service, SGLI can be converted to either Veterans' Group Life Insurance (VGLI) or a commercial plan through participating companies. SGLI coverage continues for 120 days after separation at no charge. Coverage of $10,000 is also automatically provided for dependent children of members insured under SGLI with no premium required.

Family SGLI (FSGLI) coverage is available for the spouses and dependent children of active duty service members and members of the Ready Reserve insured under Service Members' Group Life Insurance program. The service member's spouse may obtain coverage up to $100,000 or an amount equal to the service member's coverage, whichever is less. Age based premiums are charged for spouses. Each dependent child of the service member is automatically insured for $10,000 free of charge. A member can decline or elect lesser spousal coverage in increments of $10,000, but may not decline coverage for a dependent child.

For more information call toll-free 800-419-1473 or visit www.insurance.va.gov.

Veterans' Group Life Insurance

SGLI may be converted to Veterans' Group Life Insurance (VGLI), which provides renewable term coverage to:

1. Veterans who had full-time SGLI coverage upon release from active duty or the reserves.
2. Ready Reservists with part-time SGLI coverage who incur a disability or aggravate a pre-existing disability during a reserve period that renders them uninsurable at standard premium rates.
3. Members of the Individual Ready Reserve and Inactive National Guard. SGLI can be converted to VGLI up to the amount of coverage the service member had when separated from service. Veterans who submit an application and the initial premium within 120 days of leaving the service will be covered regardless of their health. After 120 days, veterans can still convert to VGLI if they submit an application, pay the initial premium, and show evidence of insurability within one year of termination of SGLI coverage.

Service members who are totally disabled at the time of separation are eligible for free SGLI Disability Extension of up to two years. Those covered under the SGLI Disability Extension are automatically converted to VGLI at the end of their extension period. VGLI is issued in increments up to a maximum $400,000 and can be converted at any time to an individual permanent (i.e., whole life or endowment) plan with any of the participating commercial insurance companies.

SGLI Disability Extension

Service members who are totally disabled at the time of separation are eligible for free SGLI Disability Extension of up to two years. Those covered under the SGLI Disability Extension are automatically converted to VGLI at the end of their extension period. VGLI is convertible at any time to a permanent plan policy with any participating commercial insurance company.

Accelerated Death Benefits

SGLI, FSGLI and VGLI policyholders who are terminally ill (prognosis of nine months or less to live) may request one time only up to 50 percent of their coverage amount in advance.

Service-Disabled Veterans Insurance (S-DVI)

A veteran who was discharged under other than dishonorable conditions and who has a service-connected disability but is otherwise in good health may apply to VA for up to $10,000 in life insurance coverage under the Service-Disabled Veterans' Insurance (S-DVI) program. Applications must be submitted within two years from the date of being notified of the approval of a new service-connected disability by VA. This insurance is limited to veterans who left service on or after April 25, 1951.

Veterans who are totally disabled may apply for a waiver of premiums and additional supplemental coverage of up to $20,000. However, premiums cannot be waived on the additional insurance. To be eligible for this type of supplemental insurance, veterans must meet all of the following three requirements:

1. Be under age 65.
2. Be eligible for a waiver of premiums due to total disability.
3. Apply for additional insurance within one year from the date of notification of waiver approval on the S-DVI policy.

Veterans can apply for basic S-DVI online at https://www.insurance.va.gov/Autoform/index.asp, or by mailing VA Form 29-4364, Application for Service-Disabled Insurance, to the Department of Veterans Affairs Regional Office and Insurance Center (RH), P.O. Box 7208, Philadelphia, PA 19101.

Veterans seeking Supplemental S-DVI can apply by mailing in an application VA Form 29-0189, Application for Supplemental Service—Disabled Veterans (RH) Life Insurance to the office above. The S-DVI forms can be downloaded from www.insurance.va.gov/gli/buying/SDVI.htm or by calling toll-free 800-669-8477.

Veterans' Mortgage Life Insurance (VMLI)

Veterans' Mortgage Life Insurance (VMLI) is available to severely disabled veterans who have been approved for a Specially Adapted Housing Grant. Maximum coverage is $90,000, and is only payable to the mortgage company. Protection is issued automatically, provided the veteran submits information required to establish a premium and does not decline coverage. Coverage automatically terminates when the mortgage is paid off. If a mortgage is disposed of through sale of the property, VMLI may be obtained on the mortgage of another home.

Insurance Dividends Issued Annually

World War I, World War II, and Korean-era veterans with active policies beginning with the letters V, RS, W, J, JR, JS, or K are issued tax-free dividends annually on the policy anniversary date. Policyholders do not need to apply for dividends, but may select from among the following dividend options:

1. Cash: The dividend is paid directly to the insured either by a mailed check or by direct deposit to a bank account.

2. Paid-Up Additional Insurance: The dividend is used to purchase additional insurance coverage.
3. Credit or Deposit: The dividend is held in an account for the policyholder with interest. Withdrawals from the account can be made at any time. The interest rate may be adjusted.
4. Net Premium Billing Options: These options use the dividend to pay the annual policy premium. If the dividend exceeds the premium, the policyholder has options to choose how the remainder is used. If the dividend is not enough to pay an annual premium, the policyholder is billed the balance.
5. Dividend Options: Dividends can also be used to repay a loan or pay premiums in advance.

Other Insurance Information

The following information applies to policies issued to World War II, Korean, and Vietnam-era veterans and any Service-Disabled Veterans Insurance policies. Policies in this group are prefixed by the letters K, V, RS, W-J, JR, JS, or RH.

Reinstating Lapsed Insurance: Lapsed term policies may be reinstated within five years from the date of lapse. A five-year term policy that is not lapsed at the end of the term is automatically renewed for an additional five years. Lapsed permanent plans may be reinstated within certain time limits and with certain health requirements. Reinstated permanent plan policies require repayment of all back premiums, plus interest.

Converting Term Policies: Term policies are renewed automatically every five years, with premiums increasing at each renewal. Premiums do not increase after age 70. Term policies may be converted to permanent plans, which have fixed premiums for life and earn cash and loan values.

Paid-up Insurance Available on Term Policies: Effective September 2000, VA provides paid-up insurance on term policies whose premiums have been capped. Veterans who have National Service Life Insurance (NSLI) term insurance (renewal age 71 or older) and stop paying premiums on their policies will be given a termination dividend. This dividend will be used to purchase a reduced amount of paid-up insurance, which insures the veteran for life and no premium payments are required. The amount of insurance remains level. This does not apply to S-DVI (RH) policies.

Disability Provisions: National Service Life Insurance (NSLI) policyholders who become totally disabled before age 65 should ask the VA about premium waivers.

Borrowing on Policies: Policyholders with permanent plan policies may borrow up to 94 percent of the cash surrender value of their insurance. Interest is compounded annually. The loan interest rate is variable and may be obtained by calling toll-free 800-669-8477.

What to Expect from Your Children

Children may be feeling the same confusing things you and your spouse feel—worry, fear, stress, happiness, and excitement. Depending on their age, they may not understand how your spouse could leave them if he/she really loved them.

They may be unsure of what to expect from your spouse. They may feel uncomfortable or think of him/her as a stranger.

It's hard for children to control their excitement. Let them give and get the attention they need from the returning parent before you try to have quiet time alone with your spouse. Children's reactions to the returning parent will differ according to their ages. Some normal reactions you can expect are:

- Infants: Cry, fuss, pull away from the returning parent, cling to you or the caregiver.
- Toddlers: Be shy, clingy, not recognize the returning parent, cry, have temper tantrums, return to behaviors they had outgrown (no longer toilet trained).
- Preschoolers: Feel guilty for making parent go away, need time to warm up to returning parent, intense anger, act out to get attention, be demanding.
- School Age: Excitement, joy, talk constantly to bring the returning parent up to date, boast about the returning parent, guilt about not doing enough or being good enough.
- Teenagers: Excitement, guilt about not living up to standards, concern about rules and responsibilities, feel too old or unwilling to change plans to meet or spend extended time with the returning parent.

Prepare children for homecoming with activities, photographs, participating in preparations, talking about dad or mom. Children are excited and tend to act out. Accept and discuss these physical, attitudinal, mental, and emotional changes. Plan time as a couple and as a family with the children.

Stay involved with your children's school and social activities.

Take Time for Yourself

Look into ways to manage stress—diet, exercise, recreation—and definitely take care of yourself! Make time to rest. Negotiate the number of social events you and your family attend. Limit your use of alcohol. Remember, alcohol was restricted during your spouse's deployment, and tolerance is lowered.

Go slowly in getting back into the swing of things. Depend on family, your spouse's unit, and friends for support.

Remember . . . go slowly—don't try to make up for lost time.

Accept that your partner may be different.

Take time to get reacquainted.

Seek help for family members, if needed.

If you feel like you are having trouble coping with adjustment, it is healthy to ask for help. Many normal, healthy people occasionally need help to handle tough challenges in their lives. Contact a counseling agency or a minister, a Military Family Center, Military Chaplain, the Veterans Administration, or one of your community support groups that has been established in your area.

Becoming a Couple Again

How to Create a Shared Sense of Purpose after Deployment

Coming together as a couple after war deployment isn't always easy or something that happens naturally. For more detailed information see *The Military Marriage Manual* published by GI. It requires effort, and an understanding that each person has grown and changed during the separation. A positive way to think about this is that both of you, service person and spouse, have developed your own sense of purpose coping with new experiences while apart. What's important now is to come together and create a "shared sense of purpose" that is essential for your well-being as a couple, that of your children and your life in the community. This won't happen overnight; it will take time, mutual compassion and a desire to do so. Here are four steps to help you create a "shared sense of purpose."

STEP #1: Understand each other's sense of purpose during separation. The returning service member's sense of purpose has been shaped by:

- Traumatic events that can be difficult to process and talk about.
- Identification and closeness with their military unit and comrades who have shared similar experiences.
- Regimentation in the form of highly structured and efficient routines.
- Heightened sensory experiences including sights, sounds and smells.
- Expanded self-importance and identity shaped by war.

The spouse's sense of purpose has been shaped by:

- New roles and responsibilities. Many spouses have assumed new or more taxing employment, oversight of finances and child rearing.
- Community support trade-offs. Some spouses and children left the military base to stay with parents and in-laws for various reasons, but will have experienced loss of connection with their military community, its familiarity and support.

- Emotional changes. Some spouses may have experienced growing independence and thrived on it; others may have found this a difficult time leading
to depression, anxiety, increased alcohol or substance use and abuse, and
other symptoms of stress.

STEP #2: Recognize that the following concerns upon return are common,
often shared or felt indirectly, and will require mutual adjustments and time:

- Home. Life at home does not have the edge and adrenaline associated with
wartime duty, which often leads to letdown, disappointment and difficulty
shifting gears.
- Children. Reconnecting with one's children is an anticipated event by service member and spouse. Children react differently depending upon their
age, and can be shy, angry, or jealous as new bonds are reestablished. Discipline will now be shared, often resulting in conflicting opinions and styles.
- Relationship. Concern about having grown apart, growing close again
without giving up individual growth and viewpoints, issues of fidelity, and
being able to discuss these issues without raising more anxiety or anger
challenge many couples.
- Public. While there has been widespread support of the service member,
the public has mixed views of the war. Protracted deployment and the po-
litical environment may polarize the public, promoting media coverage
that can undermine the pride and purpose military families feel about their
involvement.

STEP #3: Relationship breakers: Most couples argue about three things:
sex, money and children. Understanding the potential of these issues to divide
rather than unite is key to reestablishing a shared sense of purpose. These issues involve:

- Intimacy. Intimacy is a combination of emotional and physical togetherness.
It is not easily reestablished after stressful separations created an emotional
disconnect.
- Partners may also experience high or low sexual interest causing disappointment, friction or a sense of rejection. In due time, this may pass, but present
concerns may include hoping one is still loved, dealing with rumors or
concern about faithfulness, concern about medications that can affect desire
and performance, and expected fatigue and alterations in sleep cycles.
- Finances. During the deployment, most service members and families received additional income from tax breaks and combat-duty pay, as much as
$1,000 extra/month. Some families may have been able to set aside appre-
ciable savings; other families may have spent some or all of the money on

justifiable expenses and adjusted family budgets. This may create disagreement that can hamper the important work of building shared trust and financial planning as a couple essential to moving forward.

- Children. Children have grown and changed during deployment. Some returning service members will see children for the first time. It is important to build upon the positive changes in your children, and work as a couple to address issues of concern that need improvement or attention. Discipline of children will now be shared and should be viewed as something that can be built together rather than criticized or ignored.

Step #4: Relationship makers. Here are some thoughts and tips for building a shared sense of purpose and stronger family.

- Expectations. Remember that fatigue, confusion and worry, common during this transition, often lead to short tempers. In that frame of mind, it is easy to revert to the relationship breaker issues listed above. If this happens, suggest taking time out and return to discussions when both parties feel more relaxed.
- Enjoy life. Find and do activities that are pleasurable such as a movie, a family picnic, bowling or shopping. Create time in your weekly schedule to do something as a couple, as a family, and one-on-one activity that is shared between returning service member and his/her child or children.
- Give thanks. Together, thank those people, family, friends, co-workers and new service member buddies who have helped you and your family during this deployment. Showing appreciation through writing notes together, calling people or visiting them will bring a sense of fulfillment that reunites each other's experiences.
- Communicate. Talking together builds a shared sense of purpose. Desire to communicate is more important than details. Service members often prefer to discuss war stories with military buddies to protect their spouse and family from traumatic memories. Spouses should not be offended. Other ways to communicate involve physical activity. Take walks, work out together or engage in a sport. Healthy communication involves processing feelings, new information and relieving stress. Read, draw, paint, dance, sing, play an instrument, volunteer at church or in the community to keep a sense of perspective.
- Let time be your friend. Time may not mend everything, but it is often one of the most important factors in healing and solving problems.
- Be positive. A positive attitude is one of the most important gifts you can bring to each other and your family during this time. Appreciating what one has gives strength and energy to a family and a couple. Special circumstances such as physical injury and psychological problems are not

addressed in this fact sheet, and require additional support, information and resources.

- Know when to seek help. Both service member and spouse have endured a level of stress, uncertainty, worry and lonesomeness that can affect one's health and mental health. If either spouse or service member suspects they may be suffering from a health or mental health problem, it is essential to seek help. Many service members do not want to seek help for mental health problems from the military for fear of damaging their career. However, the consequences of letting a problem linger untreated can be much more damaging. There are excellent treatments including medications that can help people reclaim their lives and enjoy their families, as they should. You owe it to yourself and your family to be in good health.

THE HOME

Home Improvements and Structural Alterations for Disability Access

VA provides up to $4,100 for service-connected veterans and up to $1,200 for non-service-connected veterans to make home improvements necessary for the continuation of treatment or for disability access to the home and essential lavatory and sanitary facilities. For application information, contact the prosthetic representative at the nearest VA health care facility.

Home Modification Resources

The MSI Center (Department of Defense joint resources)
888-774-1361, 24 hours a day, 7 days a week

U.S. Army Wounded Warrior Program (AW2) (formerly called DS3)
wtc.army.mil/aw2

These two agencies can help answer questions in all areas, including home modification and can direct you to other resources as well. Some of these other resources are found below.

Department of Veterans Affairs (VA)
www.va.gov (access specific information on the programs at this website)

Depending on your service-connected disability, you may be eligible for assistance under one or more of the following programs administered by the Department of Veterans Affairs:

- Specially Adapted Housing (SAH) grants
- Special Home Adaptations (SHA) grants
- Loan Guaranty Service: VA Home Loans
- Vocational Rehabilitation and Employment (VR&E): Independent Living Services
- Veterans Health Administration (VHA) Home Improvement and Structural Alterations (HISA) grants

U.S. Department of Housing and Urban Development 203(k) Rehab Program

www.hud.gov/localoffices.cfm

ABLEDATA

800-227-0216

www.abledata.com

ABLEDATA is a comprehensive, federally funded project that provides information on assistive technology and rehabilitative equipment available sources worldwide. Offers fact sheets and consumer guides through the website or by mail.

Adaptive Environments Center, Inc.

www.adaptiveenvironments.org

The center provides consultation, workshops, courses, conferences, and other materials on accessible and adaptable design. Also offers publications through the website and by mail, including A Consumer's Guide to Home Adaptation.

Army Emergency Relief (AER)

866-878-6378

www.aerhq.org

This private nonprofit service organization provides interest-free emergency loans and grants to eligible recipients.

Center for Universal Design

800-647-6777

www.design.ncsu.edu/cud

This website is a listing of helpful advice and links, including state-by-state information.

Salute America's Heroes

www.saluteheroes.org

Salute America's Heroes provides financial assistance for wheelchair-bound or blind veterans to purchase homes that will accommodate their disabilities.

State and Local Government on the Net
Thousands of state agencies and city and county governments.

Serving Those Who Serve
www.servingthosewhoserve.org
Serving Those Who Serve is a special-needs home modification service that will be reserved exclusively for veterans who served in Operation Iraqi Freedom or Enduring Freedom, and now have loss of sight, loss of hearing, loss of mobility, or traumatic brain injury. It will not only make their homes safer, but will improve the quality of life for these brave men and women and their families by providing independence and mobility. This service is being made entirely at no cost and will be accomplished by community and military volunteers and skilled trades

EMPLOYMENT

Continuing on active duty or reserve is an option for many warriors who have experienced a severe wound, injury or illness. Indeed, many service members who have requested to stay in have been able to do so.

However, the decision whether to stay in or transition into civilian life is a difficult one and should not be taken lightly. Look at all your choices and discuss your options with qualified advisors, family and friends.

New Career Choices and Opportunities

Veterans Can Find Calendar Items, Business Opportunities on Transition Bulletin Board. To find business opportunities, a calendar of transition seminars, job fairs, information on veterans associations, transition services, training and education opportunities, as well as other announcements, visit the website at www.dmdc.osd.mil.

Educational and Vocational Counseling Services Provide Direction to Veterans. The Vocational Rehabilitation and Employment (VR&E) program provides educational and vocational counseling to service members, veterans, and certain dependents (U.S.C. Title 38, Section 3697). These counseling services are designed to help an individual choose a vocational direction, determine the course needed to achieve the chosen goal, and evaluate the career possibilities open to them.

Veterans are eligible if not more than one year has elapsed since the date the individual was last discharged or released from active duty.

Veterans and service members may apply for the counseling services using VA Form 28-8832, Application for Counseling. Veterans and service members may also write a letter expressing a desire for counseling services. Upon receipt of either type of request for counseling from an eligible individual, the VR&E Division will schedule an appointment for counseling.

Counseling services are provided to eligible persons at no charge.

Veterans' Workforce Investment Program. Recently separated veterans and those with service-connected disabilities, significant barriers to employment or who served on active duty during a period in which a campaign or expedition badge was authorized can contact the nearest state employment office for employment help through the Veterans' Workforce Investment Program. The program may be conducted through state or local public agencies, community organizations or private, nonprofit organizations.

State Employment Services. Veterans can find employment information, education and training opportunities, job counseling, job search workshops, and resume preparation assistance at state Workforce Career or One-Stop Centers. These offices also have specialists to help disabled veterans find employment.

VETS. The Department of Labor's Veterans' Employment Training Service (VETS) oversees numerous programs designed to assist job-seeking veterans. VETS provides noncompetitive grants to states to fund Disabled Veterans Outreach Program (DVOP) specialists and Local Veterans Employment Representatives (LVERs) who assist disabled veterans in finding employment.

Recovery and Employment Assistance Lifelines (REALifelines): This Department of Labor initiative provides injured and wounded service members and their families with access to a free career assistance network through One Stop Career Centers. Advisors at One Stop Career Centers throughout the country offer personal assistance with a variety of employment services including: job search, résumé writing, job placement, interviewing skills, career counseling, electronic job bank/computer access and more.

Veterans May Be Eligible for Unemployment Compensation for a Limited Time Period. Veterans who do not begin civilian employment immediately after leaving military service may receive weekly unemployment compensation for a limited period of time. The amount and duration of payments are determined by individual states. Apply by contacting the nearest state employment office listed in your local telephone directory.

Veterans Receive Preference When Applying for Federal Jobs. Since the time of the Civil War, veterans of the U.S. armed forces have been given some degree of preference in appointments to federal jobs. Veterans' preference in its present form comes from the Veterans' Preference Act of 1944, as amended, and now codified in various provisions of Title 5, United States Code. By law, veterans who are disabled or who served on active duty in the U.S. armed forces during certain specified time periods or in military campaigns are entitled to preference over others when hiring from competitive lists of eligible candidates, and also in retention during a reduction in force (RIF).

The "10-point preference" is available to veterans with a present service-connected disability rating of 10% or more, veterans receiving compensation, disability retirement or pension benefits from the VA or DoD and veterans who are Purple Heart recipients. Under certain conditions, spouses, widows/widowers and mothers of deceased or totally disabled (disability rating of 100%) veterans may be eligible for "10-point derived preference."

The "5-point preference" may be available to veterans who are not disabled, but who served in certain campaigns (including Operation Iraqi Freedom), or who served more than 180 consecutive days (other than for training), any part of which occurred after September 11, 2001.

Preference is also provided for certain widows and widowers of deceased veterans who died in service; spouses of service-connected disabled veterans; and mothers of veterans who died under honorable conditions on active duty or have permanent and total service-connected disabilities. Veterans eligible for preference now include National Guard and Reserve service members who served on active duty as defined by Title 38 at any time in the armed forces for a period of more than 180 consecutive days, any part of which occurred during the period beginning on September 11, 2001, and ending on the date prescribed by Presidential proclamation or by law as the last date of OIF.

Another recent change involves veterans who earned the Global War on Terrorism Expeditionary Medal for service in OEF. Under Title 5, service on active duty in the armed forces during a war or in a campaign or expedition for which a campaign badge has been authorized also qualifies for veterans' preference. Any Armed Forces Expeditionary medal or campaign badge qualifies for preference. Medal holders must have served continuously for 24 months or the full period called or ordered to active duty. As of December 2005, veterans who received the Global War on Terrorism Expeditionary Medal are entitled to veterans' preference if otherwise eligible. For additional information on veterans' preference, visit the Office of Personnel Management (OPM) website at opm.gov/veterans/html/vetguide.asp#2.

When applying for federal jobs, eligible veterans should claim preference on their application or resume. Veterans should apply for a federal job by contacting the personnel office at the agency in which they wish to work. For more information, visit www.usajobs.gov for job openings or help creating a federal resume.

Veterans' Employment Opportunities Act. When an agency accepts applications from outside its own workforce, the Veterans' Employment Opportunities Act (VEOA) of 1998 allows preference-eligible candidates or veterans to compete for these vacancies under merit promotion procedures. Veterans who are selected are given career or career-conditional appointments. Veterans are those who have been separated under honorable conditions from the U.S. armed forces with three or more years of continuous active service. For information, visit www.usajobs.gov.

Veterans' Recruitment Appointment. Allows federal agencies to appoint eligible veterans to jobs without competition. These appointments can be converted to career or career-conditional positions after two years of satisfactory work. Veterans should apply directly to the agency where they wish to work. For information, visit www.usajobs.gov.

Center for Veterans Enterprise Helps Veterans Form Small Businesses. VA's Center for Veterans Enterprise helps veterans interested in forming or expanding small businesses and helps VA contracting offices identify veteran-owned small businesses. For information, write the U.S. Department of Veterans Affairs (OOVE), 810 Vermont Avenue, NW, Washington, DC 20420-0001, call toll-free 866-584-2344 or visit www.vetbiz.gov.

Small Business Contracts. Like other federal agencies, the VA is required to place a portion of its contracts and purchases with small and disadvantaged businesses. The VA has a special office to help small and disadvantaged businesses get information on VA acquisition opportunities. For information, write the U.S. Department of Veterans Affairs (OOSB), 810 Vermont Avenue, NW, Washington, DC 20420-0001, call toll-free 800-949-8387 or visit www.va.gov/osdbu.

Skills Assessment

Translating military experience into civilian language is one of the most common stumbling blocks in the skills assessment process. One way to tackle this problem is to talk to friends who have already left the service. Ask them to tell you the do's and don'ts of what civilian employers want to hear. You should also consider attending workshops and seminars. Here's a good approach to assessing skills:

Step 1. Assignments: List the projects you have worked on, problems you have solved, situations you have helped clarify, and challenges you have met.
Step 2. Actions: List the actions you have taken to carry out these tasks.
Step 3. Results: List the results that your actions helped to achieve.

The skills that appear on these three lists should be incorporated into your resume and job interviews. Skill assessment for many service members and their families requires assistance. The staffs at the Transition Assistance Office and Education Center can provide that assistance. For more assistance in skills assessment, go to www.military.com/careers.

Resume Writing

In the current job market, managers receive dozens of resumes. They do not have time to read lengthy listings of skills and complete life histories. For them, "less is more." Here are some tips on creating the most effective resumes:

Know the Goal. The goal of your resume should be to motivate employers to call you in for an interview. Then during your interview, you can discuss your background in as much detail as the employer desires.

Begin with a Career Objective or a Summary? There are pros and cons to placing a career objective at the top of your resume. For example, a career objective statement clearly and unambiguously tells potential employers what you are looking for; on the other hand, it limits your flexibility by locking you into a specific position. After you have attended a Transition Assistance Program workshop, you will be able to decide what is best for you.

If you decide not to write an objective, consider using a three- to five-line summary of qualifications that concentrates on the skills and past experience you have that the employer wants. This summary can show an employer your efforts to assess your background and match it as closely as possible to his or her needs. "Targeting" your resume to the employer's current needs will increase your rate of success in getting an interview. A "one-size-fits-all" resume will not work in today's job market.

Focus on Skills. Employers are more interested in what you can do than in what you want to do. Today's resume emphasizes skills, allowing the employer to compare your skills to those required for the job. (Remember, volunteering is considered real work experience, so don't forget to include appropriate volunteer work when preparing your resume.) Writing a skills-oriented resume is easier after you have completed your skills assessment.

Don't Fuss over Format. Don't get hung up on which type of resume to use—functional, chronological, or whatever. Most employers appreciate a job history that tells them what you did and when. You should also state your accomplishments. Again, performing a skills assessment will help you do this.

Create a "Scanable" Resume. More and more, companies are scanning—rather than reading—resumes, especially if they get a great number of them. There are many books available to help you design a "scanable" resume. Research the company. Use their language where you can. There is no "perfect" resume, but you have to feel comfortable with the format you choose and be familiar with what you have written. The employer will use your resume as the basis for asking detailed questions during your interview.

Create a one-minute verbal resume that quickly highlights your experience and skills. Then, practice delivering your one-minute resume aloud until you're comfortable. This will give you the confidence to answer the "Tell me something about yourself . . ." interview question.

Workshops Help Separatees "TAP" into Good Jobs

The Department of Labor-sponsored Transition Assistance Program Employment Workshops are sponsored in conjunction with the installation Transition Assistance staffs. The DOL TAP Employment Workshops normally run 2½ days. However, some local installations may combine this workshop with other specialty workshops. During your first visit to the Transition Assistance Office, or with your Command Career Counselor, you should ask to be scheduled to attend the next available workshop (your spouse should attend if space is available). You should plan to attend employment workshops at least 180 days prior to separation.

Note: Not all installations and bases offer the Department of Labor TAP Employment Workshop. If the workshops are not available at your installation or base, the Transition Counselor will refer you to other sources where similar information is available. TAP addresses such useful subjects as the following:

* Employment and training opportunities
* Labor market information
* Civilian workplace requirements
* Resume, application, and standard forms preparation
* Job analysis, job search, and interviewing techniques
* Assistance programs offered by federal, state, local, military, and veterans' groups
* Procedures for obtaining verification of job skills and experience
* Obtaining loans and assistance for starting a small business
* Analysis of the area where you wish to relocate, including local employment opportunities, the local labor market, and the cost of living (housing, child care, education, medical and dental care, etc.)

At the TAP workshops, you will receive a participant manual. Among other valuable information, this manual contains points of contact around the nation for many of the services you will need after your separation.

Job-Hunting Workshops Provide Fresh Perspective

Besides the Department of Labor **TAP Employment Workshop**, you will find other job-hunting programs sponsored by organizations in and out of your service. Use them! By taking advantage of workshops and seminars, you will gain information about the same subject from different points of view. Different workshops emphasize different things. There are many good methods for finding a job and many good programs to teach you how.

Military Experience and Training Help You Win That Job

Verification of your military experience and training is useful in preparing your resume and establishing your capabilities with prospective employers. Verification is also helpful if you are applying to a college or vocational institution. These institutions want information on your military training and experience, as well as how this might relate to the civilian world. As a service member, you have had numerous training and job experiences, perhaps too many to recall easily and include on a job or college application. Fortunately, the military has made your life a little easier in this regard. The DD Form 2586, "Verification of Military Experience and Training," is created from your automated records on file. It lists your military job experience and training history, recommended college credit information, and civilian equivalent job titles. This document is designed to help you, but it is not a resume!

*To Obtain Your Verification of Military Experience and
Training Document*

To get your verification document, go to the VMET website at www.dmdc .osd.mil/vmet. All separating military personnel can electronically download and print their VMET document and personal cover letter from your military service from the VMET website. Simply click the "Request Document" and "Request Cover Letter" tabs and print each of these documents after they are downloaded. You can get your verification document online as long as you have a current DoD Common Access Card (CAC) or have a current DFAS myPay PIN; however, you should retrieve it within 120 days prior to your separation. If you have problems getting your VMET and need assistance, check with your local Transition Counselor.

Once You Receive Your Verification Document

Identify the items that relate to the type of work or education you are pursuing and include them in your resume. If there are problems with information listed on the form, follow the guidance indicated below for your respective service:

- **Army:** Review and follow the guidance provided by the Frequently Asked Questions (FAQs) listed on the VMET Online website.
- **Air Force:** Follow the instructions in the verification document cover letter or contact your Transition Counselor.
- **Navy:** Contact your Command Career Counselor or review and follow the guidance provided by the Frequently Asked Questions (FAQs) listed on the VMET Online website.
- **Marine Corps:** Follow the instructions in the verification document cover letter. If you need further assistance, contact your administrative office.

DoD Job Search

The Department of Defense (DoD) and the Department of Labor activated a new veterans and service member website called DoD Job Search. This website features job announcements; resume writing, and referral systems geared to transitioning military personnel and their spouses, DoD federal civilian employees and their spouses, and the spouses of relocating active-duty members. There are over 1 million jobs available on this website. Check out the website at www.dod.jobsearch.org for additional information and assistance.

Public and Community Service (PACS) Registry Program

The 1993 National Defense Authorization Act, P.L. 102-484 [10 USC, 1143 a(c)], requires the Secretary of Defense to maintain a registry of public and community service organizations. Service members selecting early retirement under the Temporary Early Retirement Act (TERA) are registered on the Public and Community Service Personnel Registry prior to release from active duty. Service members looking for employment in the public and community service arena to include those retiring under TERA, can access the PACS Organization Registry to see which organizations have registered for the purpose of hiring separating military personnel in public and community service jobs. In addition, service members with approved retirement under TERA can earn additional credit towards full retirement at age 62 by working in a public or community service job.

Employers who wish to advertise job openings in the public and community service arena on the DoD Operation Transition Bulletin Board (TBB) at https://www.dmdc.osd.mil/ot will complete DD Form 2581, "Operation Transition Employer Registration" and DD Form 2581-1, "Public and Community Service Organization Validation." Then, the organization will be included in the Operation Transition employer database and also be listed on the PACS organization registry. Completing the DD forms is a requirement for posting employment opportunities (want ads) on the TBB.

PACS employers hiring service members who retired under the TERA program are required to complete both DD Forms 2581 and 2581-1. TERA retirees who are employed by approved PACS organizations during their enhanced retirement qualification period (ERQP) enables them to earn additional retirement credit and enhanced retirement pay beginning at age 62. Retirees interested in gaining the additional credit towards full retirement can go to the TBB to look for PACS employment opportunities as well as see a list of approved PACS organizations. Please refer to the website at https://www.dmdc .osd.mil/ot.

The public and community service organizational registry program is just another tool separating service members can use to get their names in front of nonprofit, public and community service organizations such as schools, hospitals, law enforcement agencies, social service agencies and many more for employment opportunities.

Transition Bulletin Board (TBB) Makes Job Hunting Easier

Searching through the employment section of the newspaper is not the only way to find work. Internet sites provide a quick and easy way to find the latest job openings and up-to-the-minute information useful to your job search. DoD's Transition Bulletin Board lists jobs, as well as registered Public and Community Service (PACS) organizations, and a list of business opportunities. Search ads are listed by job type and/or location; jobs are located both stateside and overseas. In addition, individuals retiring under the Temporary Early Retirement Authority (TERA) can fulfill the mandatory requirement to register for Public and Community Service (PACS) online at the TBB. Simply log on to the Operation Transition/TBB website, and click "TERA Individual Registration for PACS."

Troops-to-Teachers Program

Troops to Teachers (TTT) was established in 1994 as a Department of Defense program. The National Defense Authorization Act for FY 2000 transferred the responsibility for program oversight and funding to the U.S. Department of Education but continued operation by the Department of Defense. The No Child Left Behind Act provides for the continuation of TTT as a teacher recruitment program. TTT is managed by the Defense Activity for Non-Traditional Education Support (DANTES), Pensacola, Florida.

Reflecting the focus of the No Child Left Behind Act, the primary objective of TTT is to help recruit quality teachers for schools that serve students from low-income families throughout America. TTT helps relieve teacher shortages, especially in math, science, special education and other critical subject areas, and assists military personnel in making successful transitions to second careers in teaching.

Those interested in elementary or secondary-teaching positions must have a bachelor's degree from an accredited college. Individuals who do not have a baccalaureate degree, but have experience in a vocational/technical field, may also submit an application. There is also a growing need for teachers with backgrounds in areas such as electronics, construction trades, computer technology, health services, food services and other vocational/technical fields.

A network of state TTT offices has been established to provide participants with counseling and assistance regarding certification requirements, routes to state certification, and employment leads. Pending annual appropriation of funds, financial assistance is available to eligible individuals as stipends up to $5,000 to help pay for teacher certification costs or as bonuses of $10,000 to teach in schools serving a high percentage of students from low-income families. Participants who accept the stipend or bonus must agree to teach for three years in targeted schools in accordance with the authorizing legislation. For more information go to www.proudtoserveagain.com.

Reemployment Rights Can Get You Your Old Job Back

Under certain circumstances, veterans have the right to return to their pre-service jobs after discharge or release from active duty. Your former employer must rehire you if you meet all of the following requirements:

• You must have left other-than-temporary employment to enter military service.

  AND

• You must have served in the Armed Forces (either voluntarily or involuntarily) no more than five years, unless at the request of and for the convenience of the government.

  AND

• You must have been discharged or released under honorable conditions.

  AND

• You must still be qualified to perform the duties of the job. If you became disabled while in military service, you must be able to perform some other job in your employer's organization (with comparable seniority, status, and pay).

Private Employment Agencies

Overall, private employment agencies are responsible for approximately 3 to 5 percent of all hires nationally. If your skills and experience match those fields in which the agency specializes, you can expect some assistance. For example, a separatee with computing skills should seek an agency specializing in computer-related placements. Most private employment agencies are reputable. They possess an extensive list of employers, and they charge those employers a fee for their services. Before registering with a private agency, confirm that all fees will be paid by the employer, and not by you.

Finding Federal Employment Opportunities

Opportunities for employment with the U.S. government are available in all parts of the nation as well as overseas. Here are some ways to find out about different types of federal job listings.

- Government jobs near you: Openings may be available at the installation from which you are separating. You can find out about these from your local civilian personnel office.
- You can view federal employment opportunities on the Internet at www .usajobs.gov.
- Other federal employment websites: www.fedworld.gov; www.goDefense .com; Federal Employment Portal at www.opm.gov; Army Civilian Personnel Online at www.cpol.army.mil.

Working for the DoD

The Department of Defense welcomes veterans to join the DoD civilian workforce and continue serving the Defense mission! The DoD is the nation's number one employer of veterans, offering nearly 700 challenging occupations. For more information go to www.goDefense.com or call toll-free: 888-DOD4USA (888-363-4872). TTY for Deaf/Hard of Hearing: 703-696-5436.

Veterans Get Priority at State Employment Offices

As a veteran, you receive special consideration and priority for referral, testing, and counseling from your state employment office. Your state employment office can provide many additional services. There is at least one Veterans Employment and Training Service Office in every state.

Training opportunities. State employment offices can offer you seminars on subjects such as resume writing, interviewing skills, and career changes; information on vocational training opportunities; and proficiency tests in typing and shorthand for positions requiring such certification.

Information. At your state employment office, you will find data on state training, employment, and apprenticeship programs; and statistics regarding employment availability, economic climate, and cost of living. To locate State Employment Offices visit: www.naswa.org/links.cfm.

Workshops and seminars. A variety of workshops and seminars are available through your Transition Assistance Office to help you and your spouse become more competitive in the job market.Topics include enhancing job search skills, goal setting, and preparation of standard and optional forms for federal civil service employment, resumes, and interviewing techniques. One of the most popular job-hunting workshops is sponsored by the Department of Labor. Their 2½ day Transition Assistance Employment Workshop is one component of the overall Transition Assistance Program (TAP). You can sign up for this important workshop through your Transition/ACAP Office, or through your Command Career Counselor.

Training. Some locations offer occupational skills training for those seeking entry-level classes in typing, word processing, and data entry. In addition you'll find helpful articles about writing resumes, dressing for success, interviewing techniques, and how to work a job fair at www.military.com/careers.

Employment Assistance and Credentialing Programs

Army and Navy COOL. The Army and Navy both offer Credentialing Opportunities Online (COOL). These programs give you the opportunity to find civilian credentials related to your rating, or military occupational specialty. You can learn what it takes to get the credentials and learn about programs that will help pay credentialing fees. Check out the Army COOL website at: https://www.cool.army.mil or Navy COOL website at: https://www.cool .navy.mil to learn more.

Helmets to Hardhats. The Helmets to Hardhats (H2H) program lets your military service speak for itself. The program will help you find career opportunities that match your military background. Congressionally funded, H2H is the fastest, easiest way for transitioning military, reservists, and Guardsmen to find a rewarding career in the construction industry. Visit: helmetstohardhats.org to learn more.

USMAP. USMAP (United Services Military Apprenticeship Program) is available to members of the Navy, Marine Corps, and Coast Guard who participated in this program and who are eligible to receive a Department of Labor

(DOL) Certificate of Completion, which gives them a definite advantage in getting better civilian jobs since employers know the value of apprenticeships. Visit https://usmap.cnet.navy.mil to learn more.

Library

Your local public and military libraries can be an excellent source of job search information. Most information of interest to job seekers is located in the reference section. Most public and military libraries offer access to the Internet. Helpful library resources include the following:

- Occupational Information Network the Dictionary of Occupational Titles (O*NET): This provides detailed descriptions of most occupations. Available online at online.onetcenter.org.
- The Encyclopedia of Associations: This lists the addresses of professional and industry associations. library.dialog.com/bluesheets/html/bl0114.html.
- National Trade and Professional Associations of the United States: This provides information on professional and industry associations. www.association execs.com.
- Dun and Bradstreet and Standard and Poor's Register of Corporations: Both documents offer information on individual companies and organizations. No website is available. Check the reference section of your local public library.
- The Occupational Outlook Handbook: This book addresses the projected needs for various occupations. It may help you choose a career or open the door to a new one. You can also view the handbook online at: www.bls .gov/oco/home.htm.

Libraries also offer newspapers, trade journals, magazines, audio and video cassettes, and computer software packages that aid in career identification and planning. You also may find information on state training, employment, and apprenticeship programs as well as statistics regarding employment availability, economic climate, and cost of living. Your librarian can show you where to find these resources and how to use them. Networking with others, especially other veterans, is one of the best ways to begin your search for a job.

Fraternal Military Associations and Veterans' Services Organizations

Fraternal military associations and veterans' services organizations are good sources of employment information, assistance, and services. Many provide their own job referral and registration services; others sponsor events such as job fairs to expose you to prospective employers. All provide networking opportunities to learn about job requirements and opportunities.

Your Transition Counselor can help you locate local Veteran Service Organization offices. In addition, lists of Military and Veteran Service Organizations can be found at www.mvpsoa.org.

Industry Associations

Industry associations are a source of industry-specific information. You can learn what an industry is all about from material provided by these associations. You can also learn the jargon and get insight into how people in the industry think. You also may find salary ranges, qualification requirements, locations of jobs, and the names and addresses of individual companies through these associations. More information can be found at www.bls.gov.

STARTING YOUR OWN BUSINESS

National Veteran's Business Corporation

The following information and resources will help you develop a business plan, find financing and determine if starting a franchise is your best option. This information is provided by the National Veteran Business Development Corporation, a federal contracted program for assisting veterans in starting a business or purchasing a franchise.

Many service members never consider small business ownership as a career when they transition out of the military, but you may discover that entrepreneurship is just the path for you. The skills and strengths arising from military experience, such as leadership, organization, and the ability to work under pressure, lend themselves naturally to entrepreneurship, and as a result, many veterans find themselves attracted to business ownership when they leave the military. If you are considering entrepreneurship, it is important to assess your strengths and weaknesses to determine whether you are cut out to be a business owner. Although there are no guarantees in business, successful entrepreneurs tend to share many similar characteristics.

Think about Why You Want to Be an Entrepreneur

There are many reasons people take the plunge into entrepreneurship, but not all reasons are the right reasons for opening your own business. Below are the most common reasons people consider business ownership as a career.

1. You want to be your own boss. Although this is the number one reason given by new entrepreneurs when making the change from employee to self-employed, there are a few important things to consider. Without a boss watching over you, do you have the self-discipline to get things done, to do them right, and to finish them on time? Without a boss to blame, are you willing to take responsibility for mistakes and fix problems yourself? If you eliminate the demands of your boss, will you be able to handle demands from customers and clients, suppliers and vendors, partners, and even yourself?

2. You are tired of working 9 to 5. As an entrepreneur, you can usually set your own hours, but that does not necessarily mean shorter hours. Many entrepreneurs are forced to put in 12–18 hours a day, six or seven days a week. Are you ready to work that hard, and is your drive for entrepreneurial success strong enough to get you through the long hours? You may be able to sleep in and work in the comfort of your home in your fuzzy slippers on occasion, but probably not initially and probably not all the time.

3. You are looking for an exciting challenge. Entrepreneurship is full of decisions that can affect your company's success. Every day is a new adventure, and you can learn from your mistakes as well as from your successes. Many successful entrepreneurs claim they are adrenaline junkies, motivated by the excitement of business ownership. That excitement requires risks, however, and you must know your own tolerance for risk.

   Entrepreneurship, as exciting as it may be, means putting everything on the line for your business. Sound too risky to you? Or maybe it sounds like just the adventure you are craving.

4. You want to make more money. Entrepreneurship can be an escape from structured pay charts and minimal growth opportunities, and, as a small business owner, your hard work directly benefits you. Despite the potential of big payoffs, however, entrepreneurs sometimes have to work months—even years—before they begin to see those profits. Oftentimes, entrepreneurs take a pay cut when they start out on their own. Are you willing to sacrifice your current level of pay until your business becomes a success?

5. You really want to become an entrepreneur. This is perhaps the most important reason people should enter entrepreneurship. Entrepreneurship takes time, energy, and money, but it also takes heart. It must be something you want to do in order to succeed because it takes drive and motivation, even in the face of setbacks. If you are considering entrepreneurship just because you haven't found anything else that suits you, make sure you are honest with yourself about whether or not you are ready to be an entrepreneur.

Assess Your Skills

Do your skills apply to entrepreneurial success? Many of the skills needed in entrepreneurship are those gained through military experience, including:

* Leadership
* Ability to get along with and work with all types of people
* Ability to work under pressure and meet deadlines
* Ability to give directions and delegate
* Good planning and organizational skills
* Problem-solving
* Familiarity with personnel administration and record keeping
* Flexibility and adaptability
* Self-direction
* Initiative
* Strong work habits
* Standards of quality and a commitment to excellence

Think about your other skills that might help you become a successful entrepreneur. Are you good with money with a strong credit history? Do you have a high energy level? Do you see problems as challenges and enjoy trying new methods for success? Listing your skills will not only help you assess yourself as an entrepreneur, but it might also tell you what kind of business you should start!

Define Your Personality

Your personality often helps determine what type of work best suits you. People preferring structure might find the corporate environment most suitable while creative types might enjoy flexible jobs with relaxed policies. Like any job, there are certain types of personalities that thrive in entrepreneurship.

SBA Programs and Services

What follows is a basic synopsis of the full range of SBA programs and services, designed to help you through the process of determining if small business ownership is for you, and if after you determine you do want to establish your own small business, what steps may be appropriate for you to follow, and what services are available to help you.

The U.S. Small Business Administration

Since 1953, the U.S. Small Business Administration has helped veterans start, manage and grow small businesses. Today, they provide specific programs for veterans, service-disabled veterans, and reserve and National Guard members, and they offer a full range of entrepreneurial support programs to every American, including veterans. Their job is to help you successfully transition from world's finest warrior to world's finest small business owner.

On August 17, 1999, Congress passed Public Law 106-50, the Veterans Entrepreneurship and Small Business Development Act of 1999. PL 106-50 is the most important entrepreneurial legislation for veterans since the original 1944 G.I. Bill. This law established the SBA Office of Veterans Business Development, under the guidance and direction of the Associate Administrator for Veterans Business Development, to conduct outreach, be the source of policy and program development for the government, and to act as an ombudsman for veterans within the administration.

In addition, this law created the National Veterans Business Development Corporation, set goals for federal procurement for service-disabled veterans and veterans, established the Military Reservists Economic Injury Disaster Loan, initiated new research into the success of veterans in small business, and brought focus to veterans in the full range of SBA capital, entrepreneurial, and government contracting programs.

SBA has established Veterans Business Outreach Centers, special loans and surety bonding programs for veterans and reservists, government procurement programs for Veterans, Veterans Business Development Officers in every District Office, and special outreach, counseling and training at more than 1,500 Business Development Centers.

Special Localized Programs

Special local initiatives target veterans, service-disabled veterans and reserve and National Guard members to aid in starting, managing, maintaining and growing successful small businesses.

The Patriot Express Pilot Loan Program

Patriot Express Pilot Loan is the latest program created by the SBA, which offers financial, procurement, and technical assistance programs to the military community. Patriot Express is a streamlined loan product with enhanced guarantee and interest rate characteristics. Patriot Express is available to members of the military community including veterans, service-disabled veterans, active-duty service members participating in the military's Transition Assistance Program, Reservists and National Guard members, current spouses of any of the above, and the widowed spouse of a service member or veteran who died during service, or of a service-connected disability. The new Patriot

Express Loan is offered by SBA's network of participating lenders nation-wide. It features SBA's fastest turnaround time for loan approvals. Loans are available up to $500,000 and qualify for SBA's maximum guaranty of up to 85 percent for loans of $150,000 or less and up to 75 percent for loans over $150,000 up to $500,000.

The Patriot Express Loan can be used for most business purposes, including start-up, expansion, equipment purchases, working capital, inventory or business-occupied real-estate purchases.

Patriot Express Loans feature SBA's lowest interest rates for business loans, generally 2.25 percent to 4.75 percent over prime depending upon the size and maturity of the loan. Local SBA district offices will have a listing of Patriot Express lenders in their areas. More details on the initiative can be found at www.sba.gov/patriotexpress.

District Office Veterans Business Development Officers (VBDOs)

To ensure that every aspiring veteran entrepreneur has access to the full range of SBA programs, and to receive the specific assistance and guidance you may be seeking, SBA has established a Veterans Business Development Officer (VBDO) in every one of the 68 SBA District Offices around the nation. These officers are responsible for providing prompt and direct assistance and guidance to any veteran or reservist seeking information about or access to any SBA program. To identify your local VBDO, please contact either your local SBA district office or contact OVBD at 202-205-6773 or visit www.sba .gov/VETS/reps.html.

Veterans Business Outreach Centers

OVBD provides operational funding to four Veterans Business Outreach Centers (VBOC) specifically established to offer and coordinate business development assistance to veteran, service-connected disabled veteran and reservist entrepreneurs. Services are provided include—face-to-face and online —outreach, concept development, business training, counseling and mentoring. Please contact them directly at:

The Research Foundation of the State University of New York
41 State Street
Albany, NY 12246
518-443-5398
www.nyssbdc.org/services/veterans/veterans.html
Email: brian.goldstein@nyssbdc.org

The University of West Florida in Pensacola
2500 Minnesota Avenue
Lynn Haven, FL 32444
800-542-7232 or 850-271-1108
www.vboc.org
Email: vboc@knology.net

The University of Texas—Pan American
1201 West University Drive
Edinburg, TX 78539-2999
956-292-7535
www.coserve.org/vboc
Email: vboc@panam.edu

Vietnam Veterans of California
7270 E. Southgate Drive, Suite 1
Sacramento, CA 95823
916-393-1690
www.vboc-ca.org
Email: cconley@vboc-ca.org

Small Business Development Centers

The SBA provides core funding, oversight and management to 1,100 Small Business Development Centers in all 50 states and U.S. territories. This program provides a broad range of specialized management assistance to current and prospective small business owners. SBDCs offer one-stop assistance to individuals and small businesses by providing a wide variety of information, guidance, linkages, training and counseling in easily accessible branch locations, usually affiliated with local educational institutions.

The SBDC program is designed to deliver up-to-date counseling, training and technical assistance in all aspects of small business management. SBDC services include, but are not limited to, assisting small businesses with financial, marketing, production, organization, engineering and technical problems, and feasibility studies.

To find your local SBDC: www.sba.gov/sbdc/sbdcnear.html or contact your district office VBDO.

SCORE "Counselors to America's Small Business"

SCORE is the best source of free and confidential small business advice to help you build your business—from idea to start-up, to success. The SCORE Association, headquartered in Washington, DC, is a nonprofit association dedicated to entrepreneurial education and the formation, growth and success of small businesses nationwide. More than half of SCORE's extensive, national networks of 10,500 retired and working volunteers are veterans, and they are experienced entrepreneurs and corporate manager/executives. They have worn the uniform and they have succeeded in business. They provide free business counseling and advice as a public service to all types of businesses, in all stages of development. SCORE is a resource partner with the U.S. Small Business Administration, and a resource asset for you.

- SCORE offers Ask SCORE email advice online at: www.score.org. Some SCORE e-counselors specifically target veterans, service-disabled veterans and reserve component members.
- Face-to-face small business counseling at 389 chapter offices.
- Low-cost workshops and seminars at 389 chapter offices nationwide.
- A great online web-based network.

SCORE is a nonprofit organization, which provides small business counseling and training under a grant from the U.S. Small Business Administration (SBA). SCORE members are successful, retired businessmen and women who volunteer their time to assist aspiring entrepreneurs and small business owners.

There are SCORE chapters in every state. Find your local SCORE chapter at www.score.org/findscore/chapter_maps.html.

Women's Business Centers

The Office of Women's Business Ownership provides women-focused (men are eligible as well) training, counseling and mentoring at every level of entrepreneurial development, from novice to seasoned entrepreneur, through representatives in the SBA district offices and nationwide networks of women's business centers (WBCs) and mentoring roundtables. Additionally, WBCs provide online training, counseling and mentoring.

Women's Business Centers represent a national network of more than 80 educational centers designed to assist women start and grow small businesses. WBCs operate with the mission to level the playing field for women entrepreneurs, who face unique obstacles in the world of business. To find your local WBC: www.sba.gov/wbc.html.

Financial Assistance

SBA administers three separate but equally important loan programs. The agency sets the guidelines for the loans while its partners (lenders, community development organizations, and microlending institutions) make the loans to small businesses. SBA backs those loans with a guaranty that will eliminate some of the risk to its lending partners.

Basic 7(a) Loan Guaranty. The 7(a) Loan Guaranty Program serves as the SBA's primary business loan program to help qualified small businesses obtain financing when they might not be eligible for business loans through normal lending channels. Loan proceeds can be used for most sound business purposes including working capital, machinery and equipment, furniture and fixtures, land and building (including purchase, renovation and new construction), leasehold improvements, and debt refinancing (under special conditions). Loan maturity is up to 10 years for working capital and generally up to 25 years for fixed assets. SBA does target veterans specifically in some of our loan programs. To find out more, visit www.sba.gov/financing/sbaloan/7a .html, or contact your district office, or any of the centers or chapters mentioned previously.

Certified Development Company 504 Loan Program. The Certified Development Company-504 loan program (CDC/504) loan program is a long-term financing tool for economic development within a community. The 504 program provides growing businesses with long-term, fixed-rate financing for major fixed assets, such as land and buildings. A Certified Development Company is a nonprofit corporation set up to contribute to the economic development of its community. CDCs work with the SBA and private-sector lenders to provide financing to small businesses. There are about 270 CDCs nationwide. Each CDC covers a specific geographic area. Typically, a 504 project includes a loan secured with a senior lien from a private-sector lender covering up to 50 percent of the project cost, a loan secured with a junior lien from the CDC (backed by a 100 percent SBA-guaranteed debenture) covering up to 40 percent of the cost, and a contribution of at least 10 percent equity from the small business being helped.

Microloan Program. The Microloan Program provides very small loans to start-up, newly established, or growing small business concerns. Under this program, the SBA makes funds available to nonprofit community-based lenders (intermediaries) which, in turn, make loans to eligible borrowers in amounts up to a maximum of $35,000. The average loan size is about $13,000. Applications are submitted to the local intermediary and all credit decisions are made on the local level.

Terms, Interest Rates, and Fees: The maximum term allowed for a microloan is six years. However, loan terms vary according to the size of the loan, the planned use of funds, the requirements of the intermediary lender, and the needs of the small business borrower. The maximum loan amount is $35,000; however, the average loan amount is around $13,000. Interest rates vary, depending upon the intermediary lender and costs to the intermediary from the U.S. Treasury. Generally these rates will be between 8 percent and 13 percent.

SBA's Investment Programs. In 1958 Congress created the Small Business Investment Company (SBIC) program. SBICs, licensed by the Small

Business Administration, are privately owned and managed investment firms. They are participants in a vital partnership between government and the private-sector economy. All SBICs are profit-motivated businesses. A major incentive for SBICs to invest in small businesses is the chance to share in the success of the small business if it grows and prospers. Equity (venture) capital or financing is money raised by a business in exchange for a share of ownership in the company. Ownership is represented by owning shares of stock outright or having the right to convert other financial instruments into stock of that private company. Two key sources of equity capital for new and emerging businesses are angel investors and venture capital firms.

Typically, angel capital and venture capital investors provide capital unsecured by assets to young, private companies with the potential for rapid growth. Such investing covers most industries and is appropriate for businesses through the range of developmental stages. Investing in new or very early companies inherently carries a high degree of risk. But venture capital is long term or "patient capital" that allows companies the time to mature into profitable organizations.

Surety Bond Guarantee Program. The Surety Bond Guarantee (SBG) Program was developed to provide increased bonding opportunities to small veteran and minority contractors to support contracting opportunities for which they would not otherwise bid. If your small construction, service or supply company bids or performs projects requiring surety bonds, the U.S. Small Business Administration has a program that could help make you more competitive. Small business contractors and manufacturers can overcome challenges they face in winning government or private contracts by using the SBA's Surety Bond Guarantee Program. A surety bond is a three-way agreement between the surety company, the contractor and project owner. The agreement with the SBA guarantees the contractor will comply with the terms and conditions of the contract. If the contractor is unable to successfully perform the contract, the surety assumes the contractor's responsibilities and ensures that the project is completed.

The SBA Surety Bond Guarantee Program covers four types of major contract surety bonds:

- Bid Bond—guarantees the project owner that the bidder will enter into the contract and furnish the required payment and performance bonds.
- Payment Bond—guarantees the contractor will pay all persons who furnish labor, materials, equipment or supplies for use on the project.
- Performance Bond—guarantees the contractor will perform the contract in accordance with its terms, specifications and conditions.
- Ancillary Bond—bonds that are incidental and essential to the performance of the contract.

The overall surety bond program has two programs:

- The Prior Approval Program—The SBA guarantees 80 or 90 percent of a surety's loss. Participating sureties must obtain the SBA's prior approval for each bond.
- The Preferred Surety Bond Program—Selected sureties receive a 70 percent guarantee and are authorized to issue, monitor and service bonds without the SBA's prior approval.

Program eligibility requirements: In addition to meeting the surety company's bonding qualifications, you must qualify as a small business concern, as defined by the SBA. For federal prime contracts, your company must meet the small business size standard for the North American Industry Classification System (NAICS) Code that the federal contracting officer specified for that procurement. For more information about the Surety Bond Guarantee Program, visit www.sba.gov/osg.

Business Planning and Disaster Assistance for Small Businesses Who Employ or Are Owned by Military Reservists

All of the technical assistance programs referenced above can provide pre- and post-mobilization business counseling and planning assistance to any reservist who owns their own business or to the business they work for. They also offer assistance to the caretaker of the business who may manage the business while the reservist is activated.

The Office of Disaster Assistance also offers the Military Reservist Economic Injury Disaster Loan (MREIDL) program at very favorable rates and terms. The purpose of the MREIDL is to provide funds to eligible small businesses to meet their ordinary and necessary operating expenses that they could have met, but are unable to meet, because an essential employee was "called-up" to active duty in their role as a military reservist. These loans are intended only to provide the amount of working capital needed by a small business to pay its necessary obligations as they mature until operations return to normal after the essential employee is released from active military duty. The purpose of these loans is not to cover lost income or lost profits. MREIDL funds cannot be used to take the place of regular commercial debt, to refinance long-term debt or to expand the business. Contact your district office or visit: www.sba.gov.

Government Procurement

The Office of Government Contracting (GC) works to create an environment for maximum participation by small, disadvantaged, woman, veteran and service-disabled veteran-owned small businesses in federal government contract awards and large prime subcontract awards. GC also advocates on behalf of small business in the federal procurement arena.

The federal government purchases billions of dollars in goods and services each year. To foster an equitable federal procurement policy, it is the policy of Congress and it is so stated in the Small Business Act, that all small businesses shall have the maximum practicable opportunity to participate in providing goods and services to the government. To ensure that small businesses get their fair share of federal procurements, the president has established an annual 23 percent government-wide procurement goal to small business concerns, small businesses concerns owned and controlled by service disabled veterans, qualified HUBZone small business concerns, small business concerns owned and controlled by socially and economically disadvantaged individuals and small business concerns owned and controlled by women. The individual program goals are: 5 percent of prime and subcontracts for small disadvantaged businesses; 3 percent of prime and subcontracts for HUBZone businesses; and 3 percent of prime and subcontracts for service-disabled veteran-owned small businesses. The SBA negotiates annual procurement preference goals with each federal agency and reviews each agency's results. The SBA is responsible for ensuring that the statutory government-wide goals are met in the aggregate. In addition, large business prime contractors are statutorily required to establish subcontracting goals for veteran-owned small businesses as part of each subcontracting plan submitted to the government in response to a prime federal contract opportunity. GC administers several programs and services that assist small businesses in meeting the requirements necessary to receive government contracts, either as prime contractors or subcontractors. These include the Certificate of Competency, the Non-Manufacturer Rule Waiver, and the Size Determination programs. The office also oversees special initiatives such as the Women's Procurement program, the Veteran's Procurement program, the Procurement Awards program, and the Annual Joint Industry/SBA Procurement Conference.

Resources and Opportunities: Contact your local SBA district office or visit www.sba.gov.

Federal Agency Procurement Forecast: www.sba.gov.

SBA Contacts and Representatives: Subcontracting Opportunities Directory Contains a listing of Prime Contractors doing business with the federal government: www.sba.gov.

Procurement Technical Assistance Centers (PTACS): The Defense Logistics Agency, on behalf of the Secretary of Defense, administers the DoD Procurement Technical Assistance Program (PTAC). PTA centers are a local resource available that can provide assistance to business firms in marketing products and services to the Federal, state and local governments. www.dla.mil/smallbusiness.

Procurement Center Representatives: SBA's Procurement Center Representatives (PCR), who are located in area offices, review and evaluate the small business programs of federal agencies and assist small businesses in obtaining federal contracts and subcontracts.

Traditional Procurement Center Representative: Traditional Procurement Center Representatives (TPCRs) increase the small business share of federal procurement awards by initiating small business set-asides, reserving procurements for competition among small business firms; providing small business sources to federal buying activities; and counseling small firms.

Breakout Procurement Center Representative: Breakout Procurement Center Representatives (BPCRs) advocate for the breakout of items for full and open competition to effect savings to the federal government.

Commercial Marketing Representatives: Commercial Marketing Representatives (CMRs) identify, develop and market small businesses to large prime contractors and assist small businesses in identifying and obtaining subcontracts. Contact your local SBA district office or visit www.sba.gov.

Office of Small and Disadvantaged Business Utilization: The Office of Small and Disadvantaged Business Utilization (OSDBUs) offer small business information on procurement opportunities, guidance on procurement procedures, and identification of both prime and subcontracting opportunities. OSDBUs also have Veteran Small Business Representatives. If you own, operate or represent a small business, you should contact the Small Business Specialists for marketing assistance and information. The specialists will advise you as to what types of acquisitions are either currently available or will be available in the near future. Contact your local SBA office or visit: www.osdbu.gov/members.html.

Office of Government Contracting Programs

Section 8(a) Program/Small Disadvantaged Business Certification Program: The SBA administers two particular business assistance programs for small disadvantaged businesses (SDBs). These programs are the 8(a) Business Development Program and the Small Disadvantaged Business Certification Program. While the 8(a) Program offers a broad scope of assistance to socially and economically disadvantaged firms, SDB certification strictly pertains to benefits in federal procurement. Companies which are 8(a) firms automatically qualify for SDB certification. Contact your local SBA Office or visit: www.sba.gov.

Small Disadvantaged Business: While the 8(a) Program offers a broad scope of assistance to socially and economically disadvantaged firms, SDB certification strictly pertains to benefits in federal procurement. SBA certifies SDBs to make them eligible for special bidding benefits. Evaluation credits available to prime contractors boost subcontracting opportunities for SDBs. This has become, in effect, the gateway to opportunity for small contractors and subcontractors.

Qualifications for the program are similar to those for the 8(a) Business Development Program. A small business must be at least 51% owned and controlled by a socially and economically disadvantaged individual or individuals. African Americans, Hispanic Americans, Asian Pacific Americans, Subcontinent Asian Americans, and Native Americans are presumed to qualify. Other individuals can qualify if they show by a "preponderance of the evidence" that they are disadvantaged. All individuals must have a net worth of less than $750,000, excluding the equity of the business and primary residence. Successful applicants must also meet applicable size standards for small businesses in their industry.

HUBZone Empowerment Contracting Program

The HUBZone Empowerment Contracting Program stimulates economic development and creates jobs in urban and rural communities by providing federal contracting preferences to small businesses. These preferences go to small businesses that obtain HUBZone (Historically Underutilized Business Zone) certification in part by employing staff who live in a HUBZone. The company must also maintain a "principal office" in one of these specially designated areas. A principal office can be different from a company headquarters, as explained in the section dedicated to Frequently Asked Questions.

Contact your local SBA Office or visit: https://eweb1.sba.gov/hubzone /internet or the Service-Disabled Veteran-Owned Small Business Concern Program website www.sba.gov.

On May 5, 2004, the U.S. Small Business Administration (SBA) issued regulations in the Federal Register as an Interim Final Rule implementing Section 36 of the Veterans Benefits Act of 2003 (Public Law 108-183). Section 308 of PL 108-183 amended the Small Business Act to establish a procurement program for Small Business Concerns (SBCs) owned and controlled by service-disabled veterans. This procurement program provides that contracting officers may award a sole source or set-aside contract to service-disabled veteran business owners, if certain conditions are met. Finally, the purpose of this procurement program is to assist agencies in achieving the 3 percent government-wide goal for procurement from service-disabled veteran-owned small business concerns.

Important Definitions

- **Veteran:** a person who served in the active military, naval, or air service, and who was discharged or released under conditions other than dishonorable.

- **Service-Disabled Veteran:** a person with a disability that is service-connected which was incurred or aggravated in line of duty in the active military, naval, or air service.
- **Service-Disabled Veteran with a Permanent and Severe Disability:** a veteran with a service-connected disability that has been determined by the U.S. Department of Veterans Affairs to have a permanent and total disability for purposes of receiving disability compensation or a disability pension.
- **Permanent Caregiver:** a spouse, or an individual 18 years of age or older, who is legally designated, in writing, to undertake responsibility for managing the well-being of a service-disabled veteran, to include housing, health and safety.

Service-Disabled Veteran-Owned Small Business Contracts

SDVO contracts are contracts awarded to an SDVO SBC through a sole source award or a set-aside award based on competition restricted to SDVO SBCs. The contracting officer for the contracting activity determines if a contract opportunity for SDVO competition exists.

SDVO SBC Set-Aside Contracts: The contracting officer may set-aside acquisitions for SDVO SBCs if:

- the requirement is determined to be excluded from fulfillment through award to Federal Prison Industries, Javits Wagner-O'Day, Orders under Indefinite Delivery Contracts, Orders against Federal Supply Schedules, Requirements currently being performed by 8(a) participants, and Requirements for commissary or exchange resale items;
- the requirement is not currently being performed by an 8(a) participant, and unless SBA has consented to release of the requirement from the Section 8(a) Program;
- SBA has not accepted the requirement for performance under the 8(a) authority, unless SBA has consented to release of the requirement from the Section 8(a) Program;
- there is a reasonable expectation that at least two responsible SDVO SBCs will submit offers;
- the award can be made at a fair market price.

SDVO SBC Sole Source Contracts: A contracting officer may award a sole source contract to a SDVO SBC if the contracting officer determines that none of the SDVO SBC set-aside exemptions or provisions apply and the anticipated award price of the contract, including options, will not exceed:

- $5.5 million for manufacturing requirements
- $3.5 million for all other requirements

- the SDVO SBC is a responsible contractor able to perform the contract
- award can be made at a fair and reasonable price

SDVO SBC Simplified Acquisition Contracts: If a requirement is at or below the simplified acquisition threshold, a contracting officer may set-aside the requirement for consideration among SDVO SBCs using simplified acquisition procedures or may award a sole source contract to a SDVO SBC. Contact your local SBA Office or visit: www.sba.gov.

EDUCATION

GI Bill—Sponsorships—Scholarships (VOC rehab)

Education/Training

Service members leaving the military sometimes find a gap between the civilian careers they want and the specific education or training they need to achieve it. The following section will help you identify the resources to assist you in getting the training and education needed to help close that gap.

Your Education Benefits: Montgomery GI Bill (MGIB), VEAP, and More

Several programs administered by the Department of Veterans Affairs (VA) provide financial assistance to veterans for education programs. This includes enrollment in degree programs, technical and vocational programs, correspondence courses, flight training courses, and on-the-job training and apprenticeship programs. To be eligible programs must be approved, usually by a state-approving agency, for VA purposes, before VA education program benefits are paid.

Two of these programs are the Post-Vietnam-era Veterans' Educational Assistance Program (VEAP) and the Montgomery GI Bill (MGIB). Both programs are intended to help you develop skills that will enhance your opportunities for employment. As a rule, the benefits under either of these programs must be used within 10 years of separation from active duty.

MGIB Eligibility. VA educational benefits may be used while the service member is on active duty or after the service member's separation from active duty with a fully honorable military discharge. Discharges "under honorable conditions" and "general" discharges do not establish eligibility. Eligibility generally expires 10 years after the service member's discharge. However, there are exceptions for disability, re-entering active duty, and upgraded discharges.

All participants must have a high school diploma, equivalency certificate, or completed 12 hours toward a college degree before applying for benefits.

Previously, service members had to meet the high school requirement before they completed their initial active duty obligation. Those who did not may now meet the requirement and reapply for benefits. If eligible, they must use their benefits either within 10 years from the date of last discharge from active duty or by November 2, 2010, whichever is later.

Additionally, every veteran must establish eligibility under one of the following categories.

Service after June 30, 1985: For veterans who entered active duty for the first time after June 30, 1985, did not decline MGIB in writing, and had their military pay reduced by $100 a month for 12 months. Service members can apply after completing two continuous years of service. Veterans must have completed three continuous years of active duty, or two continuous years of active duty if they first signed up for less than three years or have an obligation to serve four years in the Selected Reserve (the 2x4 program) and enter the Selected Reserve within one year of discharge.

Service members or veterans who received a commission as a result of graduation from a service academy or completion of an ROTC scholarship are not eligible under Category 1 unless they received their commission:

1. After becoming eligible for MGIB benefits (including completing the minimum service requirements for the initial period of active duty).
2. Or after September 30, 1996, and received less than $3,400 during any one year under ROTC scholarship.

Service members or veterans who declined MGIB because they received repayment from the military for education loans are also ineligible under Category 1. If they did not decline MGIB and received loan repayments, the months served to repay the loans will be deducted from their entitlement.

Early Separation from Military Service: Service members who did not complete the required period of military service may be eligible under Category 1 if discharged for one of the following:

1. Convenience of the government—with 30 continuous months of service for an obligation of three or more years, or 20 continuous months of service for an obligation of less than three years.
2. Service-connected disability.
3. Hardship.
4. A medical condition diagnosed prior to joining the military.
5. A condition that interfered with performance of duty and did not result from misconduct.
6. A reduction in force (in most cases).

Involuntary Separation/Special Separation: For veterans who meet one of the following requirements:

1. Elected MGIB before being involuntarily separated.
2. Or were voluntarily separated under the Voluntary Separation Incentive or the Special Separation Benefit program, elected MGIB benefits before being separated, and had military pay reduced by $1,200 before discharge.

Veterans Educational Assistance Program: For veterans who participated in the Veterans Educational Assistance Program (VEAP) and:

1. Served on active duty on October 9, 1996.
2. Participated in VEAP and contributed money to an account.
3. Elected MGIB by October 9, 1997, and paid $1,200.

Veterans who participated in VEAP on or before October 9, 1996, may also be eligible even if they did not deposit money in a VEAP account if they served on active duty from October 9, 1996, through April 1, 2000, elected MGIB by October 31, 2001, and contributed $2,700 to MGIB. Certain National Guard service members may also qualify under Category 4 if they:

1. Served for the first time on full-time active duty in the National Guard between June 30, 1985, and November 29, 1989, and had no previous active duty service.
2. Elected MGIB during the nine-month window ending on July 9, 1997.
3. And paid $1,200.

Payments: Effective August 1, 2011, all veterans attending public in-state schools full-time have all in-state tuition and fees paid. For those attending private and foreign schools, costs are capped at $17,500 annually.

Benefits are reduced for part-time training. Payments for other types of training follow different rules. The VA will pay an additional amount, called a "kicker" or "college fund," if directed by DOD. Visit www.gibill.va.gov for more information.

The maximum number of months veterans can receive payments is 36 months at the full-time rate or the part-time equivalent. The following groups qualify for the maximum: veterans who served the required length of active duty, veterans with an obligation of three years or more who were separated early for the convenience of the government and served 30 continuous months, and veterans with an obligation of less than three years who were separated early for the convenience of the government and served 20 continuous months.

Types of Training Available:

1. Courses at colleges and universities leading to associate, bachelor or graduate degrees, including accredited independent study offered through distance education.
2. Courses leading to a certificate or diploma from business, technical or vocational schools.
3. Apprenticeship or on-the-job training for those not on active duty, including self-employment training begun on or after June 16, 2004, for ownership or operation of a franchise.
4. Correspondence courses, under certain conditions.
5. Flight training, if the veteran holds a private pilot's license upon beginning the training and meets the medical requirements.
6. State-approved teacher certification programs.
7. Preparatory courses necessary for admission to a college or graduate school.
8. License and certification tests approved for veterans.
9. Entrepreneurship training courses to create or expand small businesses.
10. Tuition assistance using MGIB as "Top-Up" (active duty service members).

Work-Study Program: Veterans who train at the three-quarter or full-time rate may be eligible for a work-study program in which they work for the VA and receive hourly wages. The types of work allowed include:

1. Outreach services.
2. VA paperwork.
3. Work at national or state veterans' cemeteries.
4. Work at VA medical centers or state veterans' homes.
5. Other VA approved activities.

Educational and Vocational Counseling: VA counseling is available to help determine educational or vocational strengths and weaknesses and plan educational or employment goals. Additionally, individuals not eligible for the MGIB may still receive VA counseling beginning 180 days prior to separation from active duty through the first full year following honorable discharge.

Veterans' Educational Assistance Program

Eligibility: Active duty personnel could participate in the Veterans' Educational Assistance Program (VEAP) if they entered active duty for the first time after December 31, 1976, and before July 1, 1985, and made a contribution prior to April 1, 1987. The maximum contribution is $2,700. Active duty participants may make a lump-sum contribution to their VEAP account. For more information, visit the website at www.gibill.va.gov. Service members who participated in VEAP are eligible to receive benefits while on active duty if:

1. At least 3 months of contributions are available, except for high school or elementary, in which only one month is needed.
2. And they enlisted for the first time after September 7, 1980, and completed 24 months of their first period of active duty. Service members must receive a discharge under conditions other than dishonorable for the qualifying period of service. Service members who enlisted for the first time after September 7, 1980, or entered active duty as an officer or enlistee after October 16, 1981, must have completed 24 continuous months of active duty, unless they meet a qualifying exception.

Eligibility generally expires 10 years from release from active duty, but can be extended under special circumstances.

Payments: DoD will match contributions at the rate of $2 for every $1 put into the fund and may make additional contributions, or "kickers," as necessary. For training in college, vocational or technical schools, the payment amount depends on the type and hours of training pursued. The maximum amount is $300 a month for full-time training.

Training, Work-Study, Counseling: VEAP participants may receive the same training, work-study benefits and counseling as provided under the Montgomery GI Bill.

Academic Planning

Once you have identified your career goal, you may find you need a formal education to achieve it. Your Education Counselor can explore the possibilities with you. Counselors can also advise you on nontraditional educational opportunities that can make it easier for you to get a diploma, vocational certificate or college degree. These non-traditional opportunities include the following:

- **Take "challenge exams," such as a college-level equivalency exam:** You can convert knowledge learned outside the classroom into credits toward a college program. This can save you time and money.
- **Go to school part time while continuing to hold down a full-time job:** This approach might make adult education more practical.
- **See the veterans' coordinator at the college, university or vocational school of your choice:** The coordinator can help you understand your VA educational benefits and might lead you to special programs offered to former service members.

- **Determine if your military learning experiences can translate to course credit:** Check with your service Education Center, Navy College Office or Marine Corps LifeLong Learning Center well in advance of your separation date to request copies of your transcripts.
- **Take advantage of distance learning opportunities:** With today's technological advances, you can enroll in an educational program in which courses are offered by accredited educational institutions in a variety of formats, i.e., CD-ROM, the Internet, satellite TV, cable TV, and video tapes.

Vocational Services

The Education Center, Navy College Office or Marine Corps LifeLong Learning Center can tell you about vocational and technical school programs designed to give you the skills needed to work in occupations that do not require a four-year college degree. The counselors at these centers can also show you how to get course credits for non-traditional learning experience (such as military certifications and on-the-job training). The counselors can help you explore these options. The counselors may also help you find out about certification and licensing requirements—for example, how to get a journeyman card for a particular trade. The counselors can give you information on vocational and apprenticeship programs. **Note:** Local trade unions may also offer vocational training in fields that interest you.

Licensing and Certification

Your military occupational specialty may require a license or certification in the civilian workforce. There are several resources available to assist you in finding civilian requirements for licensing and certification:

- www.acinet.org: Department of Labor website. Go to "Career Tools" section to look up licenses by state, requirements for the license, and point-of-contact information for the state licensing board.
- www.dantes.doded.mil/dantes_web/danteshome.asp: DANTES website has information on certification programs.
- www.cool.army.mil: Find civilian credentials related to your military occupational specialty, learn what it takes to obtain the credentials, and see if there are available programs that will help pay credentialing fees.
- www.cool.navy.mil: Find civilian credentials related to your Navy rating, learn what it takes to obtain the credentials, and see if there are available programs that will help pay credentialing fees.

Testing Available Through Your Education Center

Testing can be an important first step in your career development. Some colleges and universities may require you to provide test results as part of your application. Prior to your departure from military service, you are encouraged to take advantage of the testing services offered by the Education Center, Navy College Office and Marine Corps LifeLong Learning Center. These services include the following:

- **Vocational interest inventories:** Most Education Centers, Navy College Offices and Marine Corps LifeLong Learning Centers offer free vocation interest inventories that can help you identify the careers most likely to interest you.
- **Academic entry exams:** Before applying for college or other academic programs, you may want to take a college admission test such as the Scholastic Aptitude Test (SAT), ACT, or the Graduate Record Examination (GRE). Some schools may require that you do so. Information on these tests is available from your Education Center, Navy College Office or Marine Corps LifeLong Learning Center. You must start early. These exams are offered only a few times each year.
- **Credit by examination:** Your Education Center, Navy College Office and Marine Corps LifeLong Learning Center offers a variety of "challenge" exams that can lead to college credit. If you score high enough, you may be exempt from taking a certain class or course requirements—resulting in a big savings of time and money as you earn your degree. The College Level Examination Program (CLEP) and the DANTES Subject Standardized Tests (DSST) are also free to service members on active duty.
- **Certification examinations:** As a service member working in an important occupational field, you have received extensive training (service schools, correspondence course, OJT) which has proved valuable in developing your professional skills. Your local Education Center, Navy College Office or Marine Corps LifeLong Learning Center can provide you information on certification examinations that "translate" military training into civilian terms. Examinations are available in many skill areas and upon successful completion the documentation you receive is readily understood and received in the professional occupational civilian community.

DoD Voluntary Education Program Website

For separating service members, the Department of Defense Voluntary Education Program website, www.voled.doded.mil, offers a wide variety of educational information of interest and use. The website was originally established to provide support for military education center staffs worldwide. As the website developed, it took on the mission of providing direct support to active and reserve components' service members and their families. This support includes information on all programs provided by the Defense Activity for Non-Traditional Educational Support (DANTES) including the Distance Learning Program, Examination Program, Certification Program, Counselor Support Program, Troops to Teachers, and a wide variety of educational catalogs and directories.

Save Time and Money: You can get up to 30 college credits by taking the five CLEP general exams. If you are currently serving in the Armed Forces, you can take these exams for free.

Contact your installation Education Center, Navy College Office, or Marine Corps LifeLong Learning Office to ensure that they have the capability to offer examinations you need in paper and pencil or computer-based-testing (CBT) format.

Links are provided to each of the services' education programs and to a wide variety of education-related resources. There is also a Directory of Education Centers on the website, which contains information on all of the services' education centers worldwide, including addresses, phone numbers and e-mail addresses.

The primary goal of the website is to provide on-site, or through links, all information for service members to select, plan and complete their program of study, either while on active duty or upon separation.

Service Unique Transcripts

Army: For everything you want to know about the free AARTS transcript (Army/American Council on Education Registry Transcript System), go to aarts.army.mil. This free transcript includes your military training, your Military Occupational Specialty (MOS), and college level examination scores with the college credit recommended for those experiences. It is a valuable asset that you should provide to your college or your employer and it is available for active army, National Guard and reserve soldiers. You can view and print your own transcript at this website.

Save Time and Money: Unless you know for sure that you need to take a particular course, wait until the school gets all your transcripts before you sign up for classes. Otherwise you may end up taking courses you don't need.

Navy and Marine Corps: Information on how to obtain the Sailor/Marine American Council on Education Registry Transcript (SMART) is available at www.navycollege.navy.mil. SMART is now available to document the American Council on Education (ACE) recommended college credit for military training and occupational experience. SMART is an academically accepted record that is validated by ACE. The primary purpose of SMART is to assist service members in obtaining college credit for their military experience. Additional information on SMART can also be obtained from your nearest Navy College Office or Marine Corps Education Center, or contact the Navy College Center.

Air Force: The Community College of the Air Force (CCAF) automatically captures your training, experience and standardized test scores. Transcript information may be viewed at the CCAF website: www.au.af.mil/au/ccaf.

Coast Guard: The Coast Guard Institute (CGI) requires each service member to submit documentation of all training (except correspondence course records), along with an enrollment form, to receive a transcript. Transcript information can be found at the Coast Guard Institute Home Page: www.uscg.mil/hq/cgi/forms.htm.

USEFUL WEBSITES

General Transition Related

A Summary of Veterans Benefits: www.vba.va.gov/bln/21/index.htm
Army Career and Alumni Program (ACAP): www.acap.army.mil
Civilian Assistance and Re-Employment (CARE): www.cpms.osd.mil/care
Department of Veterans Affairs (DVA): www.va.gov
Dept. of Veterans Affairs Locations: www2.va.gov/directory
Department of Labor: www.dol.gov
Military Home Front: www.militaryhomefront.dod.mil
Military Installation Locator: benefits.military.com/misc/installations/Landing
   _Page.jsp
Military OneSource: www.militaryonesource.com/skins/MOS/home.aspx
Operation Transition: https://www.dmdc.osd.mil/ot
National Guard Transitional Assistance Advisors: www.jointservicessupport
   .org
Air Force Airman and Family Readiness Center: www.militaryinstallations
   .dod.mil
Navy Fleet and Family Support Center: www.cnic.navy.mil
Marines Career Resource Management Center (CRMC)/Transition & Employment Assistance Program Center: www.usmc-mccs.org/tamp/index.cfm
Coast Guard Worklife Division—Transition Assistance: www.uscg.mil/work
   life/transition_assistance.asp
Family center, chaplain's office, and related resources finder: www.nvti.uc
   denver.edu/home/infoVeterans.htm

Marine for Life: www.marineforlife.org
Military Family Network: www.emilitary.org

Employment Assistance

Employer Support of the Guard and Reserve (ESGR): www.esgr.org
Department of Labor Resources:
  www.dol.gov
  www.careeronestop.org
  www.doleta.gov/programs
Transition Bulletin Board (TBB): https://www.dmdc.osd.mil/ot
Federal Job Search: www.usajobs.com
DoD Civilian Careers: www.go-defense.com
Fed World Job Resource: www.fedworld.gov
Federal Employment Portal: www.opm.gov
Army Civilian Personnel Online: www.cpol.army.mil
Troops to Cops: www.cops.usdoj.gov
Career InfoNet: www.careerinfonet.org
Careers In Government: www.careersingovernment.com
Vocational Information Center: www.khake.com
The Riley Guide: www.rileyguide.com
Veterans Employment and Training Service VETS: www.dol.gov/vets/about
  vets/contacts/main.htm
DoD Spouse Career Center: www.military.com/spouse
Helpful Career Related Resources: www.military.com/careers
Army Credentialing Opportunities Online (COOL): https://www.cool.army
  .mil
Navy Credentialing Opportunities Online (COOL): https://www.cool.navy.mil
Helmets to Hardhats (H2H): helmetstohardhats.org
Occupational Information Network (O*NET): www.onetonline.org
The Encyclopedia of Associations: library.dialog.com/bluesheets/html/bl0114
  .html
National Trade and Professional Associations of the United States: www
  .associationexecs.com
The Occupational Outlook Handbook: www.bls.gov/oco/home.htm
Military and Veteran Service Organizations: www.military.com/benefits
  /resources/military-and-veteran-associations
Skills Assessment Resources: www.military.com/careers
DD Form 2586, "Verification of Military Experience and Training" (VMET):
  www.dtic.mil/whs/directives/infomgt/forms/eforms/dd2586.pdf
Troops to Teachers (TTT): www.proudtoserveagain.com
State Employment Office Locator: www.naswa.org

Entrepreneurship and Business

U.S. Small Business Administration (SBA): www.sba.gov
SCORE "Counselors to America's Small Business:" www.score.org
Local SCORE Chapter Locator: www.score.org/findscore/chapter_maps.html
Office of Small and Disadvantaged Business Utilization: www.osdbu.gov
/members.html
Center for Veterans Enterprise (CVE): www.vetbiz.gov
Association of Small Business Development Centers (ASBDC): www.asbdc
-us.org
International Franchise Association (IFA): www.franchise.org

Education/Training

VA Education Services (GI Bill): www.gibill.va.gov
VA 22-1990 Application for Education Benefits: www.vba.va.gov/pubs/forms
/VBA-22_1990.pdf
VA Regional Office Finder: www2.va.gov/directory
The Defense Activity for Non-Traditional Education Support (DANTES):
www.dantes.doded.mil/dantes_web/danteshome.asp
Department of Defense Voluntary Education Program: apps.mhf.dod.mil/voled
Army (AARTS) Transcript: aarts.army.mil
Navy and Marine Corps (SMART) Transcript: https://www.navycollege.navy
.mil
Air Force (CCAF) Transcript: www.au.af.mil/au/ccaf
Coast Guard Institute Transcript: www.uscg.mil/hq/cgi/active_duty/go_to
_college/official_transcript.asp
Federal Financial Student Aid: www.federalstudentaid.ed.gov
Application Pell Grants or Federal Stafford Loans (FAFSA): www.fafsa.ed
.gov
Veterans' Upward Bound: www.navub.org

Relocation

Relocation Assistance Office Locator: www.militaryinstallations.dod.mil
"Plan My Move": planmymove.mhf.dod.mil
Chamber of Commerce Locator: www.chamberofcommerce.com
Military Personnel Portals:
Army Knowledge Online (AKO): www.army.mil/ako
Navy Knowledge Online (NKO): www.nko.mil
Air Force Portal: www.my.af.mil
The "It's Your Move" Pamphlet: www.move.mil
"Special Needs" Resources: www.militaryhomefront.dod.mil

Health Care

TRICARE Reserve Select (TRS): www.tricare.mil/reserve

TRICARE: www.tricare.mil

Posttraumatic Stress Disorder (PTSD) Resources:

DoD Mental Health Self-Assessment Program: www.militarymentalhealth .org

National Center for Post-Traumatic Stress Disorder (PTSD): www.ptsd.va .gov

Ameriforce Deployment Guide: www.ameriforce.net/deployment

Courage to Care: www.usuhs.mil/psy/courage.html

Returning Reservists Resources: www.usuhs.mil/psy/GuardReserveReentry Workplace.pdf

Continued Health Care Benefit Program (CHCBP): www.humana-military .com/chcbp/main.htm

VA Home Page: www.va.gov

TRICARE Dental Program: www.tricaredentalprogram.com

TRICARE Retiree Dental Program: www.trdp.org

Life Insurance

VA Office of Service Members' Group Life Insurance (OSGLI): www .insurance.va.gov/sgliSite/SGLI/SGLI.htm

Form SGLV 8286, "Service Members' Group Life Insurance Election & Certificate": www.insurance.va.gov/sgliSite/forms/8286.htm

Form SGLV 8286A, "Family Coverage Election (FSGLI)": www.insurance .va.gov/sgliSite/forms/8286A.htm

Form SGLV 8714, "Application for Veterans' Group Life Insurance": www .insurance.va.gov/sgliSite/forms/8714.htm

VA OSGLI FAQs: www.insurance.va.gov/sgliSite/SGLI/deployFAQ.htm

Finance

Military Installation Finder: www.militaryinstallations.dod.mil

Military One Source: militaryonesource.com

AnnualCreditReport.Com: www.annualcreditreport.com

Experian National Consumer Assistance: www.experian.com

Equifax Credit Information Service: www.equifax.com

TransUnion: www.transunion.com

VA Form 26-1880, "Request for Certificate of Eligibility": www.vba.va.gov /pubs/forms/vba-26-1880-are.pdf

Get your W-2 from myPay: https://mypay.dfas.mil/mypay.aspx

Veterans Benefits

Department of Veterans Affairs: www.va.gov
Vet Center Directory: www.va.gov
State Veterans Benefits Directory: www.military.com
Health Care Benefits: www.va.gov/health
Health Care Enrollment—Priority Groups: www.va.gov/healtheligibility
Education Benefits: www.gibill.va.gov
Compensation and Pension: www.vba.va.gov/bln/21
Vocational Rehabilitation and Employment (VR&E): www.vba.va.gov/bln/vre
DVA Life Insurance Programs: www.insurance.va.gov

Note: In June 2011, the Pentagon launched a program to encourage companies to employ service member spouses. The DoD initiative—dubbed the "Military Spouse Employment Partnership"—includes 79 Fortune 500 plus companies and is intended to make hiring military spouses attractive to employers by offering them good public exposure while highlighting spouses as a potential workforce solution.

"We're really holding their feet to the fire with this," said Robert Gordon, the Pentagon's chief of military community and family policy. "We want documentation—who they're hiring, how many they're hiring, in terms of what kind of jobs our spouses are getting."

Military spouses have an unemployment rate of 26 percent and a wage gap of 25 percent compared to their civilian counterparts, Gordon said during an interview with military bloggers. The partnership is attempting to fix both of those problems.

Military spouses—particularly those with higher education and those holding licenses for specific jobs—often face difficulties finding quality employment. Frequent moves make building and maintaining an attractive resume difficult. And too often employers are hesitant to hire someone who is at risk of being transferred, officials admit.

Additionally, the federal government does not provide tax incentives to employers for hiring military spouses or block them from discriminating against spouses based on their military affiliation.

To become part of the MSEP program companies must fill out an application and undergo a vetting process from the DoD and the Commerce Department, Gordon said. Available jobs are then posted to the MSEP website where spouses can register and submit their information. Spouse resumes are sent directly to the appropriate human resource department.

6

Benefits, Taxes, and Legal Issues

INCOME AND FINANCES

Pay

The military will continue to pay 100% of a service member's pre-injury salary for line-of-duty injuries until the service member is (1) found fit to return to service, (2) placed on a temporary disabled list or (3) released from service through separation or retirement. Generally, deployed active duty service members return to their unit in a backup capacity when they are ill or injured and thus continue to draw their regular pay.

However, reservist service members have no similar unit to return to and thus must take additional steps to continue receiving their active duty salary. DoD guidelines call for an MEB disability determination to occur within a year. However, there is no time limit for how long the service member may continue to draw his or her salary if the medical evaluation process takes longer than a year.

Injured reservists who wish to continue receiving their regular service salary and benefits must apply for either the Medical Retention Processing (MRP) program or the Active Duty Medical Extension (ADME) program. The MRP program applies specifically to Reserve Component service members mobilized in support of Global War on Terror (GWOT) contingency operations and who are wounded, incur an injury, or aggravate a previous illness or disease in the line of duty. To remain on active duty pending evaluation of an injury, all other Reserve Component service members (i.e., those not mobilized in support of GWOT contingency operations) must apply through the Active Duty Medical Extension (ADME) program.

Under the MRP program, an injured reservist who is not expected to return to duty within 60 days of being injured must consent to reassignment to a

Army:
Department of the Army
U.S. Army Physical Disability
  Agency (USAPDA)
Traumatic SGLI (TSGLI)
200 Stovall St.
Alexandria, VA 22332-0470
Fax: 866-275-0684
Email: TSGLI@hoffman.army.mil

Coast Guard:
Commandant, US Coast Guard
Attn: CG-12222
100 2nd St, NW
Washington, DC 20593-0001
Email: twalsh@comdt.uscg.mil
Fax: 202-267-4823

Marine Corps:
Headquarters, U.S. Marine
  Corps
MI-TSGLI
3280 Russell Rd.
Quantico, VA 22134
Email: t-sgli@usmc.mil
Fax: 888-858-2315

Navy:
Navy Personnel Command
Attn: PERS62
5720 Integrity Drive
Millington, TN 38055-6200
Email: MILL_TSGLI@navy.mil
Fax: 901-874-2265

Medical Retention Processing Unit (MRPU) in order to continue to receive his or her regular service salary and benefits. The injured reservist will remain on active duty with the MRPU until he or she is determined to be fit to return to duty or the medical evaluation is completed through his or her branch's disability evaluation system. The reassignment orders last 179 days. Injured reservists may request extensions in order to remain on active duty for medical treatment.

Those reservists injured not in connection with GWOT contingency operations must apply through the ADME program to remain on active duty while continuing to receive medical treatment for their injuries. Like the MRP program, ADME is a voluntary program: the service member must consent to participation by applying through his or her branch of service. Members of the Reserve Components must apply for the MRP and ADME programs by submitting an MRP or ADME packet to their respective branch of service.

Combat-Related Special Compensation

The 2008 National Defense Authorization Act (NDAA) was signed into law on January 29, 2008. It expanded Combat-Related Special Compensation (CRSC) eligibility to include those who were medically retired under Chapter 61 with less than 20 years of service, effective January 1, 2008.

A Chapter 61 retiree is anyone who was medically retired from military service. Chapter 61 is a new component for CRSC. Medically retired veterans must still provide documentation that shows a causal link between a current VA disability and a combat-related event.

Submitting a Claim

CRSC will not begin processing claims until the DoD provides program implementation instructions. However, potentially eligible retirees can begin to gather the required documentation (VA rating decision, DD214, medical records) needed to submit their claim. Required documentation includes:

- a signed claim form
- copy of Chapter 61 Board results (Chapter 61 claimants only)
- copies of ALL VA rating decisions which include the letter and the narrative summaries
- copies of ALL DD214's
- medical records that support *how* the injury occurred for each claimed disability that meets the criteria for combat-related

The CRSC website will be kept updated with program guidance and claim information:

https://www.hrc.army.mil/site/crsc/index.html
Call center: 866-281-3254

Social Security Disability Benefits

Military service members can receive expedited processing of disability claims from Social Security. Benefits available through Social Security are different than those from the VA and require a separate application.

The expedited process is used for military service members who become disabled while on active military duty on or after October 1, 2001, regardless of where the disability occurs. Wounded warriors can now qualify while on active duty as part of the expedited process and active duty status and receipt of military pay does not, in itself, necessarily prevent payment of Social Security disability benefits. Receipt of military payments should never stop you from applying for disability benefits from Social Security. If you are receiving treatment at a military medical facility and working in a designated therapy program or on limited duty, the SSA will evaluate your work activity to determine your eligibility for benefits.

Monthly retirement, disability and survivor benefits under Social Security are payable to veterans and dependents if the veteran has earned enough work credits under the program. Upon the veteran's death, a one-time payment of

$255 also may be made to the veteran's spouse or child. In addition, a veteran may qualify at age 65 for Medicare's hospital insurance and medical insurance. Medicare protection is available to people who have received Social Security disability benefits for 24 months, and to insured people and their dependents who need dialysis or kidney transplants, or who have amyotrophic lateral sclerosis (more commonly known as Lou Gehrig's disease).

Since 1957, military service earnings for active duty (including active duty for training) have counted toward Social Security and those earnings are already on Social Security records. Since 1988, inactive duty service in the Reserve Component (such as weekend drills) has also been covered by Social Security. Service members and veterans are credited with $300 in additional earnings for each calendar quarter in which they received active duty basic pay after 1956 and before 1978.

Veterans who served in the military from 1978 through 2001 are credited with an additional $100 in earnings for each $300 in active duty basic pay, up to a maximum of $1,200 a year. No additional Social Security taxes are withheld from pay for these extra credits. If veterans enlisted after September 7, 1980, and did not complete at least 24 months of active duty or their full tour of duty, they may not be able to receive the additional earnings. Check with Social Security for details. Additional earnings will no longer be credited for military service periods after 2001.

Also, noncontributory Social Security earnings of $160 a month may be credited to veterans who served after September 15, 1940, and before 1957, including attendance at service academies. For information, call 800-772-1213 or visit www.socialsecurity.gov. (**Note:** Social Security cannot add these extra earnings to the record until an application is filed for Social Security benefits.)

Although VA compensation and pension benefits are counted in determining income for SSI purposes, some other income is not counted. Also, not all resources count in determining eligibility. For example, a person's home and the land it is on do not count. Personal effects, household goods, automobiles and life insurance may not count, depending upon their value. Information and help is available at any Social Security office or by calling 800-772-1213.

The Social Security Administration (SSA) offers two kinds of benefits for disabled individuals: Social Security Disability Insurance (SSDI) and Supplemental Security Income (SSI). SSDI functions as an insurance program that makes payments to those who become unable to work due to a disability. SSDI payments vary based on an individual's previous income and the amount of Social Security (or FICA) taxes he or she paid in the past. SSI is a federal program that provides monthly assistance to the elderly, blind and disabled who have low income and limited resources. SSI payments vary based on income.

Disabled service members may qualify for one or both of these sources of assistance, depending on their individual situation.

To qualify for SSDI, an individual must (1) have worked for several years in jobs covered by social security (i.e., had Social Security taxes withheld from his or her pay), and (2) be disabled. The amount of time an individual needs to have worked in order to receive SSDI varies with the age at which he or she becomes disabled. SSDI benefits are only available to those who are totally disabled (i.e., unable to work); no benefits are payable for partial disabilities or for short-term disabilities.

To qualify as disabled, an individual must have a medical condition that is expected to prevent him or her from engaging in "substantial gainful activity" (SGA) for at least one year, or to result in death. SGA means working and earning above a certain amount of income per month. The threshold for SGA is higher for individuals suffering from blindness than it is for individuals with other disabilities. For current SGA amounts, visit www.ssa.gov/OACT/COLA/sga.html. For more information on what constitutes disability, see the Social Security Red Book, available at www.ssa.gov/redbook.

Disability status for Social Security benefits is determined separately from an individual's DoD and VA disability ratings. Once SSA determines that an individual meets the basic requirements for benefits, they forward the individual's application to his or her state's disability determination services (DDS) office. The DDS office will determine if his or her medical condition qualifies as a disability for purposes of Social Security. SSA maintains a list of medical conditions severe enough to automatically qualify. This list is available at www.ssa.gov/dibplan/dqualify.htm. If the applicant's condition is not on the list, then the DDS office will determine, based on his or her medical records, whether he or she is capable of returning to a previous job or of doing another type of work. In some cases, the DDS office asks an individual to undergo further physical examination in order to obtain further information.

SSDI payments are determined based on an individual's lifetime average earnings covered by Social Security (i.e., how much Social Security tax he or she paid over his or her lifetime). SSDI payments may be reduced if an individual receives worker's compensation payments or other government disability benefits, such as DoD or VA disability compensation. Benefit calculators that provide an estimate of an individual's SSDI payments are available on the SSA website at www.ssa.gov/planners/calculators.htm.

In addition to monthly payments, SSDI recipients will usually become eligible for Medicare coverage after 24 months.

Individuals who qualify for SSDI become eligible to receive benefits beginning the sixth full month after the date their disability began. Since each month's benefits are paid the following month, recipients will not receive payment until the seventh month. For example, an individual who becomes disabled in January will be eligible for benefits beginning in July. He or she will receive a check for July benefits in August.

Benefits last a minimum of 24 months and usually continue until it is determined that an individual is no longer totally disabled, either because of medical improvement or a return to work. DDS periodically reviews disability cases to see if an individual's condition has improved. Once an individual's disability ceases he or she will receive SSDI benefits for a 3-month grace period: the month in which the determination was made plus two months afterwards. Under certain circumstances, an individual may continue to receive SSDI payments beyond the grace period if he or she is enrolled in an approved program for vocational rehabilitation, employment services or other support services. See the Social Security Red Book at www.ssa.gov/redbook for more information on employment support services to help SSDI recipients reenter the workforce.

In order to receive SSDI benefits, an individual must complete an Application for Social Security Benefits and a Disability Report, which contains information about his or her disabling condition and its effects on his or her ability to work. Individuals may either complete these forms online at www .socialsecurity.gov/applyfordisability or through an interview with a claims representative. Interviews may be conducted in person or over the phone. Individuals may contact an SSA claims representative at 800-772-1213 (TTY: 800-325-0778) to schedule an interview.

Applicants for SSDI should be prepared to submit proof of identity and evidence of disability, including:

- Social Security number;
- birth certificate (or other proof of age);
- contact information for doctors and medical facilities where they received treatment;
- names and prescribed dosages of medications they are taking;
- medical records and test results;
- a work history for the past 16 years, including contact information for previous employers and the type of work done;
- copies of W-2 forms (or federal tax returns for self-employed individuals);
- bank account numbers;
- emergency contact information: name, address and phone number of a designated emergency contact person; and
- original or certified copies of military discharge papers (Form DD 214) for all periods of active duty.

For a complete checklist of items to prepare, visit www.ssa.gov/disability/ Adult_Starterkit_checklist.pdf.

Individuals have the right to be represented by an attorney or other qualified representative throughout the application and appeals process. Represented applicants must submit a Form SSA-1696-U4, Appointment of Representative, available at www.ssa.gov/online/ssa-1696.pdf. See www.ssa.gov/pubs/10075.pdf for more information on the right to representation.

An individual who disagrees with an SSA determination regarding disability benefits can appeal a decision by filing a Request for Appeal and an Appeal Disability Report with SSA within 65 days of the date on his or her notice of decision from SSA. For more information on appeals, visit https://secure.ssa.gov/apps6z/iAppeals/ap001.jsp, or call the toll-free number listed above.

Supplemental Security Income (SSI)

An individual may qualify for supplemental security income if he or she (1) is over age 65, blind or disabled; (2) is a low-income earner; and (3) owns assets worth less than $2,000 (or $3,000 for a couple). The disability determination process and the standard for finding a disability are the same as those discussed above for SSDI. In determining whether an individual is a low-income earner, the SSA considers earned income, unearned income and government benefits such as VA and DoD disability compensation and other Social Security benefits (e.g., SSDI). When determining whether an individual has assets in excess of the maximum threshold amount, SSA generally does not include an individual's home and the land it is on, a car, life insurance policies worth $1,500 or less, burial plots and up to $1,500 each in burial funds for a recipient and his or her spouse. However, other assets such as cash, stock, retirement accounts and similar items are considered.

SSI payments are determined based on the amount of "countable income" an applicant receives and his or her living arrangement/family status. An eligible applicant will receive the basic monthly payment known as the Federal Benefit Rate (FBR) minus any countable income. Countable income includes earned income, unearned income and government benefits. Most states provide an additional monthly payment or "state supplement" to SSI. States each set their own qualifications and amounts for state supplements. SSI recipients may also be eligible to receive Medicaid.

Applicants for SSI must call SSA at 800-772-1213 to speak with a claims representative and schedule an interview. In order to receive SSI benefits, an individual will have to complete and submit a Disability Report to SSA. Individuals may complete this form online at www.socialsecurity.gov/applyfor disability.

In addition to the documents required for SSDI benefits (see above), applicants for SSI also may need:

- information about their home: either mortgage information or a lease;
- financial records: payroll slips, bank records, insurance policies, car registrations and other information about assets; and
- proof of citizenship or noncitizen status: birth certificate, passport or immigration documents.

The appeals process for individuals who disagree with SSA's determination regarding SSI benefits is the same as for SSDI benefits.

Commissary and Exchange Privileges for Veterans and Family Members

Unlimited exchange and commissary store privileges in the United States are available to honorably discharged veterans with a service-connected disability rated at 100 percent, unremarried surviving spouses of members or retired members of the armed forces, recipients of the Medal of Honor, and their dependents and orphans. Certification of total disability is done by the VA. Reservists and their dependents also may be eligible. Privileges overseas are governed by international law and are available only if agreed upon by the foreign government concerned.

Though these benefits are provided by the DoD, the VA does provide assistance in completing DD Form 1172, "Application for Uniformed Services Identification and Privilege Card." For detailed information, contact the nearest military installation.

Thrift Savings Plan

The Thrift Savings Plan (TSP) is a retirement savings plan with special tax advantages for federal government employees and service members. Participation is optional, and service members must join TSP while they are still serving in the military. TSP is similar to traditional 401(k) plans often sponsored by private employers; contributions to TSP accounts are not taxed at the time they are made, but distributions from the accounts generally are subject to income tax at the time the distributions are withdrawn. Veterans who did not sign up for TSP while in service cannot join the plan after leaving the military. Contributions to TSPs are subject to certain limitations. Detailed information about TSP is available at www.tsp.gov.

There are three basic ways for service members to access funds in their TSP accounts: in-service withdrawals, TSP loans, and post-separation withdrawals.

In-Service Withdrawals: Most service members can borrow against the contributions and earnings made to his or her TSP account. These loans generally have no tax consequences. However, the loan must be paid back with interest, usually within five years. Payments usually take the form of payroll deductions. Therefore, service members who do not receive monthly pay (i.e., reservists with irregular training intervals) may not be eligible for TSP loans.

TSP Loans: Service members may also withdraw money from their TSP account under what is known as a financial hardship withdrawal. Financial hardship withdrawals generally are subject to a 10% penalty, in addition to the income tax on the withdrawal. However, this 10% penalty generally does not apply if the withdrawal is made because of a permanent and total disability or if the money is used to pay for deductible medical expenses that exceed 7.5% of the service member's adjusted gross income.

The 10% penalty does not apply to any portion of a distribution which represents tax exempt contributions from pay earned in a combat zone. Also, Combat Zone Exclusion pay contributed to a TSP account is not taxable when withdrawn, unlike regular pay. However, the interest earned on amounts contributed to a TSP account that were exempt from tax because of the Combat Zone Exclusion is taxable. If a service member receives a distribution from an account that has both Exclusion and non-Exclusion contributions, the distribution will be paid in the same proportions as the service member's Exclusion and non-Exclusion contributions.

TSP participants may withdraw money from their accounts if either they are at least 59½ years old or they have a verifiable financial hardship. For instance, a disabled service member may face financial hardship in connection with his or her medical condition. In such a case, a financial hardship withdrawal may be permitted.

Post-Separation Withdrawals: After separation from military service, TSP participants may access the money in their TSP accounts in a number of ways, including transferring the money into an IRA or a qualifying employer-sponsored retirement plan (like a 401(k) plan) and receiving the money directly in the form of a lump-sum payment or monthly payments or as an annuity. Each of these options has a different tax consequence, and payments received directly before the age of 59½ may still be subject to a 10% early withdrawal penalty in addition to income tax at the time the money is received.

Service members should consult their TSP plan administrator and a tax advisor when contemplating a withdrawal from a TSP in order to determine which option is best suited for their financial needs and to assess the tax consequences of a withdrawal.

HOUSING

VA Home Loan Guaranty

VA home loan guaranties are issued to help eligible service members, veterans, reservists and unmarried surviving spouses obtain homes, condominiums, residential cooperative housing units, and manufactured homes, and to refinance loans. For additional information or to obtain VA loan guaranty forms, visit www.homeloans.va.gov.

Loan Uses: A VA guaranty helps protect lenders from loss if the borrower fails to repay the loan. It can be used to obtain a loan to:

1. Buy or build a home.
2. Buy a residential condominium.
3. Buy a residential cooperative housing unit.
4. Repair, alter or improve a home.
5. Refinance an existing home loan.
6. Buy a manufactured home with or without a lot.
7. Buy and improve a manufactured home lot.
8. Install a solar heating or cooling system or other weatherization improvements.
9. Buy a home and install energy-efficient improvements.

Eligibility

In addition to the periods of eligibility and conditions of service requirements, applicants must have a good credit rating, sufficient income, a valid Certificate of Eligibility (COE), and agree to live in the property in order to be approved by a lender for a VA home loan. To obtain a COE, complete VA Form 26-1880—"Request for a Certificate of Eligibility for VA Home Loan"—and mail to: VA Loan Eligibility Center, P.O. Box 20729, Winston-Salem, NC 27120.

It is also possible to obtain a COE from your lender. Most lenders have access to VA's "WebLGY" system. This Internet-based application can establish eligibility and issue an online COE in seconds. Not all cases can currently be processed online—only those for which VA has sufficient data in its records. However, veterans are encouraged to ask their lenders about this method of obtaining a certificate before sending an application to the Eligibility Center. For more information, visit www.homeloans.va.gov/eligibility.htm.

Relevant Periods of Eligibility

Post-Vietnam Period: (1) active duty after May 7, 1975, and prior to August 2, 1990; (2) active duty for 181 continuous days, all of which occurred after May 7, 1975; and (3) discharge under conditions other than dishonorable or early discharge for service-connected disability.

24-Month Rule: If service was between September 8, 1980 (October 16, 1981, for officers) and August 1, 1990, veterans must generally complete 24 months of continuous active duty service or the full period (at least 181 days) for which they were called or ordered to active duty, and be discharged under conditions other than dishonorable. Exceptions are allowed if the veteran completed at least 181 days of active duty service but was discharged earlier than 24 months for (1) hardship, (2) the convenience of the government, (3) reduction-in-force, (4) certain medical conditions, or (5) service-connected disability.

Gulf War: Veterans of the Gulf War era—August 2, 1990, to a date to be determined—must generally complete 24 months of continuous active duty service or the full period (at least 90 days) for which they were called to active duty, and be discharged under other than dishonorable conditions.

Exceptions are allowed if the veteran completed at least 90 days of active duty but was discharged earlier than 24 months for (1) hardship, (2) the convenience of the government, (3) reduction-in-force, (4) certain medical conditions, or (5) service-connected disability. Reservists and National Guard members are eligible if they were activated after August 1, 1990, served at least 90 days, and received an honorable discharge.

Active Duty Personnel: Until the Gulf War era is ended, persons on active duty are eligible after serving 90 continuous days.

VA Guaranty Varies with Size and Type of Loan

The VA guaranty varies with the size of the loan, and is issued to protect lenders so they may make loans to eligible borrowers. Because the lenders are able to obtain this guaranty from the VA, borrowers do not need to make a down payment, provided they have enough home loan entitlement. The maximum guaranty amount is equal to 25 percent of the Freddie Mac conforming loan limit for a single-family home. This limit changes yearly, but for 2011 ranges from $431,000 to $1,000,000 depending on which state you live in.

The total loan amount may include the funding fee, as well as up to $6,000 of home improvements to make the home more energy efficient. An eligible borrower who wishes to use a VA-guaranteed loan to refinance an existing mortgage generally can borrow up to 90 percent of the home's appraised value. However, a loan to reduce the interest rate on an existing VA-guaranteed loan may include the entire outstanding balance of the prior loan, the costs of energy-efficient improvements, as well as closing costs, including up to two discount points. An eligible borrower who wishes to obtain a VA-guaranteed loan to purchase a manufactured home or lot can borrow up to 95 percent of the home's purchase price.

Table 6.1. VA 2014 Funding Fees

Type of Veteran	Down Payment	Percentage for First Time Use	Percentage for Subsequent Use
Regular Military	None	2.15%	3.3%*
	5% or more (up to 10%)	1.50%	1.50%
	10% or more	1.25%	1.25%
Reserves/National Guard	None	2.4%	3.3%*
	5% or more (up to 10%)	1.75%	1.75%
	10% or more	1.5%	1.5%

Cash-Out Refinancing Loans

Type of Veteran	Percentage for First Time Use	Percentage for Subsequent Use
Regular Military	2.15%	3.3%*
Reserves/National Guard	2.4%	3.3%*

Other Types Of Loans

Type of Loan	Percentage for Either Type of Veteran Whether First Time or Subsequent Use
Interest Rate Reduction Refinancing Loans	.50%
Manufactured Home Loans	1.00%
Loan Assumptions	.50%

* The higher subsequent use fee does not apply to these types of loans if the veteran's only prior use of entitlement was for a manufactured home loan.

VA Appraisals

No loan can be guaranteed by the VA without first being appraised by a VA-assigned fee appraiser. A buyer, seller, real estate agent or lender can request a VA appraisal by completing VA Form 26-1805, "Request for Determination of Reasonable Value." The requester pays for the appraisal upon completion, according to a fee schedule approved by the VA. This VA appraisal estimates the value of the property. It is not an inspection and does not guarantee the house is free of defects. The VA guarantees the loan, not the condition of the property.

Closing Costs

For purchase home loans, payment in cash is required on all closing costs, including title search and recording fees, hazard insurance premiums and prepaid taxes. For refinancing loans, all such costs may be included in the loan, as long as the total loan does not exceed 90 percent of the reasonable value of the property. Interest rate reduction loans may include closing costs, including a maximum of two discount points.

All veterans, except those receiving VA disability compensation and un-married surviving spouses of veterans who died in service or as a result of a service-connected disability, are charged a VA funding fee. For all types of loans, the loan amount may include this funding fee.

Required Occupancy

To qualify for a VA purchase home loan, a veteran or the spouse of a service member must certify that he or she intends to occupy the home. When refinancing a VA-guaranteed loan solely to reduce the interest rate, a veteran need only certify to prior occupancy.

Financing, Interest Rates and Terms

Veterans obtain VA-guaranteed loans through the usual lending institutions, including banks, savings and loan associations and mortgage brokers. VA-guaranteed loans can have either a fixed interest rate or an adjustable rate, where the interest rate may adjust up to one percent annually and up to five percent over the life of the loan. VA does not set the interest rate. Interest rates are negotiable between the lender and borrower on all loan types.

Veterans may also choose a different type of adjustable rate mortgage called a hybrid ARM, where the initial interest rate remains fixed for three to 10 years. If the rate remains fixed for less than five years, the rate adjustment cannot be more than one percent annually and five percent over the life of the loan. For a hybrid ARM with an initial fixed period of five years or more, the initial adjustment may be up to two percent. The secretary has the authority to determine annual adjustments thereafter. Currently annual adjustments may be up to two percentage points and six percent over the life of the loan. If the lender charges discount points on the loan, the veteran may negotiate with the seller as to who will pay points or if they will be split between buyer and seller. Points paid by the veteran may not be included in the loan (with the exception that up to two points may be included in interest rate reduction loans). The term of the loan may be for as long as 30 years and 32 days.

Loan Assumption Requirements and Liability

VA loans are not assumable without the prior approval of the VA or its autho-rized agent (usually the lender collecting the monthly payments). To approve the assumption, the lender must ensure that the assumer is a satisfactory credit risk and will assume all of the veteran's liabilities on the loan. If approved, the assumer will have to pay a funding fee that the lender sends to the VA, and the veteran will be released from liability to the federal government.

A release of liability does not mean that a veteran's guaranty entitlement is restored. That occurs only if the assumer is an eligible veteran who agrees to substitute his or her entitlement for that of the seller. If a veteran allows assumption of a loan without prior approval, then the lender may demand immediate and full payment of the loan, and the veteran may be liable if the loan is foreclosed and the VA has to pay a claim under the loan guaranty.

Loans made prior to March 1, 1988, are generally freely assumable, but veterans should still request the VA's approval in order to be released of liability. Veterans whose loans were closed after December 31, 1989, usually have no liability to the government following a foreclosure, except in cases involving fraud, misrepresentation, or bad faith, such as allowing an unapproved assumption. However, for the entitlement to be restored, any loss suffered by the VA must be paid in full.

VA Acquires Property Foreclosures

The VA acquires properties as a result of foreclosures. Ocwen Loan Servicing, LLC, under contract with the VA, is currently marketing the properties through listing agents using local Multiple Listing Services. A listing of "VA Properties for Sale" may be found at www.ocwen.com/reo/home.cfm. Contact a real estate agent for information on purchasing a VA acquired property.

Loans for Native American Veterans

Eligible Native American veterans can obtain a loan from the VA to purchase, construct or improve a home on Federal Trust land, or to reduce the interest rate on such a VA loan. The maximum loan amount is equal to the Freddie Mac conforming loan limit for a single-family home. This limit changes yearly. In 2008, the limit is $417,000 for the continental United States and $625,500 for Hawaii, Alaska, Guam, and the U.S. Virgin Islands.

Veterans who are not Native American, but who are married to Native American non-veterans, may be eligible for a direct loan under this program. To be eligible for such a loan, the qualified non-Native American veteran and the Native American spouse must reside on Federal Trust land, and both the veteran and spouse must have a meaningful interest in the dwelling or lot.

A funding fee must be paid to the VA unless the veteran is exempt from such a fee because he or she receives VA disability compensation. The fee, which is 1.25 percent for loans to purchase, construct or improve a home, and 0.5 percent to refinance an existing VA loan, may be paid in cash or included in the loan. Closing costs such as VA appraisal, credit report, loan processing fee, title search, title insurance, recording fees, transfer taxes, survey charges or hazard insurance may not be included in the loan.

Safeguards Established to Protect Veterans

The following safeguards have been established to protect veterans:

1. The VA may suspend from the loan program those who take unfair advantage of veterans or discriminate because of race, color, religion, sex, disability, family status or national origin.
2. The builder of a new home (or manufactured home) is required to give the purchasing veteran either a one-year warranty or a 10-year insurance-backed protection plan.
3. The borrower obtaining a loan may only be charged closing costs prescribed by the VA as allowable.
4. The borrower can prepay without penalty the entire loan or any part not less than one installment or $100.
5. The VA encourages holders to extend forbearance if a borrower becomes temporarily unable to meet the terms of the loan.

Housing Grants

Veterans with service-connected disabilities may be eligible to receive a VA grant to assist in building a new specially adapted home or modifying an existing home to meet their disability-related needs.

The VA provides grants for veterans who need to build or renovate their homes to adapt to severe disabilities connected with their military service. There are two types of grants administered by the VA: the Specially Adapted Housing grant (up to $50,000) and the Special Adaptations grant (up to $10,000). Eligibility for one grant or the other depends on the veteran's type of disability.

The VA offers grants of up to $50,000 (or 50% of the cost of the home or repairs, whichever is less) to cover the cost of building or buying a specially adapted home or adapting an existing home. Alternatively, the grant may be applied against any unpaid balance of a mortgage on a specially adapted home already purchased.

Veterans are eligible to receive the Specially Adapted Housing grant if they are eligible to receive VA compensation for a permanent and total service disability due to one of the following:

- loss or loss of use of both legs, such as to preclude movement without the aid of crutches, a wheelchair, or other assistive devices;
- loss or loss of use of both upper arms at or above the elbow;
- blindness in both eyes, having only light perception, plus loss or loss of use of one lower leg; or

- loss or loss of use of one leg together with (a) residual effects of organic disease or injury, or (b) the loss or loss of use of one arm, which so affects the functions of balance or propulsion as to preclude movement without the aid of assistive devices.

Additionally, the house must meet all three of the following requirements:

1. It must be medically feasible for the veteran to reside in the house.
2. The house must be adapted to be suitable to the veteran's needs for living purposes, both now and in the future.
3. It must be financially feasible for the veteran to acquire the house or make the adaptations, with the assistance provided by the grant.

The VA will provide assistance to a veteran temporarily residing in a family member's home to adapt the family member's home to meet his or her special needs. The grant is limited to a maximum of $14,000.

The **Special Home Adaptations grant** is a VA grant of up to $10,000 to cover the costs of special housing adaptations to accommodate the needs of certain eligible veterans.

This grant is available to veterans with a service-connected disability entitling them to compensation for permanent and total disability due to:

- Blindness in both eyes with 5/200 visual acuity or less; or
- The anatomical loss, or the loss of use of, both hands or arms below the elbow.

The veteran may apply the grant towards the purchase or adaptation of a home in which he or she resides or intends to reside, including the adaptation of a home owned by a member of the veteran's family.

The VA may approve a grant of up to $2,000 to cover the costs of adapting a family member's home in which the veteran is temporarily residing. A veteran may receive the grants up to three times. However, the aggregate amount of the assistance cannot exceed the maximum amounts allowable for either grant.

Other Benefits

USDA Provides Loans for Farms and Homes

The U.S. Department of Agriculture (USDA) provides loans and guarantees to buy, improve or operate farms. Loans and guarantees are available for housing in towns generally up to 20,000 in population. Applications from veterans have preference. For further information, contact Farm Service Agency or Rural Development, USDA, 1400 Independence Ave., SW, Washington, DC 20250, or apply at local Department of Agriculture offices, usually located in county seats.

Housing and Urban Development Veteran Resource Center (HUDVET)

Housing and Urban Development (HUD) sponsors the Veteran Resource Center (HUDVET), which works with national veterans service organizations to serve as a general information center on all HUD-sponsored housing and community development programs and services. To contact HUDVET, call 800-998-9999, TDD 800-483-2209, or visit www.hud.gov/offices/cpd /about/hudvet/helping.cfm.

EMPLOYMENT

Veterans have the right under USERRA to be reemployed at the civilian jobs they held prior to their military service provided they meet certain criteria (see chapter 5). The Americans with Disabilities Act (ADA) requires employers with more than 15 employees to make reasonable accommodations for employees with disabilities and prohibits discrimination against qualified individuals with disabilities when making hiring, promotion, compensation and training decisions.

Employment Benefits

Transition Assistance Program (TAP)

The Transition Assistance Program (TAP) helps veterans make the transition from military service to the civilian workplace by providing employment and training information within 12 months of separation and within 24 months of retirement. TAP programs, sponsored by the VA and DoD, are free.

Disabled Transition Assistance Program (DTAP) provides information and assistance to veterans who believe they have a disability qualifying them for the VA's Vocational Rehabilitation and Employment (VR&E) program.

Vocational Rehabilitation & Employment (VR&E) Service

The Vocational Rehabilitation and Employment Service (VR&E, sometimes referred to as VRES), a division of the VA, helps veterans with service-connected disabilities gain and maintain suitable employment. VR&E offers the following services:

- comprehensive rehabilitation evaluation to determine abilities, skills, interests and needs;
- vocational counseling and rehabilitation planning;
- employment services, such as job-seeking skills and résumé development;
- on the job training, apprenticeships and nonpaid work experiences;
- post-secondary training at a college, vocational, technical or business school; and
- supportive rehabilitation services, including case management, counseling and referral.

Veterans who have received or will receive a discharge that is other than dishonorable and who have a service-connected disability rating of 10% or more may be eligible for assistance from VR&E. Those with a disability of 20% or higher are automatically eligible, provided they have an "employment handicap." The VA will find an employment handicap where a veteran has an impairment stemming from a service-connected disability affecting his or her ability to train for, find and retain suitable employment given his or her abilities, aptitudes and interests. Those with a 10% rating must show a "serious employment handicap," or a significant impairment of his or her ability to train for, find and retain suitable employment given his or her abilities, aptitudes and interests, in order to receive assistance from VR&E.

Applicants must complete VA Form 28-1900, Disabled Veterans Application for Vocational Rehabilitation, available at www.va.gov/vaforms. A copy of the application also may be obtained by mail by calling 800-827-1000.

Once a VRC determines that a veteran applicant is entitled to assistance from VR&E, the counselor will work with the applicant to identify employment options, determine what training requirements may be necessary, address any physical demands of a chosen profession and develop an individualized vocational plan.

Depending upon the individualized vocational plan chosen, the VRC and veteran may decide that additional education is appropriate for the achievement of the veteran's vocational goals. Veterans who are enrolled in a vocational school, a special rehabilitation facility, or a 2- or 4-year degree program at a college or university may be eligible for an education benefit to cover tuition, fees, books, tools or other necessary supplies. In addition, subsistence allowances vary based on the type of training undertaken, rate of attendance (full-time or part-time), and number of dependents. A veteran who receives VR&E benefits may also be eligible for a monthly subsistence allowance to cover living expenses.

Disabled veterans whose service-connected disabilities render them unable to seek and maintain employment may be eligible for VR&E's Independent Living Program (ILP). ILP seeks to ensure that eligible veterans are able to live independently, participate in family and community life and, over time, return to work. ILP benefits may include assistive technology, independent living skills-training and collaboration with community-based support services. To be eligible for ILP benefits, veterans must submit the same application as for other VR&E benefits.

TAXES

Federal taxes must be paid on all income, including wages, interest earned on bank accounts and so on. However, some tax benefits may arise as a result of a service member serving in a combat zone, while other benefits—such as exclusions, deductions and credits—may arise as a result of certain expenses incurred by the service member. The Combat Zone Exclusion, for instance, is tax-free and does not have to be reported on tax returns.

Expenses incurred in modifying a home to accommodate a disability are normally tax deductible as deductions if the modification does not increase the property's value. An example would be constructing entrance or exit ramps.

Credits directly offset the amount owed in tax. If a service member receives a $2,000 Disabled Tax Credit he will owe $1,000 less in taxes, or receive a refund of $1,000 after filing a tax return.

Tax Returns

The deadline for filing tax returns and paying any tax due is automatically extended for those serving and those hospitalized as a result of injuries incurred while serving in the Armed Forces in a combat zone, in a qualified hazardous duty area or on deployment outside of the United States while participating in a contingency operation.

Combat zones are designated by an executive order from the president as areas in which the U.S. Armed Forces are engaging or have engaged in combat. There are currently three such combat zones (including the airspace above each):

- Arabian Peninsula Areas, beginning January 17, 1991—the Persian Gulf, Red Sea, Gulf of Oman, the part of the Arabian Sea north of 10° North latitude and west of 68° East longitude, the Gulf of Aden, and the countries of Bahrain, Iraq, Kuwait, Oman, Qatar, Saudi Arabia and the United Arab Emirates.
- Kosovo area, beginning March 24, 1999—Federal Republic of Yugoslavia (Serbia and Montenegro), Albania, the Adriatic Sea and the Ionian Sea north of the 39th Parallel.
- Afghanistan, beginning September 19, 2001.

In general, the deadlines for performing certain actions applicable to taxes are extended for the period of the service member's service in the combat zone, plus 180 days after the last day in the combat zone. This extension applies to the filing and paying of income taxes that would have been due April 15.

Members of the U.S. Armed Forces who perform military service in an area outside a combat zone qualify for the suspension of time provisions if their service is in direct support of military operations in the combat zone, and they receive special pay for duty subject to hostile fire or imminent danger as certified by the Department of Defense.

The deadline extension provisions apply not only to members serving in the U.S. Armed Forces (or individuals serving in support thereof) in the combat zone, but to their spouses as well, with two exceptions. First, if you are hospitalized in the United States as a result of injuries received while serving in a combat zone, the deadline extension provisions would not apply to your spouse. Second, the deadline extension provisions for a spouse do not apply for any tax year beginning more than 2 years after the date of the termination of the combat zone designation.

Filing individual income tax returns for your dependent children is not required while your husband is in the combat zone. Instead, these returns will be timely if filed on or before the deadline for filing your joint income tax return under the applicable deadline extensions. When filing your children's individual income tax returns, put "COMBAT ZONE" in red at the top of those returns.

Tax Exclusions

The Combat Zone Exclusion

If you serve in a combat zone as an enlisted person or as a warrant officer (including commissioned warrant officers) for any part of a month, all your military pay received for military service that month is excluded from gross income. For commissioned officers, the monthly exclusion is capped at the highest enlisted pay, plus any hostile fire or imminent danger pay received.

Military pay received by enlisted personnel who are hospitalized as a result of injuries sustained while serving in a combat zone is excluded from gross income for the period of hospitalization, subject to the 2-year limitation provided below. Commissioned officers have a similar exclusion, limited to the maximum enlisted pay amount per month. These exclusions from gross income for hospitalized enlisted personnel and commissioned officers end 2 years after the date of termination of the combat zone.

Annual leave payments to enlisted members of the U.S. Armed Forces upon discharge from service are excluded from gross income to the extent the annual leave was accrued during any month in any part of which the member served in a combat zone. If your wife is a commissioned officer, a portion of

THRIFT SAVINGS PLANS

Withdrawals from TSP accounts generally must be included in income. As a result, withdrawals are subject to withholding. State and local taxes are not withheld from TSP distributions. However, the distributions are reported by the IRS to the service member's state of residence at the time of the payment. Consequently, a service member generally will be required to pay state and local income taxes on the withdrawal unless an exception applies. Consult a state or local tax official or a tax advisor for more information.

the annual leave payment she receives for leave accrued during any month in any part of which she served in a combat zone may be excluded. The annual leave payment is not excludable to the extent it exceeds the maximum enlisted pay amount for the month of service to which it relates less the amount of military pay already excluded for that month.

The reenlistment bonus is excluded from gross income although received in a month that you were outside the combat zone, because you completed the necessary action for entitlement to the reenlistment bonus in a month during which you served in the combat zone.

A recent law change makes it possible for members of the military to count tax-free combat pay when figuring how much they can contribute to a Roth or traditional IRA. Before this change, members of the military whose earnings came from tax-free combat pay were often barred from putting money into an IRA, because taxpayers usually must have taxable earned income. Taxpayers choosing to put money into a Roth IRA don't need to report these contributions on their individual tax return. Roth contributions are not deductible, but distributions, usually after retirement, are normally tax-free. Income limits and other special rules apply.

Deductions and Credits

Medical Care

Many medical expenses may be deducted, including artificial limbs, wheelchairs, psychiatric care and therapy, long-term care, and many other expenses. For a list of allowable deductions, see IRS Publication 502, Medical and Dental Expenses.

Disability-Related Home Modifications

Expenses incurred in modifying a home to accommodate a disability are considered medical expenses. Permanent improvements are deductible if they do not increase the value of the property. Improvements that increase a home's value, if the main purpose is medical care, may be partly included as a medical expense.

The difference between the cost of the improvement and the amount that the value of the property increased is the deductible medical expense. However, many common disability-related improvements do not generally increase the value of a property, and, in such a case, the full cost can be included as a medical expense. For a list of examples, see IRS Publication 502, Medical and Dental Expenses. The cost of maintaining disability-related home modifications also qualify as medical expenses.

Tax Credits

Depending on their income, those service members who (1) are U.S. citizens or residents, (2) have retired on permanent and total disability and (3) if under age 65, receive taxable disability benefits, may be eligible for a disability tax credit. It is important to note that because VA and DoD disability benefits are *not* taxable, these payments cannot make a service member eligible for a credit; he or she will need some other source of disability benefits.

Individuals seeking to claim the disability tax credit must provide a physician's statement certifying that they are disabled with their tax return. Disabled service members can substitute VA Form 21-0172, Certification of Total and Permanent Disability, for the physician's statement. VA Form 21-0172 can be obtained from VA regional offices.

Service members applying for the disability credit can either choose to calculate the amount of the credit themselves or have the IRS do so for them. Service members wishing to calculate the credit themselves must complete Schedule R (if filing Form 1040) or Schedule 3 (if filing Form 1040A) of their tax return form. Alternately, service members can return the above forms with "CFE" printed on the dotted line next to line 49 on Form 1040 or line 30 on Form 1040A and the IRS will figure their credit for them. For more information on this credit see IRS Publication 524, Credit for the Elderly or the Disabled.

Impairment-Related Work Expenses

Any service member with a physical or mental disability that limits his or her ability to be employed or substantially limits one or more major life activities can deduct impairment-related work expenses. Impairment-related work expenses are expenses that are necessary for a service member to be able to work, such as attendant care services. Generally, to qualify as impairment-related, an expense must be (1) necessary for a disabled service member to perform their work satisfactorily, (2) not used for the service member's personal activities, and (3) not be specifically covered under any other tax provision. An example of a qualifying expense would be a reader for a blind service member who assists the service member in doing his or her work, where the service member pays for the reader's services. In this example, the service member is permitted to deduct the cost of the reader. Service members wishing to deduct impairment-related work expenses must complete IRS Form 2106, Employee Business Expenses, or 2106-EZ, Unreimbursed Employee Business Expenses.

Financial Assistance Programs

Generally, VA disability pay is not taxable. Under certain circumstances DoD disability pay is not taxable, including disability pay received by a service member as a result of combat-related injury. This includes the Individual Unemployability (IU) Program and Combat-Related Special Compensation (CRSC) benefits received from veterans' programs administered by the VA, which are not taxable.

Benefits received from traumatic injury protection under Service Members' Group Life Insurance (TSGLI) are not subject to tax. Social Security Disability Insurance benefits are only subject to taxation where the service member's additional income exceeds a certain threshold amount.

Education and Employment Benefits

Generally, benefits received under the GI Bill are not taxable and should not be reported as income to the IRS. Benefits (whether monetary or services) received as a part of a VA administered program, including VA Work-Study programs, the Transition Assistance Program, and the Employment Readiness Program, likewise should not be reported as income to the IRS. See IRS Publication 970, Tax Benefits for Education, for more information.

Disability-Related Expenses and Retirement Funds

Medical Expenses: Distributions from IRAs for deductible medical expenses (i.e., medical expenses in excess of 7.5% of adjusted gross income) are not subject to the 10% penalty. For further information on what constitutes deductible medical expenses, see IRS Publication 502, "Medical and Dental Expenses."

Disability: Service members who are disabled before the age of 59½ and unable to engage in any substantial gainful activity because of the disability "incurred" are permitted to make withdrawals from an IRA without penalty.

Many 401(k) plans also permit early withdrawal if the money is used for medical purposes or in cases of financial hardship.

LEGAL ISSUES

The Uniformed Services Employment and Reemployment Rights Act (USERRA)

The Uniformed Services Employment and Reemployment Rights Act (USERRA) clarifies and strengthens the Veterans' Reemployment Rights (VRR) Statute. USERRA protects civilian job rights and benefits for veterans and members of reserve components. USERRA also makes major improvements in protecting service member rights and benefits by clarifying the law, improving enforcement mechanisms, and adding federal government employees to those employees already eligible to receive Department of Labor assistance in processing claims.

USERRA establishes the cumulative length of time that an individual may be absent from work for military duty and retain reemployment rights to five years (the previous law provided four years of active duty, plus an additional year if it was for the convenience of the government). There are important exceptions to the five-year limit, including initial enlistments lasting more than five years, periodic National Guard and reserve training duty, and involuntary active duty extensions and recalls, especially during a time of national emergency. USERRA clearly establishes that reemployment protection does not depend on the timing, frequency, duration, or nature of an individual's service as long as the basic eligibility criteria are met.

USERRA provides protection for disabled veterans, requiring employers to make reasonable efforts to accommodate the disability. Service members convalescing from injuries received during service or training may have up to two years from the date of completion of service to return to their jobs or apply for reemployment.

USERRA provides that returning service members are reemployed in the job that they would have attained had they not been absent for military service (the long-standing "escalator" principle), with the same seniority, status and pay, as well as other rights and benefits determined by seniority. USERRA also requires that reasonable efforts (such as training or retraining) be made to enable returning service members to refresh or upgrade their skills to help them qualify for reemployment. The law clearly provides for alternative reemployment positions if the service member cannot qualify for the "escalator" position. USERRA also provides that while an individual is performing military service, he or she is deemed to be on a furlough or leave of absence and is entitled to the non-seniority rights accorded other individuals on non-military leaves of absence.

Health and pension plan coverage for service members is provided for by USERRA. Individuals performing military duty of more than 30 days may elect to continue employer-sponsored health care for up to 24 months; however, they may be required to pay *up to* 102 percent of the full premium. For military service of less than 31 days, health care coverage is provided as if the service member had remained employed. USERRA clarifies pension plan coverage by making explicit that all pension plans are protected.

The period an individual has to make application for reemployment or report back to work after military service is based on time spent on military duty. For service of less than 31 days, the service member must return at the beginning of the next regularly scheduled work period on the first full day after release from service, taking into account safe travel home plus an eight-hour rest period. For service of more than 30 days but less than 181 days, the service member must submit an application for reemployment within 14 days of release from service. For service of more than 180 days, an application for reemployment must be submitted within 90 days of release from service.

USERRA also requires that service members provide advance written or verbal notice to their employers for all military duty unless giving notice is impossible, unreasonable, or precluded by military necessity. An employee should provide notice as far in advance as is reasonable under the circumstances. Additionally, service members are able (but are not required) to use accrued vacation or annual leave while performing military duty.

The Department of Labor, through the Veterans' Employment and Training Service (VETS), provides assistance to all persons having claims under USERRA, including federal and Postal Service employees.

If resolution is unsuccessful following an investigation, the service member may have his or her claim referred to the Department of Justice for consideration of representation in the appropriate district court, at no cost to the claimant. Federal and Postal Service employees may have their claims referred to the Office of Special Counsel for consideration of representation before the Merit Systems Protection Board (MSPB). If violations under USERRA are shown to be willful, the court may award liquidated damages. Individuals who pursue their own claims in court or before the MSPB may be awarded reasonable attorney and expert witness fees if they prevail.

Service member employees of intelligence agencies are provided similar assistance through the agency's Inspector General.

For more information about U.S. Department of Labor employment and training programs for veterans, contact the Veterans' Employment and Training Service office nearest you, listed in the phone book in the United States

Government under the Labor Department, or visit www.dol.gov/vets/about
vets/contacts/main.htm.

The Family and Medical Leave Act (FMLA)

Eligible employees are entitled to up to 12 weeks of leave because of "any
qualifying exigency" arising out of the fact that the spouse, son, daughter, or
parent of the employee is on active duty, or has been notified of an impend-
ing call to active duty status, in support of a contingency operation. By the
terms of the statute, this provision requires the Secretary of Labor to issue
regulations defining "any qualifying exigency." In the interim, employers are
encouraged to provide this type of leave to qualifying employees.

New Leave Entitlement: An eligible employee who is the spouse, son,
daughter, parent, or next of kin of a covered service member who is recovering from a serious illness or injury sustained in the line of duty on active duty
is entitled to up to 26 weeks of leave in a single 12-month period to care for
the service member. This provision became effective immediately upon en-
actment. This military caregiver leave is available during "a single 12-month
period" during which an eligible employee is entitled to a combined total of
26 weeks of all types of FMLA leave.

Additional information on the amendments and a version of Title I of the
FMLA with the new statutory language incorporated are available on the
FMLA amendments website at www.dol.gov/esa/whd/fmla/NDAA_fmla.htm.

The Service Members Civil Relief Act (SCRA)

The purpose of the SCRA is to strengthen and expedite national defense by
giving service members certain protections in civil actions. By providing for
the temporary suspension of judicial and administrative proceedings and
transactions that may adversely affect service members during their military
service, the SCRA enables service members to focus their energy on the
defense of the United States. Among other things, the SCRA allows for forbearance and reduced interest on certain obligations incurred prior to military
service, and it restricts default judgments against service members and rental
evictions of service members and all their dependents. The SCRA applies to
all members of the United States military on active duty, and to U.S. citizens
serving in the military of United States allies in the prosecution of a war or
military action. The provisions of the SCRA generally end when a service
member is discharged from active duty or within 90 days of discharge, or
when the service member dies. Portions of the SCRA also apply to reservists
and inductees who have received orders but not yet reported to active duty or
induction into the military service.

There are three primary areas of coverage under the SCRA: (1) protection against the entry of default judgments; (2) stay of proceedings where the service member has notice of the proceeding; and (3) stay or vacation of execution of judgments, attachments and garnishments. For more information, go to https://www.dmdc.osd.mil/appj/scra/scraHome.do.

The Americans with Disabilities Act (ADA)

The ADA is a federal civil rights law that prohibits discrimination based on a person's disability. It applies to all employers with 15 or more employees, including state and local governments, employment agencies and labor unions. The primary purpose of the ADA is to prohibit workplace discrimination and require employers to make reasonable accommodations for employees with disabilities. The act also covers disabled persons' access to certain government services, public transport, public parks and recreational areas, sports stadiums and state and local government websites.

Any individual who believes his or her rights under the ADA have been violated can bring an action against his or her employer. However, before bringing a lawsuit under the ADA, the individual must generally file a complaint with the Equal Employment Opportunity Commission (EEOC) no more than 180 days after the violation has occurred. The EEOC then conducts an investigation and if it cannot resolve the claim it may file suit on the individual's behalf in federal court, or the individual may file independently.

Veterans Receive Naturalization Preference

Honorable active-duty service in the U.S. armed forces during a designated period of hostility allows an individual to naturalize without being required to establish any periods of residence or physical presence in the United States. A service member who was in the United States, certain territories, or aboard an American public vessel at the time of enlistment, re-enlistment, extension of enlistment or induction, may naturalize even if he or she is not a lawful permanent resident.

On July 3, 2002, the president issued Executive Order 13269 establishing a new period of hostility for naturalization purposes beginning September 11, 2001, and continuing until a date designated by a future executive order. Qualifying members of the armed forces who have served at any time during a specified period of hostility may immediately apply for naturalization using the current application—Form N-400—"Application for Naturalization." Additional information about filing and requirement fees and designated period of hostility are available on the U.S. Citizenship and Immigration Services (USCIS) website at www.uscis.gov.

Individuals who served honorably in the U.S. Armed Forces, but were no longer serving on active duty status as of September 11, 2001, may still be naturalized without having to comply with the residence and physical presence requirements for naturalization if they filed Form N-400 while still serving in the U.S. Armed Forces or within six months of termination of their active duty service. An individual who files the application for naturalization after the six-month period following termination of active-duty service is not exempt from the residence and physical presence requirements, but can count any period of active-duty service towards the residence and physical presence requirements. Individuals seeking naturalization under this provision must establish that they are lawful permanent residents (such status not having been lost, rescinded or abandoned) and that they served honorably in the U.S. Armed Forces for at least one year.

If a service member dies as a result of injury or disease incurred or aggravated by service during a time of combat, the service member's survivor(s) can apply for the deceased service member to receive posthumous citizenship at any time within two years of the service member's death. The issuance of a posthumous certificate of citizenship does not confer U.S. citizenship on surviving relatives. However, a non-U.S. citizen spouse or qualifying family member may file for certain immigration benefits and services based upon their relationship to a service member who died during hostilities or a noncitizen service member who died during hostilities and was later granted posthumous citizenship. For additional information, visit the USCIS website at www.uscis.gov.

LEGAL ASSISTANCE

The military offers free legal assistance to active duty and retired service members, including medically retired service members and their dependents, through legal assistance attorneys located in the Judge Advocate General (JAG) office on most bases. This should usually be the first place the disabled service member seeks legal assistance for military issues. Individuals whose legal needs cannot be met by a military legal assistance attorney or who are not eligible for a military assistance attorney should consider contacting a civilian attorney. Pro bono legal services are often provided through local bar associations or private law firms by attorneys who donate their time to work for eligible clients. Generally, these legal services are only available to those who are extremely needy.

The American Bar Association's Operation Enduring LAMP program provides legal services to military service members and their families through a network of state and local bar associations. For more information about Operation Enduring LAMP and a directory of participating bar associations, visit www.abanet.org/legalservices/helpreservists.

Air Force

Air Force Legal Services Agency
150 Chennault Circle
Maxwell Air Force Base, AL 36112
334-953-4179
www.afjag.af.mil

Army

US Army Legal Assistance Policy Division, Client Services Branch
1777 North Kent St., Suite 9001
Rosslyn, VA 22209
703-696-1477
www.jagcnet.army.mil/Legal

Coast Guard

Legal and Defense Services
4200 Wilson Blvd., Suite 750
Ballston, VA 22203
202-493-1745
www.uscg.mil/legal

Marine Corps

Commandant of the Marine Corps (JAL)
HQMC
2 Navy Annex
Washington, DC 20380
703-614-1266, 703-614-3880, 703-614-3886
www.marines.mil/unit/judgeAdvocate

Navy

Legal Assistance Division
1322 Patterson Ave., Suite 3000
Washington Navy Yard, DC 20374
202-685-4642
www.jag.navy.mil

EDUCATION

The Montgomery GI Bill is a federal program that provides monthly educational assistance to military veterans, reservists and National Guard enrolled in qualified education programs or career training programs. For more information, refer to chapter 5.

The Reserve Educational Assistance Program (REAP) provides educational assistance to reservists and National Guard members who were called up for at least 90 days of active duty since September 11, 2001. It provides up to 36 months of education benefits, which vary based on type of education or training, type of enrollment (full-time or part-time) and length of service. It is not necessary for the reservist to have enrolled in or contributed to the GI Bill program to receive REAP benefits.

The procedure for claiming REAP benefits is similar to the procedure used to claim benefits under the GI Bill. Eligible reservists and guard members must enroll in a qualifying educational or training program, apply for benefits using a VA Form 22-1990. For more information about REAP, see www.gibill.va.gov/pamphlets/CH1607/REAP_FAQ.htm, or call 888-GI-BILL-1.

Note: A veteran may only receive benefits from one program at a time. Veterans who believe they may be eligible for multiple benefits should contact their local VA office for assistance in choosing which benefits program, or combination of successive benefits programs, is right for them.

Student Work-Study Allowance Program

An exception to the above is the Student Work-Study Allowance Program. Veterans enrolled at least three-quarter time in a degree, professional or vocational program and receiving VA education benefits still may be eligible for the VA Work-Study Allowance Program. Further information regarding the Student Work-Study Allowance program is available at www.gibill.va.gov/resources/education_resources/programs/work_study_program.html.

State Educational Benefits

Many states offer free or subsidized tuition to state-sponsored institutions of higher learning (such as state universities) to eligible applicants. Veterans and service members should contact their state's veterans' affairs office, which will often oversee military service-related education benefits for the state. However, some states administer their education benefits through a higher education agency instead of the state veterans' affairs office.

Educational Programs for Service Members' Families

Dependents' Educational Assistance (DEA) provides education and training opportunities to eligible dependents of certain veterans. The program offers up to 45 months of education benefits. These benefits may be used for degree and certificate programs, apprenticeship, and on-the-job training. If you are a spouse, you may take a correspondence course. Remedial, deficiency, and refresher courses may be approved under certain circumstances. You must be the son, daughter, or spouse of:

- A veteran who died or is permanently and totally disabled as the result of a service-connected disability. The disability must arise out of active service in the Armed Forces.
- A veteran who died from any cause while such service-connected disability was in existence.
- A service member missing in action or captured in the line of duty by a hostile force.
- A service member forcibly detained or interned in the line of duty by a foreign government or power.
- A service member who is hospitalized or receiving outpatient treatment for a service-connected permanent and total disability and is likely to be discharged for that disability. This change is effective December 23, 2006.

If you are a son or daughter and wish to receive benefits for attending school or job training, you must be between the ages of 18 and 26. In certain instances, it is possible to begin before age 18 and to continue after age 26. Marriage is not a bar to this benefit. If you are in the Armed Forces, you may not receive this benefit while on active duty. To pursue training after military service, your discharge must not be under dishonorable conditions. The VA can extend your period of eligibility by the number of months and days equal to the time spent on active duty. This extension cannot generally go beyond your 31st birthday, although there are some exceptions.

If you are a spouse, benefits end 10 years from the date the VA finds you eligible or from the date of death of the veteran. For surviving spouses (spouses of service members who died on active duty) benefits end 20 years from the date of death. You should make sure that your selected program is approved for VA training. If you are not clear on this point, the VA will inform you and the school or company about the requirements.

Obtain and complete VA Form 22-5490, Application for Survivors' and Dependents' Educational Assistance. Send it to the VA regional office with jurisdiction over the state where you will train. If you are a son or daughter, under legal age, a parent or guardian must sign the application.

If you have started training, take your application to your school or employer. Ask them to complete VA Form 22-1999, Enrollment Certification, and send both forms to the VA.

Scholarships

There are many scholarships available for dependents of disabled veterans. Each scholarship has its own set of criteria to determine eligibility. Scholarship providers include:

Air Force Aid Society: www.afas.org/Education/ScholarshipLinks.cfm
Army Emergency Relief: www.aerhq.org/education.asp
Marine Corps Scholarship Foundation: www.marine-scholars.org
Military.com: www.military.com/education-home
Navy League of the United States: www.navyleague.org/corporate/donate /scholarship.html
Navy Marine Corps Relief Society: www.nmcrs.org/education.html
Scholarships for Military Children: www.MilitaryScholar.org
Society of the Daughters of the U.S. Army: www.dodea.edu/students/dusa .htm

TRANSPORT

Automobile and Special Adaptive Equipment Grants

The VA provides grants to qualifying disabled veterans to purchase new or used automobiles or special adaptive equipment for currently owned vehicles. Eligible veterans do not receive money from the VA. Rather, the grant of up to $11,000 is paid directly to the seller of the automobile. A grant for adaptive equipment may be used to purchase power steering, power brakes, power window lifts, power seats, and special equipment necessary to assist the eligible person into and out of the vehicle, among other things, and may be paid either to the claimant or the seller. Claimants should consider applying for the grant prior to purchasing equipment in order to ensure receipt of the maximum benefit allowable.

Veterans and service members with disabilities resulting from an injury or disease incurred or aggravated during active military service are eligible for the automobile grant. Specifically, the veteran or service member must have one of the following types of disabilities to qualify: (1) loss, or permanent loss of use, of one or both feet; (2) loss, or permanent loss of use, of one or both hands; or (3) permanent loss of vision in both eyes, to a certain extent. Additionally, veterans and service members with service-connected ankylosis (immobility of the joint) of one or both knees or hips qualify for adaptive equipment grants.

7

The DoD and VA

The DoD and VA continue to examine the continuum of care they provide from the point of injury through rehabilitation to community reintegration. The objectives are to improve the timeliness, effectiveness, and transparency by integrating DoD and VA processes, eliminating duplication, and improving information provided to service members and their families.

To ensure a seamless transition of our wounded, ill, and injured from the care, benefits, and services of the DoD to the VA system, they continue to test enhanced case management methods and identify opportunities to improve the flow of information and identification of additional resources to the service member and family. Key features include one medical examination and a single-sourced disability rating. One goal is to enable service members to more effectively transition to veteran status and provide them with their VA benefits and compensation.

This includes all non-clinical care and administrative activities, such as case management and counseling requirements, associated with disability case processing from the point of service member referral to a military department medical evaluation board to the point of compensation and provision of benefits to veterans by the VA.

This is part of a larger effort to improve care and services to our wounded, injured and ill. Some of the other ongoing initiatives include improved information technology and data sharing, facility enhancements, recruitment and retention of care professionals, new methods to care for brain injuries and mental health concerns including posttraumatic stress disorder, and the use of lifelong care plans to fully support wounded, ill, and injured service members from recovery through rehabilitation to community integration.

MEDICAL

The Military Health System

The Military Health System (MHS) comprises the entire breadth of the Department of Defense military medical system. Serving over 9 million Americans— active duty and Reserve Component service members; military families; retirees, survivors and their families—the MHS has more than 150,000 medical personnel, both military and civilian, providing medical services in combat theaters and in facilities worldwide.

The MHS operates over 70 hospitals and 400 clinics around the world, conducts global aeromedical evacuation, shipboard and undersea medicine, and delivers humanitarian and other medical crisis response capabilities. The MHS conducts ground-breaking medical research through many DoD research organizations focused on activities from breakthrough technologies that save lives on the battlefield, to advanced research in cancer treatment; traumatic brain injury, posttraumatic stress disorder and the full range of clinical conditions. It supplements its services to the 9 million beneficiaries through a global network of health care providers, and offers the most comprehensive health benefit in the country to its people. The delivery system, research programs, and civilian network of health professionals provides over $45 billion worth of medical value to service members and the Nation.

Partnership for Health

The MHS achieves its mission by creating a partnership for health that brings the service member and family, the military leader and the medical provider/ planner together with the objective of patient-focused health care. The success of the partnership for health depends on each partner accepting their role in shaping a healthy, fit, high performance military force.

On the battlefield, the responsibility of the service member is completing the mission, and that mission becomes getting medical attention when ill or injured. At home, the role of the service member and family is to take action to promote their health and, in the event of illness or injury, to provide their medical care providers with complete information to ensure early assessment and treatment.

The responsibility of the military medical community is to promote healthy lifestyles and provide the highest quality care for each and every service member who becomes ill or injured.

The role of the leadership is supporting the service member getting medical care and using the timetable provided by the medical personnel to plan the reintegration of the service member into the unit.

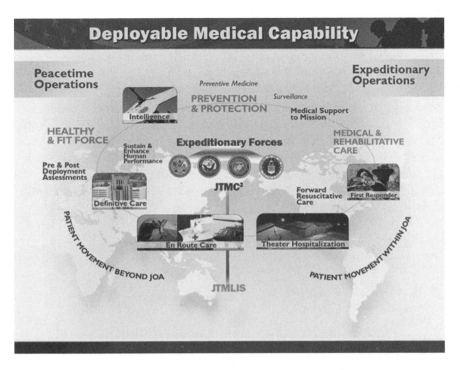

The role of the medical care provider is diagnosing and treating the illness or injury and keeping the service member and family, as well as the line leadership, informed of the expected outcome.

The shared expectation in this partnership for health is returning the ill or injured service member to health and to duty.

Patient-Centered Care

The strategic theme for patient-centered care is to manage and deliver the health benefit. To effectively accomplish this, involves building partnerships with beneficiaries and an integrated health delivery system that encompasses MTFs, private-sector care and other federal health care facilities, including the Veterans Administration. This is particularly important as 70% of care for DoD beneficiaries is now delivered by civilian partners through Managed Care Support Contracts (Humana Military Health Services, TRIWEST and Health Net Federal Services).

By working more closely with VA, MHS is able to provide a better service for our wounded warriors and their families and a smoother segue either transitioning back into the service once recovered or continuing in care with the VA.

THE VA AND BENEFITS

The Department of Veterans Affairs is responsible for ensuring that disabled veterans receive the care, support, and recognition that they have earned. Eligibility for most VA benefits is based upon discharge from active military service under other than dishonorable conditions. Active service means full-time service, other than active duty for training, as a member of the Army, Navy, Air Force, Marine Corps, Coast Guard, or as a commissioned officer of the Public Health Service, Environmental Science Services Administration or National Oceanic and Atmospheric Administration, or its predecessor, the Coast and Geodetic Survey. Generally, men and women veterans with similar service may be entitled to the same VA benefits.

VA PHONE NUMBERS

Education: 888-442-4551
Headstones and Markers: 800-697-6947
Health Care Revenue Center: 877-222-8387
Life Insurance: 800-669-8477
National Suicide Prevention Lifeline: 800-273-8255
Special Health Issues: 800-749-8387
Telecommunication Device for the Deaf (TDD): 800-829-4833
VA Benefits: 800-827-1000

VA WEBSITES

Burial and Memorial Benefits: www.cem.va.gov
Department of Defense: www.defenselink.mil
Education Benefits: www.gibill.va.gov
Federal Jobs: www.usajobs.gov
Health Care Eligibility: www.va.gov/healtheligibility
Home Loan Guaranty: www.homeloans.va.gov
Life Insurance: www.insurance.va.gov
Mental Health: www.mentalhealth.va.gov
Records: www.archives.gov/st-louis/military-personnel
Returning Veterans: www.seamlesstransition.va.gov
Veterans Employment and Training: www.dol.gov/vets
Veterans Preference: www.opm.gov/veterans/index.asp
Voc. Rehabilitation & Employment: www.vetsuccess.gov
VA Benefit Payment Rates: www.vba.va.gov/bln/21/rates
VA Home Page: www.va.gov
VA Forms: www.va.gov/vaforms

Important Documents

To expedite benefits delivery, veterans seeking a VA benefit for the first time must submit a copy of their service discharge form (DD-214, DD-215, or for World War II veterans, a WD form), which documents service dates and type of discharge, or give their full name, military service number, and branch and dates of service. The veteran's service discharge form should be kept in a safe location accessible to the veteran and next of kin or designated representative.

The following documents will be needed for claims processing related to a veteran's death:

1. Veteran's marriage certificate for claims of a surviving spouse or children.
2. Veteran's death certificate if the veteran did not die in a VA health care facility.
3. Children's birth certificates or adoption papers to determine children's benefits.
4. Veteran's birth certificate to determine parents' benefits.

Vet Centers

Vet Centers are open to any veteran who served in the military in a combat theater during wartime or anywhere during a period of armed hostilities.

Vet Centers provide readjustment counseling and outreach services to all veterans who served in any combat zone. Services are also available for their family members for military related issues. Veterans have earned these benefits through their service and all are provided at no cost to the veteran or family. Readjustment counseling is a wide range of services provided to combat veterans in the effort to make a satisfying transition from military to civilian life. Services include:

- Individual counseling
- Group counseling
- Marital and family counseling
- Bereavement counseling
- Medical referrals
- Assistance in applying for VA benefits
- Employment counseling
- Guidance and referral
- Alcohol/drug assessments
- Information and referral to community resources
- Military sexual trauma counseling and referral
- Outreach and community education

MEDICAL CARE

Perhaps the most visible of all VA benefits and services is health care. VA's health care system now includes 152 medical centers, with at least one in each state, Puerto Rico and the District of Columbia. VA operates more than 1,400 sites of care, including 872 ambulatory care and community-based outpatient clinics, 135 nursing homes, 45 residential rehabilitation treatment programs, 209 Veterans Centers and 108 comprehensive home-care programs. VA health care facilities provide a broad spectrum of medical, surgical and rehabilitative care for over 5.5 million veterans each year.

VA manages the largest medical education and health professions training program in the United States. VA facilities are affiliated with 107 medical schools, 55 dental schools and more than 1,200 other schools across the country. Each year, about 90,000 health professionals are trained in VA medical centers. More than half of the physicians practicing in the United States had some of their professional education in the VA health care system.

Contact your nearest Vet Center through the Vet Center Directory at www2 .va.gov/directory or listings in your local blue pages. The Vet Center staff is available toll free during normal business hours at 800-905-4675 (Eastern) and 866-496-8838 (Pacific).

Programs and Services

Veterans of the U.S. Armed Forces may be eligible for a broad range of programs and services provided by the federal Department of Veterans Affairs (VA). These benefits are legislated in Title 38 of the United States Code.

Recent laws passed by Congress have made several changes in veterans' eligibility for VA medical care. Basically, these laws ensure that VA care will be continued for disabled veterans with service-connected disabilities. Veterans with non-service-connected disabilities will also continue to receive VA medical care, but on a space-available basis and a co-payment may be charged. Laws are subject to change, and there are many applicable details. For additional information, visit the VA website at www.va.gov.

Basic Eligibility

A person who served in the active military, naval, or air service and who was discharged or released under conditions other than dishonorable may qualify for VA health care benefits. Reservists and National Guard members may also qualify for VA health care benefits if they were called to active duty (other than for training only) by a federal order and completed the full period for which they were called or ordered to active duty.

Minimum Duty Requirements: Veterans who enlisted after September 7, 1980, or who entered active duty after October 16, 1981, must have served 24 continuous months or the full period for which they were called to active duty in order to be eligible. This minimum duty requirement may not apply to veterans discharged for hardship, early out or a disability incurred or aggravated in the line of duty.

Enrollment

For most veterans, entry into the VA health care system begins by applying for enrollment. To apply, complete VA Form 10-10EZ, Application for Health Benefits, which may be obtained from any VA health care facility or regional benefits office, at www.va.gov/1010ez.htm or by calling 877-222-VETS (8387).

Once enrolled, veterans can receive health care at VA health care facilities anywhere in the country. Veterans enrolled in the VA health care system are afforded privacy rights under federal law. VA's Notice of Privacy Practices, which describes how VA may use and disclose veterans' medical information, is also available at www.va.gov/vhapublications/View-Publication.asp?pub _ID=1089. The following four categories of veterans are not required to enroll, but are urged to do so to permit better planning of health resources:

1. Veterans with a service-connected disability of 50 percent or more.
2. Veterans seeking care for a disability the military determined was incurred or aggravated in the line of duty, but which VA has not yet rated, within 12 months of discharge.
3. Veterans seeking care for a service-connected disability only.
4. Veterans seeking registry examinations (Ionizing Radiation, Agent Orange, Gulf War/Operation Iraqi Freedom and Depleted Uranium).

Priority Groups

During enrollment, each veteran is assigned to a priority group. VA uses priority groups to balance demand for VA health care enrollment with resources. Changes in available resources may reduce the number of priority groups VA can enroll. If this occurs, VA will publicize the changes and notify affected enrollees. A description of priority groups follows:

Group 1: Veterans with service-connected disabilities rated 50 percent or more and/or veterans determined by the VA to be unemployable due to service-connected conditions.

Group 2: Veterans with service-connected disabilities rated 30 or 40 percent.

Group 3: Veterans with service-connected disabilities rated 10 and 20 percent, veterans who are former prisoners of war (POW) or were awarded a Purple Heart medal, veterans awarded special eligibility for disabilities incurred in treatment or participation in a VA Vocational Rehabilitation program and veterans whose discharge was for a disability incurred or aggravated in the line of duty.

Group 4: Veterans receiving aid and attendance or housebound benefits and/or veterans determined by VA to be catastrophically disabled.

Group 5: Veterans receiving VA pension benefits or eligible for Medicaid programs, and non-service-connected veterans and non-compensable, zero percent service-connected veterans whose gross annual household income and net worth are below the established VA means test thresholds.

Group 6: Veterans of World War I; veterans seeking care solely for certain conditions associated with exposure to radiation; for any illness associated with combat service in a war after the Gulf War or during a period of hostility after November 11, 1998; for any illness associated with participation in tests conducted by the Department of Defense (DoD) as part of Project 112/Project SHAD; and veterans with zero percent service-connected disabilities who are receiving disability compensation benefits.

Group 7: Non-service-connected veterans and non-compensable, zero-percent service-connected veterans with household income and/or net worth above VA's national income threshold, but whose household income is below the geographically based income threshold for their resident location.

Group 8: All other non-service-connected veterans and zero percent, non-compensable service-connected veterans who agree to pay copays. (**Note:** Effective January 17, 2003, VA no longer enrolls new veterans into priority group 8).

Special Access to Care

Service Disabled Veterans: Veterans who are 50 percent or more disabled from service-connected conditions, unemployable due to service-connected conditions, or receiving care for a service-connected disability receive priority in scheduling of hospital or outpatient medical appointments.

Combat Veterans: Veterans discharged from active duty on or after January 28, 2003, are eligible for enhanced enrollment placement into Priority Group 6 (unless eligible for higher enrollment Priority Group placement) for 5 years post-discharge. Veterans with combat service after November 11, 1998, who were discharged from active duty before January 28, 2003, and who apply for enrollment on or after January 28, 2008, were eligible for this enhanced enrollment benefit through January 27, 2011.

Veterans exposed to herbicides while serving in Vietnam and other areas now have an easier path to access quality health care and qualify for disability compensation under a final regulation published on August 31, 2010, in the Federal Register by the Department of Veterans Affairs (VA). The rule expands the list of health problems VA will presume to be related to Agent Orange and other herbicide exposures.

VA has added Parkinson's disease and ischemic heart disease and expanded chronic lymphocytic leukemia to include all chronic B-cell leukemias, such as hairy cell leukemia. In practical terms, veterans who served in Vietnam during the war and who have a "presumed" illness don't have to prove an association between their medical problems and their military service. By helping veterans overcome evidentiary requirements that might otherwise present significant challenges, this "presumption" simplifies and speeds up the application process and ensures that veterans receive the benefits they deserve.

Veterans who served in Vietnam any time during the period beginning January 9, 1962, and ending on May 7, 1975, are presumed to have been exposed to herbicides. The VA is reviewing approximately 90,000 previously denied claims by Vietnam veterans for service connection for these conditions. All those awarded service-connection who are not currently eligible for enrollment into the VA health care system are now eligible.

Veterans, including activated reservists and members of the National Guard, are eligible if they served on active duty in a theater of combat operations after November 11, 1998, and have been discharged under other than dishonorable conditions. Veterans who enroll with VA under this "Combat Veteran" authority will retain enrollment eligibility even after their five-year post-discharge period ends. At the end of their post-discharge period, the VA will reassess the veteran's information (including all applicable eligibility factors) and make a new enrollment decision. For additional information, call 877-222-VETS (8387).

Reserve and National Guard

Reservists who serve on active duty establish veteran status and may be eligible for the full range of VA benefits, depending on the length of active military service and a discharge or release from active duty under conditions other than dishonorable. In addition, reservists not activated may qualify for some VA benefits. National Guard members can establish eligibility for VA benefits if activated for federal service during a period of war or domestic emergency. Activation for other than federal service does not qualify guard members for all VA benefits. Claims for VA benefits based on federal service filed by members of the National Guard should include a copy of the military orders, presidential proclamation or executive order that clearly demonstrates the federal nature of the service.

Qualifying for VA Health Care

Veterans discharged from active duty on or after January 28, 2003, are eligible for enhanced enrollment placement into Priority Group 6 (unless eligible for higher Priority Group placement) for 5 years post-discharge. Veterans with combat service after November 11, 1998, who were discharged from active duty before January 28, 2003, and who apply for enrollment on or after January 28, 2008, are eligible for this enhanced enrollment benefit through January 27, 2011. Activated reservists and members of the National Guard are eligible if they served on active duty in a theater of combat operations after November 11, 1998, and, have been discharged under other than dishonorable conditions.

Veterans who enroll with VA under this "Combat Veteran" authority will retain enrollment eligibility even after their five-year post-discharge period ends. At the end of their post-discharge period, the VA will reassess the veteran's information (including all applicable eligibility factors) and make a new enrollment decision. For additional information, call 877-222-VETS (8387).

Disability Benefits

The VA pays monthly compensation benefits for service-connected disabilities —those incurred or aggravated during active duty and active duty for training, and for residuals of heart attack or stroke that occurred during inactive duty for training.

Montgomery GI Bill—Selected Reserve

Members of reserve elements of the Army, Navy, Air Force, Marine Corps and Coast Guard, and members of the Army National Guard and the Air National Guard, may be entitled to up to 36 months of educational benefits under the Montgomery GI Bill (MGIB)—Selected Reserve. To be eligible, the participant must:

1. Have a six-year obligation in the Selected Reserve or National Guard signed after June 30, 1985, or, if an officer, agree to serve six years in addition to the original obligation.
2. Complete initial active duty for training.
3. Have a high school diploma or equivalency certificate before applying for benefits.
4. Remain in good standing in a Selected Reserve or National Guard unit.

Reserve components determine eligibility for benefits. The VA does not make decisions about eligibility and cannot make payments until the reserve component has determined eligibility and notified the VA.

Period of Eligibility: Benefits generally end the day a reservist or National Guard member separates from the military. However, if you leave the Selected Reserve, you may still be eligible for a full 10 years from the date of eligibility (if eligible before October 1, 1992), or a full 14 years from the date of eligibility on or after October 1, 1992. Veterans may be eligible if separated because of a disability that was not caused by misconduct, the unit was inactivated, or otherwise involuntarily separated during October 1, 1991, through December 31, 2001. If in the Selected Reserve and called to active duty, the VA can generally extend the eligibility period by the length of time on active duty plus four months. Once this extension is granted, it will not be taken away if you leave the Selected Reserve.

Payments: The rate for full-time training effective October 1, 2007, is $317 a month for 36 months. Part-time benefits are reduced proportionately. For complete current rates, visit www.gibill.va.gov. DoD may make additional contributions.

Training: Participants may take undergraduate or technical training at colleges and universities. Those who have a six-year commitment beginning after September 30, 1990, may also take the following training: graduate courses; state licensure and certification; courses for a certificate or diploma from business, technical or vocational schools; cooperative training; apprenticeship or on-the-job training; correspondence courses; independent study programs; flight training; entrepreneurship training; or remedial, deficiency or refresher courses needed to complete a program of study.

Work-Study: Participants may be eligible for a work-study program in which they work for the VA and receive hourly wages. Veterans must train at the three-quarter or full-time rate. The work allowed includes:

1. Outreach services for VA.
2. VA paperwork.
3. Work at national or state veterans' cemeteries.
4. Work at VA medical centers or state veterans homes.
5. Other VA approved activities.

Counseling: VA counseling is available to help determine educational or vocational strengths and weaknesses and plan education or employment goals. Additionally, those ineligible for MGIB may still receive VA counseling beginning 180 days prior to separation from active duty through the first full year following honorable discharge.

Table 7.1. 2011 Reserve Educational Assistance Rates

Time Reserve Member Serves on Active Duty	Full-Time Rate (effective Oct. 1, 2010)
90 days but less than one year	$688.80
One year but less than two years	$1,030.20
Two years or more	$1,373.60

Reserve Educational Assistance Program

This program provides educational assistance to members of National Guard and reserve components—Selected Reserve and Individual Ready Reserve (IRR)—who are called or ordered to active duty service in response to a war or national emergency as declared by the president or Congress. Visit www .gibill.va.gov for more information.

Eligibility: Eligibility is determined by DoD or the Deptartment of Homeland Security. Generally, a service member who serves on active duty on or after September 11, 2001, for at least 90 consecutive days is eligible.

Payments: The educational payment rate is based on the number of continuous days of active duty service performed by the reservist or National Guard service member. Full-time students receive payments on a monthly basis.

Training: Approved training includes graduate and undergraduate degrees, vocational/technical training, on-the-job or apprenticeship training, correspondence training, and flight training. Licensing and certification test reimbursement is effective January 6, 2006.

Period of Eligibility: Members of the Selected Reserve called to active duty are eligible as long as they continue to serve in the Selected Reserve. They lose eligibility if they go into the IRR. Members of the IRR called to active duty are eligible as long as they stay in the IRR or Selected Reserve. Members who separate from the IRR or Selected Reserve for a disability which was not the result of willful misconduct are entitled to benefits for 10 years after date of eligibility.

Home Loan Guaranty

National Guard members and reservists are eligible for a VA home loan if they have completed at least six years of honorable service, are mobilized for active duty service for a period of at least 90 days, or were discharged because of a service-connected disability. Reservists who do not qualify for VA housing loan benefits may be eligible for loans on favorable terms insured by the Federal Housing Administration (FHA), part of HUD. See information on Home Loan Guaranty.

Life Insurance

National Guard members and reservists are eligible to receive Service Members' Group Life Insurance, Veterans' Group Life Insurance, and Family Service members' Group Life Insurance. They may also be eligible for Traumatic Service members' Group Life Insurance or Service-Disabled Veterans Insurance if called to active duty and injured with a service-connected disability, and Veterans' Mortgage Life Insurance if approved for a Specially Adapted Housing Grant.

Re-employment Rights

A person who left a civilian job to enter active duty in the armed forces is entitled to return to the job after discharge or release from active duty if they:

1. Gave advance notice of military service to the employer.
2. Did not exceed five years cumulative absence from the civilian job (with some exceptions).
3. Submitted a timely application for re-employment.
4. Did not receive a dishonorable or other punitive discharge.

The law calls for a returning veteran to be placed in the job as if they had never left, including benefits based on seniority such as pensions, pay increases and promotions. The law also prohibits discrimination in hiring, promotion or other advantages of employment on the basis of military service. Veterans seeking re-employment should apply, verbally or in writing, to the company's hiring official and keep a record of their application. If problems arise, contact the Department of Labor's Veterans' Employment and Training Service (VETS) in the state of the employer.

Federal employees not properly re-employed may appeal directly to the Merit Systems Protection Board. Non-federal employees may file complaints in U.S. District Court. For information, visit www.dol.gov/vets/programs/userra/main.htm.

Army Reserve Warrior and Family Assistance Center

The Army Reserve Warrior and Family Assistance Center (ARWFAC) provides Army reserve soldiers, veterans, families, and units with a single source to resolve situations related to medical issues and education on programs available to Army reserve soldiers. The center was established in 2007 to ensure that reservists receive appropriate support under the Army Medical Action Plan. The center provides a sponsor to each Army reserve soldier and family currently assigned to a Warrior Transition Unit, Community Based

Health Care Organization, or VA PolyTrauma center. The ARWFAC also assists Army reserve commands at all echelons with the resolution of medical and other issues and provides education on programs and benefits available to Army reserve soldiers. For information, call 866-436-6290 or visit www .arfp.org/wfac.

National Guard Transition Assistance Advisors

The Transition Assistance Advisor (TAA) program places a National Guard/VA-trained expert at each National Guard State Joint Forces Headquarters to act as an advocate for Guard members and their families within the state. They also serve as an advisor on Veterans Affairs issues for the Family Programs and Joint Forces Headquarters staffs. TAAs receive annual training by VA experts in health benefits for both Department of Defense and Department of Veterans Affairs and help Guard members and their families access care at VA and TRICARE facilities in their state or network. The TAA works with the State Director of Veterans Affairs and other state coalition partners to integrate the delivery of VA and community services to Guard and Reserve veterans. You can reach your TAA through your state National Guard Joint Forces Headquarters.

Financial Assessment

Most veterans not receiving VA disability compensation or pension payments must provide information on their gross annual household income and net worth to determine whether they are below the annually adjusted financial thresholds. Veterans who decline to disclose their information or have income above the thresholds must agree to pay copays in order to receive certain health benefits, effectively placing them in Priority Group 8. The VA is currently not enrolling new applicants who decline to provide financial information unless they have a special eligibility factor.

This financial assessment includes all household income and net worth, including Social Security, retirement pay, unemployment insurance, interest and dividends, workers' compensation, black lung benefits and any other income. Also considered are assets such as the market value of property that is not the primary residence, stocks, bonds, notes, individual retirement accounts, bank deposits, savings accounts and cash.

The VA also compares veterans' financial assessment with geographically based income thresholds. If the veteran's gross annual household income is above the VA's national means test threshold and below the VA's geographic means test threshold, or is below both the VA national threshold and the VA geographically based threshold, but their gross annual household income plus net worth exceeds the VA's ceiling the veteran is eligible for an 80% reduction in inpatient copay rates.

VA Medical Services and Supplies Requiring Copays

Some veterans must make copays to receive VA health care.

Inpatient Care: Priority Group 7 and certain other veterans are responsible for paying 20 percent of the VA's inpatient copay or $226.40 for the first 90 days of inpatient hospital care during any 365-day period. For each additional 90 days, the charge is $113.20. In addition, there is a $2 per diem charge. Priority Group 8 and certain other veterans are responsible for VA's inpatient copay of $1,132 for the first 90 days of care during any 365-day period and $10 per day. For each additional 90 days, the charge is $566 plus a $10 per diem charge.

Extended Care: For extended care services, veterans may be subject to a copay determined by information supplied by completing VA Form 10-10EC. VA social workers can help veterans interpret their eligibility and copay requirements. The copay amount is based on each veteran's financial situation and is determined upon application for extended care services and will range from $0 to $97 a day.

Medication: Most veterans are currently charged $8 for each 30-day or less supply of medication provided by VA for treatment of conditions that are not service-connected. For veterans enrolled in Priority Groups 2 through 6, the maximum copay for medications that will be charged in a calendar year is $960. The following groups of veterans are not charged medication copays: veterans with a service-connected disability of 50 percent or more; veterans receiving medication for service-connected conditions; veterans whose annual income does not exceed the maximum annual rate of the VA pension; veterans enrolled in Priority Group 6 who receive medication under their special authority; veterans receiving medication for conditions related to sexual trauma related to service on active duty; certain veterans receiving medication for treatment of cancer of the head or neck; veterans receiving medication for a VA-approved research project; and former POWs.

Note: Copays apply to prescription and over-the-counter medications, such as aspirin, cough syrup or vitamins, dispensed by a VA pharmacy. However, veterans may prefer to purchase over-the-counter drugs, such as aspirin or vitamins, at a local pharmacy rather than making the copay. Copays are not charged for medications injected during the course of treatment or for medical supplies, such as syringes or alcohol wipes.

Outpatient Care: A three-tiered copay system is used for all outpatient services. The copay is $15 for a primary care visit and $50 for some specialized care. Certain services are not charged a copay.

Outpatient Visits Not Requiring Copays

Copays do not apply to publicly announced VA health fairs or outpatient visits solely for preventive screening and/or immunizations, such as immunizations for influenza or screening for hypertension, hepatitis C, tobacco, alcohol, hyperlipidemia, breast cancer, cervical cancer, colorectal cancer by fecal occult blood testing, education about the risks and benefits of prostate cancer screening, and smoking cessation counseling (individual and group). Laboratory tests, flat film radiology, and electrocardiograms are also exempt from copays.

Private Health Insurance Billing

The VA is required to bill private health insurance providers for medical care, supplies and prescriptions provided for treatment of veterans' non-service-connected conditions. Generally, the VA cannot bill Medicare, but can bill Medicare supplemental health insurance for covered services.

All veterans applying for VA medical care are required to provide information on their health insurance coverage, including coverage provided under policies of their spouses. Veterans are not responsible for paying any remaining balance of the VA's insurance claim not paid or covered by their health insurance, and any payment received by the VA may be used to offset "dollar for dollar" a veteran's VA copay responsibility.

Reimbursement of Travel Costs

Certain veterans may be provided special-mode travel (e.g., wheelchair van, ambulance) or reimbursed for travel costs when traveling for approved VA medical care. Reimbursement is paid at 41.5 cents per mile and is subject to a deductible of $3 for each one-way trip and $6 for a round trip, with a maximum deductible of $18 per calendar month. Two exceptions to the deductible are travel for a C&P exam and special modes of transportation, such as an ambulance or a specially equipped van. These deductibles may be waived when their imposition would cause a severe financial hardship.

Eligibility: Payments may be made to the following:

1. Veterans whose service-connected disabilities are rated 30 percent or more.
2. Veterans traveling for treatment of service-connected conditions.
3. Veterans who receive a VA pension.
4. Veterans traveling for scheduled compensation or pension examinations.
5. Veterans whose gross household income does not exceed the maximum annual VA pension rate.
6. Veterans whose medical condition requires a special mode of transportation, if they are unable to defray the costs and travel is pre-authorized.

Advance authorization is not required in an emergency if a delay would be hazardous to life or health.

VA MEDICAL PROGRAMS

Veteran Health Registries

Certain veterans can participate in a VA health registry and receive free medical examinations, including laboratory and other diagnostic tests deemed necessary by an examining clinician. VA maintains health registries to provide special health examinations and health-related information. To participate, contact the nearest VA health care facility or visit www.va.gov/environagents.

Gulf War Registry: For veterans who served in the Gulf War and Operation Iraqi Freedom (OIF).

Depleted Uranium Registries: The VA maintains two registries for veterans possibly exposed to depleted uranium. The first is for veterans who served in the Gulf War, including Operation Iraqi Freedom. The second is for veterans who served elsewhere, including Bosnia and Afghanistan.

Agent Orange Registry: For veterans possibly exposed to dioxin or other toxic substances in herbicides used during the Vietnam War, while serving in Korea in 1968 or 1969, or as a result of testing, transporting, or spraying herbicides for military purposes.

Ionizing Radiation Registry: For veterans possibly exposed to atomic radiation during the following activities: atmospheric detonation of a nuclear device; occupation of Hiroshima or Nagasaki from August 6, 1945, through July 1, 1946; internment as a prisoner of war in Japan during World War II; serving in official military duties at the gaseous diffusion plants at Paducah, KY, Portsmouth, OH, or the K-25 area at Oak Ridge, TN, for at least 250 days before February 1, 1992, or in Longshot, Milrow or Cannikin underground nuclear tests at Amchitka Island, AK, before January 1, 1974; or treatment with nasopharyngeal (NP) radium during military service.

Readjustment Counseling Services

The VA provides readjustment counseling services through 207 community-based Vet Centers located in all 50 states, the District of Columbia, Guam, Puerto Rico, and the U.S. Virgin Islands. Counseling is designed to help combat veterans readjust to civilian life.

Eligibility: Veterans are eligible if they served on active duty in a combat theater during World War II, the Korean War, the Vietnam War, the Gulf War, or the campaigns in Lebanon, Grenada, Panama, Somalia, Bosnia, Kosovo, Afghanistan, Iraq and the global war on terror. Veterans who served in the active military during the Vietnam era, but not in the Republic of Vietnam, must have requested services at a Vet Center before January 1, 2004.

Services Offered: Vet Center staff provide individual, group, family, military sexual trauma, and bereavement counseling. Services include treatment for posttraumatic stress disorder (PTSD) or help with any other military-related issue that affects functioning within the family, work, school or other areas of everyday life. Other services include outreach, education, medical referral, homeless veteran services, employment, VA benefit referral, and the brokering of non-VA services.

Prosthetic and Sensory Aids

Veterans receiving VA care for any condition may receive VA prosthetic appliances, equipment and services, such as home respiratory therapy, artificial limbs, orthopedic braces and therapeutic shoes, wheelchairs, powered mobility, crutches, canes, walkers, and other durable medical equipment and supplies.

The VA will provide hearing aids and eyeglasses to veterans who receive an increased pension based on the need for regular aid and attendance or being permanently housebound, receive compensation for a service-connected disability or are former POWs. Otherwise, hearing aids and eyeglasses are provided only in special circumstances, and not for normally occurring hearing or vision loss. For additional information, contact the prosthetic representative at your nearest VA health care facility.

Home Improvements and Structural Alterations

VA provides grants for service-connected veterans and non-service-connected veterans to make home improvements necessary for the continuation of treatment or for disability access to the home and essential lavatory and sanitary facilities.

For application information, contact the prosthetic representative at the nearest VA health care facility.

Services for Blind Veterans

Blind and visually impaired veterans may be eligible for services at a VA medical center or for admission to a VA blind rehabilitation center. In addition, blind veterans enrolled in the VA health care system may receive:

1. A total health and benefits review.
2. Adjustment to blindness training and counseling.
3. Home improvements and structural alterations.
4. Specially adapted housing and adaptations.

5. Automobile grant.
6. Low-vision devices and training in their use.
7. Electronic and mechanical aids for the blind, including adaptive computers and computer-assisted devices such as reading machines and electronic travel aids.
8. Guide dogs, including cost of training for the veteran to learn to work with the dog.
9. Talking books, tapes and Braille literature.

Eligible visually impaired veterans (who are not blind) enrolled in the VA health care system may receive:

1. A total health and benefits review.
2. Adjustment to vision loss counseling and training.
3. Low-vision devices and training in their use.
4. Electronic and mechanical aids for the visually impaired, including adaptive computers and computer-assisted devices such as reading machines and electronic travel aids, and training in their use.

Mental Health Care Treatment

Veterans eligible for VA medical care may apply for general mental health treatment including specialty services such as PTSD and substance abuse treatment. Contact the nearest VA health care facility to apply.

Suicide Prevention Hotline. Veterans experiencing an emotional crisis or who need to talk to a trained mental health professional may call the National Suicide toll-free hotline number, 800-273-TALK (8255). The hotline is available 24 hours a day, 7 days a week. Callers are immediately connected with a qualified and caring provider who can help.

Work Restoration Programs

VA provides vocational assistance and therapeutic work opportunities through several programs for veterans receiving VA health care. Each program offers treatment and rehabilitation services to help veterans live and work in their communities. Participation in the following VA Work Restoration Programs cannot be used to deny or discontinue VA compensation or pension benefits.

Incentive Therapy is a pre-vocational program available at 70 VA Medical Centers and frequently serves as a mainstay for seriously disabled veterans for whom employment is not considered viable in the foreseeable future. Participants receive a token payment for services provided.

Compensated Work Therapy (CWT) is a vocational program available at 141 VA Medical Centers. Veterans receive an individualized vocational assessment, rehabilitation planning and work experience with the goal of job placement in the community. The program works closely with community-based organizations, employers and state and federal agencies to establish transitional work experiences, supported employment opportunities, direct job placement and supportive follow-up services.

CWT/Transitional Residence provides work-based, residential treatment in a stable living environment. This program differs from other VA residential bed programs in that participants use their earnings to contribute to the cost of their residences and are responsible for planning, purchasing and preparing their own meals. The program offers a comprehensive array of rehabilitation services including home, financial and life skills management.

Domiciliary Care

Domiciliary care provides rehabilitative and long-term health care for veterans who require minimal medical care but do not need the skilled nursing services provided in nursing homes. A Domiciliary also provides rehabilitative care for veterans who are homeless.

Eligibility: The VA may provide domiciliary care to veterans whose annual gross household income does not exceed the maximum annual rate of VA pension or to veterans the Secretary of Veterans Affairs determines have no adequate means of support. The copays for extended-care services apply to domiciliary care. Call your nearest benefits or health care facility to obtain the latest information.

Outpatient Dental Treatment

VA outpatient dental treatment includes the full spectrum of diagnostic, surgical, restorative and preventive procedures. The extent of care provided may be influenced by eligibility category.

Eligibility: The following veterans are eligible to receive dental care:

1. Veterans with service-connected, compensable dental conditions.
2. Former POWs.
3. Veterans with service-connected, non-compensable dental conditions as a result of combat wounds or service injuries.
4. Veterans with non-service-connected dental conditions determined by the VA to be aggravating a service-connected medical problem.
5. Veterans with service-connected conditions rated permanently and totally disabling or 100 percent by reason of permanent unemployability.
6. Veterans in a VA vocational rehabilitation program.
7. Certain enrolled homeless veterans.

8. Veterans with non-service-connected dental conditions who received dental treatment while an inpatient in a VA facility.
9. Veterans requiring treatment for dental conditions clinically determined to be complicating a medical condition currently under treatment.

Recently discharged veterans who served on active duty 90 days or more and who apply for VA dental care within 180 days of separation from active duty, may receive a one-time dental treatment if their certificate of discharge does not indicate that they received necessary dental care within the 90-day period prior to discharge.

Nursing Home Care

The VA provides nursing home services to veterans through three national programs: VA owned and operated nursing homes, state veterans' homes owned and operated by the states, and the community nursing home program. Each program has admission and eligibility criteria specific to the program.

VA Nursing Homes: VA owned and operated nursing homes typically admit patients requiring short-term care, in need of placement for a service-connected disability, or those who have a 70 percent or greater service-connected disability. All other admissions are based on available resources.

State Veterans' Home Program: The state veterans' home program is a cooperative venture between the states and VA whereby the states petition the VA for matching construction grants and, once granted, the VA pays a portion of the per diem. States establish eligibility criteria for short- and long-term care. Specialized services offered are dependent upon the capability of the home to render them.

Community Nursing Home Program: The VA maintains contracts with community nursing homes through every VA medical center. The purpose of this program is to meet the nursing home needs of veterans who require long-term nursing home care in their own community, close to their families.

Admission Criteria: The general admission criteria for nursing home placement requires that a resident must be medically stable, i.e., not acutely ill, have sufficient functional deficits to require inpatient nursing home care, and is assessed by an appropriate medical provider to be in need of institutional nursing home care. Furthermore, the veteran must meet the required VA eligibility criteria for nursing home care or the contract nursing home program and the eligibility criteria for the specific state veterans home.

Long-Term Care Services: In addition to nursing home care, VA offers a variety of other long-term care services either directly or by contract with community-based agencies. Such services include adult day health care, inpatient or outpatient respite care, inpatient or outpatient geriatric evaluation and management, hospice and palliative care, and home-based primary care. Veterans receiving these services may be subject to a copay.

Emergency Medical Care in Non-VA Facilities

VA may reimburse or pay for medical care provided to certain enrolled or otherwise eligible veterans by non-VA facilities only in cases of medical emergencies where VA or other federal facilities were not feasibly available. Other conditions also apply. To determine eligibility or initiate a claim, contact the VA medical facility nearest to where the emergency service was provided.

Disability Compensation

Disability compensation is a monetary benefit paid to veterans who are disabled by an injury or illness that was incurred or aggravated during active military service. These disabilities are considered to be service-connected. Disability compensation varies with the degree of disability and the number of veteran's dependents, and is paid monthly. Veterans with certain severe disabilities may be eligible for additional special monthly compensation. The benefits are not subject to federal or state income tax.

The payment of military retirement pay, disability severance pay and separation incentive payments known as SSB (Special Separation Benefits) and VSI (Voluntary Separation Incentives) affects the amount of VA compensation paid to disabled veterans.

To be eligible, the service of the veteran must have been terminated through separation or discharge under conditions other than dishonorable.

For additional details, visit the website at www.vba.va.gov/bln/21.

Receiving Disability Benefit Payments

VA offers three disability benefit payment options. Most veterans receive their payments by direct deposit to a bank, savings and loan or credit union account. In some areas, veterans who do not have a bank account can open a federally insured Electronic Transfer Account, which costs about $3 a month, provides a monthly statement and allows cash withdrawals. Other veterans may choose to receive benefits by check. To choose a payment method, call toll-free 877-838-2778, Monday–Friday, 7:30 a.m.–4:50 p.m. CST.

Presumptive Conditions for Disability Compensation

Certain veterans are eligible for disability compensation based on the presumption that their disability is service-connected.

DISABILITY COMPENSATION RATES FOR VETERANS

Veteran's Disability Rating	Monthly Rate
10 percent	$130.94
20 percent	$258.83
30 percent*	$400.93
40 percent*	$577.54
50 percent*	$822.15
60 percent*	$1,041.39
70 percent*	$1,312.40
80 percent*	$1,525.55
90 percent*	$1,714.34
100 percent*	$2,858.24

*Veterans with disability ratings of at least 30 percent are eligible for additional allowances for dependents, including spouses, minor children, children between the ages of 18 and 23 who are attending school, children who are permanently incapable of self-support because of a disability arising before age 18, and dependent parents. The additional amount depends on the disability rating and the number of dependents.

Prisoners of War: For former POWs who were imprisoned for any length of time, the following disabilities are presumed to be service-connected if they are rated at least 10 percent disabling any time after military service: psychosis, any of the anxiety states, dysthymic disorder, organic residuals of frostbite, post-traumatic osteoarthritis, heart disease or hypertensive vascular disease and their complications, and stroke and residuals of stroke.

For former POWs who were imprisoned for at least 30 days, the following conditions are also presumed to be service-connected: avitaminosis, beriberi, chronic dysentery, helminthiasis, malnutrition (including optic atrophy), pellagra and/or other nutritional deficiencies, irritable bowel syndrome, peptic ulcer disease, peripheral neuropathy and cirrhosis of the liver.

Veterans Exposed to Agent Orange and Other Herbicides: A veteran who served in the Republic of Vietnam between January 9, 1962, and May 7, 1975, is presumed to have been exposed to Agent Orange and other herbicides used in support of military operations. Eleven illnesses are presumed by the VA to be service-connected for such veterans: chloracne or other acneform disease similar to chloracne, porphyria cutanea tarda, soft-tissue sarcoma (other than osteosarcoma, chondrosarcoma, Kaposi's sarcoma or mesothelioma), Hodgkin's disease, multiple myeloma, respiratory cancers (lung, bronchus, larynx, trachea), non-Hodgkin's lymphoma, prostate cancer, acute and subacute peripheral neuropathy, diabetes mellitus (Type 2) and chronic lymphocytic leukemia.

Veterans Exposed to Radiation: For veterans who participated in "radiation risk activities" as defined in VA regulations while on active duty, the following conditions are presumed to be service-connected: all forms of leukemia (except for chronic lymphocytic leukemia); cancer of the thyroid, breast, pharynx, esophagus, stomach, small intestine, pancreas, bile ducts, gall bladder, salivary gland, urinary tract (renal pelvis, ureter, urinary bladder and urethra), brain, bone, lung, colon, and ovary, bronchiolo-alveolar carcinoma, multiple myeloma, lymphomas (other than Hodgkin's disease), and primary liver cancer (except if cirrhosis or hepatitis B is indicated). To determine service-connection for other conditions or exposures not eligible for presumptive service-connection, the VA considers factors such as the amount of radiation exposure, duration of exposure, elapsed time between exposure and onset of the disease, gender and family history, age at time of exposure, the extent to which a non-service-related exposure could contribute to disease, and the relative sensitivity of exposed tissue.

Gulf War Veterans with Chronic Disabilities: May receive disability compensation for chronic disabilities resulting from undiagnosed illnesses, medically unexplained chronic multi-symptom illnesses defined by a cluster of signs or symptoms. A disability is considered chronic if it has existed for at least six months. The undiagnosed illnesses must have appeared either during active service in the Southwest Asia Theater of Operations during the Gulf War or to a degree of at least 10 percent at any time since then through December 31, 2011.

The following are examples of symptoms of an undiagnosed illness: chronic fatigue syndrome, fibromyalgia, skin disorders, headache, muscle pain, joint pain, neurological symptoms, neuropsychological symptoms, symptoms involving the respiratory system, sleep disturbances, gastrointestinal symptoms, cardiovascular symptoms, abnormal weight loss, and menstrual disorders. Amyotrophic Lateral Sclerosis (ALS), also known as Lou Gehrig's disease, may be determined to be service-connected if the veteran served in the Southwest Asia Theater of Operations anytime during the period of August 2, 1990, to July 31, 1991. This Theater of Operations includes Iraq, Kuwait, Saudi Arabia, the neutral zone between Iraq and Saudi Arabia, Bahrain, Qatar, the United Arab Emirates, Oman, the Gulf of Aden, the Gulf of Oman, the Persian Gulf, the Arabian Sea, the Red Sea, and the airspace above these locations.

Concurrent Retirement and Disability Payments

Concurrent Retirement and Disability Payments (CRDP) restores retired pay on a graduated 10-year schedule for retirees with a 50 to 90 percent VA-rated disability. Concurrent retirement payments increase 10 percent per year through

2013. Veterans rated 100% disabled by the VA are entitled to full CRDP without being phased in. Veterans receiving benefits at the 100% rate due to individual unemployability are entitled to full CRDP in 2009.

Eligibility: To qualify, veterans must also meet all three of the following criteria:

1. Have 20 or more years on active duty, or be a reservist age 60 or older with 20 or more creditable years.
2. Be in a retired status.
3. Be receiving retired pay (must be offset by VA payments).

Retirees do not need to apply for this benefit. Payment is coordinated between the VA and the Department of Defense (DoD).

Combat-Related Special Compensation

Combat-Related Special Compensation (CRSC) provides tax-free monthly payments to eligible retired veterans with combat-related injuries. With CRSC, veterans can receive both their full military retirement pay and their VA disability compensation, if the injury is combat-related.

Eligibility: Retired veterans with combat-related injuries must meet all of the following criteria to apply for CRSC:

1. Active, reserve, or medically retired with 20 years of creditable service.
2. Receiving military retired pay.
3. Have a 10% or greater VA-rated injury.
4. Military retired pay is reduced by VA disability payments (VA waiver).

In addition, veterans must be able to provide documentary evidence that their injuries were a result of one of the following:

- Training that simulates war (e.g., exercises, field training)
- Hazardous duty (e.g., flight, diving, parachute duty)
- An instrumentality of war (e.g., combat vehicles, weapons, Agent Orange)
- Armed conflict (e.g., gunshot wounds, Purple Heart)

For information, visit http://prhome.defense.gov, or call the toll-free phone number for the veteran's branch of service: (Army) 866-281-3254; (Air Force) 800-616-3775; (Navy) 877-366-2772. The Army has its own website at https://www.hrc.army.mil/site/crsc/index.html.

Programs for Veterans with Service-Connected Disabilities

Vocational Rehabilitation and Employment

The Vocational Rehabilitation and Employment (VR&E) Program assists veterans who have service-connected disabilities with obtaining and maintaining suitable employment. Independent living services are also available for severely disabled veterans who are not currently ready to seek employment. Additional information is available on VA's website at www.vba.va .gov/bln/vre.

Eligibility: A veteran must have a VA service-connected disability rated at least 20 percent with an employment handicap, or rated 10 percent with a serious employment handicap, and be discharged or released from military service under other than dishonorable conditions. Service members pending medical separation from active duty may also apply if their disabilities are reasonably expected to be rated at least 20 percent following their discharge.

Entitlement: A VA counselor must decide if the individual has an employment handicap based upon the results of a comprehensive evaluation. After an entitlement decision is made, the individual and counselor will work together to develop a rehabilitation plan. The rehabilitation plan will specify the rehabilitation services to be provided.

Services: Rehabilitation services provided to participants in the VR&E program are under one of five tracks. VA pays the cost of all approved training programs. Subsistence allowance may also be provided. The five tracks are:

1. Reemployment with Previous Employer: For individuals who are separating from active duty or in the National Guard or reserves and are returning to work for their previous employer.
2. Rapid Access to Employment: For individuals who either wish to obtain employment soon after separation or who already have the necessary skills to be competitive in the job market in an appropriate occupation.
3. Self-Employment: For individuals who have limited access to traditional employment, need flexible work schedules, or who require more accommodation in the work environment due to their disabling conditions or other life circumstances.
4. Employment Through Long-Term Services: For individuals who need specialized training and/or education to obtain and maintain suitable employment.
5. Independent Living Services: For veterans who are not currently able to work and need rehabilitation services to live more independently.

Period of a Rehabilitation Program: Generally, veterans must complete a program within 12 years from their separation from military service or within 12 years from the date VA notifies them that they have a compensable service-connected disability. Depending on the length of program needed, veterans may be provided up to 48 months of full-time services or their part-time equivalent. These limitations may be extended in certain circumstances.

Work-Study: Veterans training at the three-quarter or full-time rate may participate in VA's work-study program and provide VA outreach services, prepare/process VA paperwork, work at a VA medical facility, or perform other VA-approved activities. A portion of the work-study allowance equal to 40 percent of the total may be paid in advance.

Specially Adapted Housing Grants

Certain veterans and service members with service-connected disabilities may be entitled to a Specially Adapted Housing (SAH) grant from the VA to help build a new specially adapted house, to adapt a home they already own, or buy a house and modify it to meet their disability-related requirements. Eligible veterans or service members may now receive up to three grants, with the total dollar amount of the grants not to exceed the maximum allowable. Previous grant recipients who had received assistance of less than the current maximum allowable may be eligible for an additional SAH grant.

Eligible veterans who are temporarily residing in a home owned by a family member may also receive a grant to help the veteran adapt the family member's home to meet his or her special needs. Those eligible for a $50,000 grant would be permitted to use up to $14,000 and those eligible for a $10,000 grant would be permitted to use up to $2,000. (See eligibility requirements for different grant amounts.) However, the VA is not authorized to make such grants available to assist active duty personnel.

Eligibility for up to $50,000: The VA may approve a grant of not more than 50 percent of the cost of building, buying, or adapting existing homes or paying to reduce indebtedness on a currently owned home that is being adapted, up to a maximum of $50,000. In certain instances, the full grant amount may be applied toward remodeling costs. Veterans and service members must be determined eligible to receive compensation for permanent and total service-connected disability due to one of the following:

1. Loss or loss of use of both lower extremities, such as to preclude locomotion without the aid of braces, crutches, canes or a wheelchair.
2. Loss or loss of use of both upper extremities at or above the elbow.
3. Blindness in both eyes, having only light perception, plus loss or loss of use of one lower extremity.
4. Loss or loss of use of one lower extremity together with (a) residuals of organic disease or injury, or (b) the loss or loss of use of one upper extremity which so affects the functions of balance or propulsion as to preclude locomotion without the use of braces, canes, crutches or a wheelchair.

Eligibility for up to $10,000: The VA may approve a grant for the cost, up to a maximum of $10,000, for necessary adaptations to a veteran's or service member's residence or to help them acquire a residence already adapted with special features for their disability, to purchase and adapt a home, or for adaptations to a family member's home in which they will reside.

To be eligible for this grant, veterans and service members must be entitled to compensation for permanent and total service-connected disability due to:

1. Blindness in both eyes with 5/200 visual acuity or less.
2. Or anatomical loss or loss of use of both hands.

Supplemental Financing: Veterans and service members with available loan guaranty entitlement may also obtain a guaranteed loan or a direct loan from the VA to supplement the grant to acquire a specially adapted home. Amounts with a guaranteed loan from a private lender will vary, but the maximum direct loan from the VA is $33,000.

Adapting an Automobile

Veterans and service members may be eligible for a one-time payment of not more than $11,000 toward the purchase of an automobile or other conveyance if they have service-connected loss or permanent loss of use of one or both hands or feet, permanent impairment of vision of both eyes to a certain degree, or ankylosis (immobility) of one or both knees or one or both hips. They may also be eligible for adaptive equipment, and for repair, replacement, or reinstallation required because of disability or for the safe operation of a vehicle purchased with VA assistance. To apply, contact a VA regional office at 800-827-1000 or the nearest VA medical center.

Clothing Allowance

Any veteran who is service-connected for a disability for which he or she uses prosthetic or orthopedic appliances may receive an annual clothing allowance. This allowance also is available to any veteran whose service-connected skin condition requires prescribed medication that irreparably damages outer garments. To apply, contact the prosthetic representative at the nearest VA medical center.

Aid and Attendance or Housebound Veterans

A veteran who is determined by the VA to be in need of the regular aid and attendance of another person, or a veteran who is permanently housebound, may be entitled to additional disability compensation or pension payments. A veteran evaluated at 30 percent or more disabled is entitled to receive an additional payment for a spouse who is in need of the aid and attendance of another person.

Vocational Rehabilitation and Employment Rates

In some cases, a veteran requires additional education or training to become employable. A subsistence allowance is paid each month during training and is based on the rate of attendance (full-time or part-time), the number of dependents, and the type of training. The tables below show the rates as of October 1, 2010. Subsistence allowance is paid at the following monthly rates for training in an institution of higher learning (table 7.2).

Subsistence allowance is paid for full-time training only, in the following training programs: Non-pay or nominal-pay on-job training in a federal, state, local, or federally recognized Indian tribe agency; training in the home; vocational course in a rehabilitation facility or sheltered workshop; institutional non-farm cooperative (table 7.3).

The following rates are paid for Work Experience programs: Non-pay or nominal-pay work experience in a federal, state, local or federally recognized Indian tribe agency (table 7.4).

Subsistence allowance is paid for full-time training only in the following training programs: Farm Cooperative, Apprenticeship, or other On-Job Training (table 7.5).

Table 7.2. Monthly Subsistence Allowance Paid for Training in an Institution of Higher Learning

Number of Dependents	Full-Time	Three-Quarter Time	One-Half Time
No Dependents	$594.47	$446.67	$298.88
One Dependent	$737.39	$553.85	$370.30
Two Dependents	$868.96	$649.68	$435.27
Each Additional Dependent	$63.34	$48.72	$32.50

Table 7.3. Monthly Subsistence Allowance Paid for Full-Time Training Only in Non-Pay or Nominal Pay On-the-Job Training

Number of Dependents	Full-Time
No Dependents	$594.47
One Dependent	$737.39
Two Dependents	$868.96
Each Additional Dependent	$63.34

Table 7.4. Monthly Subsistence Paid for Non-Pay or Nominal-Pay Work Experience

Number of Dependents	Full-Time	Three-Quarter Time	One-Half Time
No Dependents	$594.47	$446.67	$298.88
One Dependent	$737.39	$553.85	$370.30
Two Dependents	$868.96	$649.68	$435.27
Each Additional Dependent	$63.34	$48.71	$32.50

Table 7.5. Monthly Subsistence Allowance Paid for Full-Time Training Only in Farm Cooperative, Apprenticeship, and Other On-Job Training

Number of Dependents	Full-Time
No Dependent	$519.77
One Dependent	$628.55
Two Dependents	$724.41
Each Additional Dependent	$47.12

Table 7.6. Monthly Subsistence Allowance Paid for Greater Than Half-Time Training Programs

Number of Dependents	Institutional Greater Than One-Half	On-the-Job Greater Than One-Half
No Dependent	$594.47	$519.77
One Dependent	$737.39	$628.55
Two Dependents	$868.96	$724.41
Each Additional Dependent	$63.34	$47.12

Subsistence allowance is paid at the following rates for combined training programs: Combination of Institutional and On-Job Training (full-time rate only) (table 7.6).

Subsistence Allowance is paid at the following rates for Non-farm Cooperative Training: Non-farm Cooperative Institutional Training and Non-farm Cooperative On-Job Training (full-time rate only) (table 7.7).

Subsistence Allowance is paid at the following rates for Independent Living programs: A subsistence allowance is paid each month during the period of enrollment in a rehabilitation facility when a veteran is pursuing an approved Independent Living Program plan. Subsistence allowance paid during a period of Independent Living Services is based on rate of pursuit and number of dependents. Independent Living subsistence allowance rates (table 7.8).

Subsistence allowance is paid at the following rates for Extended Evaluation programs: A subsistence allowance is paid each month during the period

Table 7.7. Monthly Subsistence Allowance for Full-Time Training Only for Non-Farm Cooperative Institutional Training and Non-Farm Cooperative On-Job Training

Number of Dependents	FT Non-Farm Coop/Institutional	FT Non-Farm Coop/On-the-Job
No Dependent	$594.47	$519.77
One Dependent	$737.39	$628.55
Two Dependents	$868.96	$724.41
Each Additional Dependent	$63.34	$47.12

Table 7.8. Monthly Subsistence Allowance Paid During the Period of Enrollment in a Rehab Facility When a Veteran Is Pursuing an Approved Independent Living Program Plan

Number of Dependents	Full-Time	Three-Quarter Time	One-Half Time
No Dependents	$594.47	$446.67	$298.88
One Dependent	$737.39	$553.85	$370.30
Two Dependents	$868.96	$649.68	$435.27
Each Additional Dependent	$63.34	$48.71	$32.50

Table 7.9. Monthly Subsistence Allowance Paid During the Period of Enrollment in a Rehab Facility When a Veteran Requires This Service for the Purpose of Extended Evaluation

Number of Dependents	Full-Time	Three-Quarter Time	One-Half Time	One-Quarter Time
No Dependents	$594.47	$446.67	$298.88	$149.41
One Dependent	$737.39	$553.85	$370.30	$185.17
Two Dependents	$868.96	$649.68	$435.27	$217.64
Each Additional Dependent	$63.34	$48.71	$32.50	$16.21

of enrollment in a rehabilitation facility when a veteran requires this service for the purpose of extended evaluation. Subsistence allowance during a period of extended evaluation is paid based on the rate of attendance and the number of dependents. Extended Evaluation program subsistence allowance rates (table 7.9).

VA PENSIONS

Eligibility for Disability Pension

Veterans with low incomes who are permanently and totally disabled, or are age 65 and older, may be eligible for monetary support if they have 90 days or more of active military service, at least one day of which was during a period of war. (Veterans who entered active duty on or after September 8, 1980, or officers who entered active duty on or after October 16, 1981, may have to meet a longer minimum period of active duty.) The veteran's discharge must have been under conditions other than dishonorable and the disability must be for reasons other than the veteran's own willful misconduct.

Payments are made to bring the veteran's total income, including other retirement or Social Security income, to a level set by Congress. Unreimbursed medical expenses may reduce countable income for VA purposes.

Improved Disability Pension

Congress establishes the maximum annual improved disability pension rates. Payments are reduced by the amount of countable income of the veteran, spouse or dependent children. When a veteran without a spouse or a child is furnished nursing home or domiciliary care by VA, the pension is reduced to an amount not to exceed $90 per month after three calendar months of care. The reduction may be delayed if nursing-home care is being continued to provide the veteran with rehabilitation services.

Additional information can be found in the Compensation and Pension Benefits section of the VA's website at www.vba.va.gov/bln/21/index.htm.

Protected Pension Programs

Pension beneficiaries who were receiving a VA pension on December 31, 1978, and do not wish to elect the Improved Pension will continue to receive the pension rate they were receiving on that date. This rate generally continues as long as the beneficiary's income remains within established limits, his

Table 7.10. 2008 VA Improved Disability Pension Rates

Status	Maximum Annual Rate
Veteran without dependent	$12,256
With one dependent	16,051
Veteran permanently housebound	14,978
With one dependent	18,773
Veteran needing regular aid and attendance	20,447
With one dependent	24,239
Two veterans married to one another	16,051
Veterans of World War I and Mexican Border Period, addition to the applicable annual rate	2,783
Increase for each additional dependent child	2,093

or her net worth does not bar payment, and the beneficiary does not lose any dependents.

These beneficiaries must continue to meet basic eligibility factors, such as permanent and total disability for veterans, or status as a surviving spouse or child. The VA must adjust rates for other reasons, such as a veteran's hospitalization in a VA facility.

Medal of Honor Pension

VA administers pensions to recipients of the Medal of Honor. The monthly pension is $1,194.

Vet Centers

Vet Centers provide readjustment counseling and outreach services to all veterans who served in any combat zone. Services are also available for their family members for military-related issues. Veterans have earned these benefits through their service and all are provided at no cost to the veteran or family.

Readjustment counseling is wide range of services provided to combat veterans in the effort to make a satisfying transition from military to civilian life. Services include:

- Individual counseling
- Group counseling
- Marital and family counseling
- Bereavement counseling
- Medical referrals
- Assistance in applying for VA benefits
- Employment counseling
- Guidance and referral
- Alcohol/drug assessments
- Information and referral to community resources
- Military sexual trauma counseling and referral
- Outreach and community education.

The VA's readjustment counseling is provided at community-based Vet Centers located near veterans and their families. There is no cost for Vet Center readjustment counseling. Find your nearest Vet Center www2.va .gov/directory or check your local blue pages. The Vet Center staff is available toll-free during normal business hours at 800-905-4675 (Eastern) and 866-496-8838 (Pacific).

DD Form 214, "Certificate of Release or Discharge from Active Duty": This form is one of the most important documents the service will ever give you. It is your key to participation in all Department of Veterans Affairs (VA) programs as well as several state and federal programs. Keep your original in a safe, fireproof place and have certified photocopies available for reference. You can replace this record, but that takes a long time—time that you may not have. Be safe. In most states, DD Form 214 can be registered/recorded just like a land deed or other significant document. So, immediately after you separate, register your DD Form 214 with your county recorder or town hall. If you register your documents, they can later be retrieved quickly for a nominal fee. You should check whether state or local law permits public access to the recorded document. If public access is authorized and you register DD Form 214, others could obtain a copy for an unlawful purpose (e.g., to obtain a credit card in your name). If public access is permitted and you choose not to register your DD Form 214, you still should take steps to protect it as you would any other sensitive document (wills, marriage and birth certificates, insurance policies). You may wish to store it in a safe deposit box or at some other secure location.

In addition, your local Vet Center can certify your DD214 and have a copy placed on file. Find your nearest Vet Center online at www2.va.gov/directory.

DisabilityInfo.gov: The Online Disability Resource

The federal government has created the www.disabilityinfo.gov website, which is designed to give people with disabilities and many others access to the information and resources they need to live full and independent lives in the workplace and in their communities. Managed by the U.S. Department of Labor's Office of Disability Employment Policy (www.dol.gov/odep), DisabilityInfo.gov offers a broad range of valuable information, not only for people with disabilities, but also their family members, health care professionals, service providers and many others.

Easy to navigate, DisabilityInfo.gov is organized by subject areas that include benefits, civil rights, community life, education, employment, health, housing, technology and transportation. By selecting a category from the tabs at the top of the home page, users are directed to valuable information covering state and local resources, news and events, grants and funding, laws and regulations and more. Several sections of the site link to disability-related programs geared toward veterans and the military community.

With 21 federal agencies contributing content to this website DisabilityInfo .gov contains extensive, frequently updated information on a host of crosscutting topics. Areas of particular interest to the military community and their families include information on the availability of assistive technologies for DoD employees and service members with disabilities, links to employment programs for transitioning wounded service members in addition to information on benefits, compensation and health care programs, links to relocation and employment services as well as special needs programs for military families, and many other Department of Defense programs serving troops and their families.

DisabilityInfo.gov also offers a free subscription service where you can sign up to receive *Disability Connection,* the quarterly newsletter, as well as other e-mail alerts covering information tailored to your individual interests. Just visit service.govdelivery.com/service/user.html?code=USODEP to sign up.

Special Groups of Veterans

Women Veterans

Women veterans are eligible for the same VA benefits as male veterans, but can also receive additional gender-specific services, including breast and pelvic examinations and other reproductive health care services.

VA provides preventive health care counseling, contraceptive services, menopause management, Pap smears and mammography. Referrals are made for services that the VA is unable to provide. Women Veterans' Program Managers are available in a private setting at all VA facilities to help women veterans seeking treatment and benefits.

For information, visit www.va.gov/womenvet. VA health care professionals provide counseling and treatment to help veterans overcome psychological issues resulting from sexual trauma that occurred while serving on active duty, or active duty for training if service was in the National Guard or reserves. Veterans who are not otherwise eligible for VA health care may still receive these services and do not need to enroll. Appropriate services are provided for any injury, illness or psychological condition resulting from such trauma.

VA Benefits for Veterans Living or Traveling Overseas

VA will pay for medical services for service-connected disabilities and related conditions or medical services needed as part of a vocational rehabilitation program for veterans living or traveling outside the United States. Veterans living in the Philippines should register with the U.S. Veterans Affairs office in Pasay City, telephone 011-632-833-4566. All other veterans living or planning to travel outside the U.S. should register with the Denver Foreign Medical

Program office, P.O. Box 65021, Denver, CO 80206-9021, USA; telephone 303-331-7590. For information visit: www.va.gov/hac/forbeneficiaries/fmp/ fmp.asp.

Some veterans traveling or living overseas can telephone the Foreign Medical Program toll free from these countries: Germany 0800-1800-011; Australia 1800-354-965; Italy 800-782-655; United Kingdom (England and Scotland) 0800-032-7425; Mexico 001-877-345-8179; Japan 00531-13-0871; Costa Rica 0800-013-0759; and Spain 900-981-776. (**Note:** Veterans in Mexico or Costa Rica must first dial the United States country code.)

VA monetary benefits, including disability compensation, pension, educational benefits, and burial allowances, generally are payable overseas. Some programs are restricted. Home loan guaranties are available only in the United States and selected U.S. territories and possessions. Educational benefits are limited to approved, degree granting programs in institutions of higher learning. Beneficiaries living in foreign countries should contact the nearest American embassy or consulate for help. In Canada, contact an office of Veterans Affairs Canada. For information, visit www.vba.va.gov/bln/21/ foreign/index.htm.

Appeals of VA Claims Decisions

Veterans and other claimants for VA benefits have the right to appeal decisions made by a VA regional office or medical center. Typical issues appealed are disability compensation, pension, education benefits, recovery of overpayments, and reimbursement for unauthorized medical services.

A claimant has one year from the date of the notification of a VA decision to file an appeal. The first step in the appeal process is for a claimant to file a written notice of disagreement with the VA regional office or medical center that made the decision.

Following receipt of the written notice, the VA will furnish the claimant a "Statement of the Case" describing what facts, laws and regulations were used in deciding the case. To complete the request for appeal, the claimant must file a "Substantive Appeal" within 60 days of the mailing of the Statement of the Case, or within one year from the date the VA mailed its decision, whichever period ends later.

Board of Veterans' Appeals

The Board of Veterans' Appeals makes decisions on appeals on behalf of the Secretary of Veterans Affairs. Although it is not required, a veteran's service organization, an agent or an attorney may represent a claimant. Appellants may present their cases in person to a member of the board at a hearing in Washington, DC, at a VA regional office, or by videoconference. Decisions made by the board can be found on the website at www.va.gov/vbs/bva. The pamphlet, "Understanding the Appeal Process," is available on the website or may be requested by writing: Hearings and Transcription Unit (014HRG), Board of Veterans' Appeals, 811 Vermont Avenue, NW, Washington, DC 20420.

U.S. Court of Appeals for Veterans Claims

A final Board of Veterans' Appeals decision that does not grant a claimant the benefits desired may be appealed to the U.S. Court of Appeals for Veterans Claims, an independent court, not part of the Department of Veterans Affairs.

Notice of an appeal must be received by the court with a postmark that is within 120 days after the Board of Veterans' Appeals mailed its decision. The court reviews the record considered by the Board of Veterans' Appeals. It does not hold trials or receive new evidence. Appellants may represent themselves before the court or have lawyers or approved agents as representatives. Oral argument is held only at the direction of the court. Either party may appeal a decision of the court to the U.S. Court of Appeals for the Federal Circuit and may seek review in the Supreme Court of the United States. Published decisions, case status information, rules and procedures, and other special announcements can be found on the court's website at www.vetapp.gov. The court's decisions can also be found in West's *Veterans Appeals Reporter,* and on the Westlaw and LEXIS online services. For questions, write the Clerk of the Court, 625 Indiana Avenue NW, Suite 900, Washington, DC 20004, or call 202-501-5970.

8

Success Stories

LANCE CPL. COLIN SMITH

On October 30, 2006, Lance Cpl. Colin Smith was a USMC machine gunner in his vehicle's turret when he was shot through the skull by a single shot just as the Marines were leaving a rural settlement on the western edge of Karma, a city near Falluja in Anbar Province. "Every time before we go out, we say a prayer," said a fellow Marine. "It is a prayer for serenity. It says a lot about things that do pertain to us in this kind of environment."

His family spent Christmas, New Year's and weeks in a Minneapolis hospital until finally, they saw some promising signs. Lance Cpl. Smith was not going to give up this fight for his life.

Because of damage to areas of the brain that control speech, Mr. Smith said it was not clear how fully Lance Cpl. Smith would recover his ability to converse. Similarly, he has extremely limited movement on the right side of his body.

"You never know when the healing process will plateau," Mr. Smith said, but added, "Every day you can see him improve."

Colin's father, Bob Smith, contacted Hope For The Warriors™ in the late fall of 2006 with a request for assistance in purchasing a home that would provide a safe and adaptive haven for Colin to continue down his amazing path of recovery. Staff at Hope For The Warriors™ were honored to provide a $100,000 home grant to the Smiths and wish them the best in their future. Lance Cpl. Colin Smith and his family proudly purchased a new home fully adapted to accommodate Colin's injuries.

Lance Cpl. Colin Smith is the epitome of a hero and the spirit of American pride. His family stands behind him with admiration, love and the utmost respect for the choices and the sacrifices he has made. They are truly role models to all families.

A PERSONAL STORY

My name is Daniel Acosta and I was born on June 18, 1984, in Joliet, IL. I resided in Joliet, IL, for eighteen years and attended Joliet Central High School. Post-graduation, I joined the U.S. Air Force on 10 December 2002. In October of 2003 I graduated from Naval Explosive Ordnance Disposal School, which is one of the toughest schools in the military. Upon graduation I was stationed at Hill AFB, UT. There I spent the next 3 years working and training for combat. On June 17, 2004, I got married to Sandra Sanchez and became stepfather of daughter Alexis. On March 7, 2004, my wife gave birth to our daughter Sophia.

In September of 2005 I deployed to Baghdad, Iraq. My job on a daily basis was to go on missions throughout Baghdad to render safe IED's (improvised explosive devices) by disarming, countercharging, or neutralizing by other means. On a routine mission to render safe a roadside IED, my teammate and I disarmed two IED's and were getting ready to leave but I had a gut feeling that there was another IED at that scene. I told my teammate that we cannot leave without at least searching the area, "I don't feel like dying today."

For us time on scene was critical because it allows time for insurgents to counter-attack us. As I was sweeping the area with the mine detector I looked back at my security team member and told him to get back on the road because he was too close to me; if something happens you don't need to get hurt. That was the last thing I remember, the date was December 7, 2005.

An IED meant for a vehicle went off 20 feet to my left side. The IED was two 122-mm projectiles with a wooden pressure plate containing a micro switch as the initiator. The post-blast analysis determined that IED was set off by me stepping on the pressure plate and was undetectable because the wooden pressure plate and the projectile were separated by 20 feet.

The injuries I sustained were a traumatic left arm amputation, 18% third degree burns to both legs, damage to right femoral artery, shrapnel damage to abdomen, and severe blood loss. The doctor gave me a 25% chance of living and if I made it through the first surgery I'll have a 50% chance of living.

I beat the odds and the next memory I have was waking up on December 11, 2005 at Brooke Army Medical Center, San Antonio, Texas. The first person I saw was my wife. She was the one to tell me what happened, where I was, and the true extent of my traumatic injuries. That very moment my road to recovery began and is currently ongoing. The first significant progress in my recovery was learning to walk and since then it's been all uphill.

When I got to the point in my recovery to where I felt my normal self minus the physical losses, I realized what is important in life and what I want to do with it. The most important part of it was my family and there was a chance that I would never see them again. My wife and I wanted to complete our family with trying to have a boy, well we were blessed. On January 19, 2007, my wife gave birth to our son Mario Daniel.

I separate from the Air Force within the next 6 months, so my immediate goal is to find a house in San Antonio that will be affordable and comfortable. Once we have a home and are established I will concentrate on finishing college and graduate with a degree in business. From there I will continue to work and provide for my family.

My goals are ones that will be met because of my determination to move on from what happened to me. The way I see it, I have been given a second chance with a new outlook on life to become the person I want to be and provide for my wife and children to give them the opportunities I did not have growing up.

Please assist me and my family making out dreams become a true reality, any support given would be greatly appreciated and will take me and my family to another level in life. Hope For The Warriors™ assisted with $5000 toward the down payment on the Acosta's new home and $5000 towards furnishings. It is a privilege to provide help to a family whose outlook on their future is bright despite the challenges they face.

2ND LIEUTENANT ANDREW KINARD, USMC

On Sunday, April 1, 2007, 2nd Lt. Andrew Kinard was flown in a private jet to Ellis Albert Airport in Jacksonville, NC. In August of 2006, Lt. Kinard deployed to Iraq with Alpha Co., 2ndLAR. He was severely wounded in October of 2006, losing both legs and suffering from many internal injuries. He deployed as an ambitious healthy Marine. He returned more motivated and inspiring, bearing the battle scars of a promise to the American way of life he vowed to uphold, regardless of the sacrifices required.

That Sunday was the first time Andrew has been out of the hospital since October 2006, his wish . . . to be at Camp Lejeune when his fellow Marines returned from their 7-month deployment. Andrew needed to welcome them home and get some answers to the questions that have haunted him since he was injured. What happened on that day in October? Andrew's homecoming was that befitting of the sacrifices he has made—the airport runway was flanked by a 40-man Patriot Guard welcome, all proudly hailing American flags.

A newly donated van escorted Andrew aboard Camp Lejeune. The caravan was received by well-respected salutes as they passed through the front

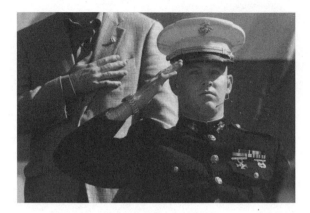

2nd Lt. Andrew Kinard

gate. Upon reaching Warrior House™, Andrew was greeted by friends and fellow Marines—all anxious to hug this amazing young man, whose spirit and courage epitomizes that of a hero. He was presented with a new "Humvee" of a wheelchair that suits his personality and his wish to be more mobile and active.

On Monday, April 2, 2007, Alpha Co. returned in typical homecoming style with tents and bouncy houses, children and families carrying flags and waving signs. Andrew, in his new wheelchair was right up front. His charismatic smile told a story to all—this day was more therapeutic than any amount of hospital rehabilitation could ever provide.

SERGEANT SHURVON PHILLIP, USMC

On May 7, 2005, while on maneuvers and patrol in Al Anbar, Iraq, the Humvee that Sgt. Phillip was riding in was struck by an improvised explosive device. Sgt. Phillip suffered a multitude of critical injuries in the explosion, including traumatic brain injury. From the very start, consistent with his dedication, Sgt. Phillip has absolutely refused to quit. During his stay in various hospitals, and facing various surgeries and infections, Sgt. Phillip has fought off death's doorstep on at least three different occasions. He now zealously fights the daily challenges of complete paralysis.

His dedication has touched the lives of many persons, including his family, complete strangers, those charged with his care, and even President Bush, who visited Sgt. Phillip's bedside at Naval Medical Center Bethesda. Since his injuries, Sgt. Phillip's proudest moments involve obtaining his U.S. citizenship in August 2005 and his Welcome Home ceremony in June 2006 upon his arrival in Cleveland, Ohio. Indeed, when he is most proud and appreciative, Sgt. Phillip exercises all his energy to slightly raise his left hand to express immense joy and gratitude.

In September 2006, Sgt. Phillip left the VA Hospital in Cleveland, Ohio, and he returned to the family's apartment in East Cleveland, Ohio. Although the apartment is not conducive for his medical conditions, Sgt. Phillip has remained strong, dedicated and brave. Severe brain injuries, a craniotomy, a tracheotomy, and feeding tubes will not stop Sgt. Phillip. His eyes, which serve as his only means of communication, are focused and express his courage. He is thankful for the daily accomplishments and he ever so slightly cracks a smile knowing that he is home and that so many have rallied to now support him and his family.

ED SALAU, NATIONAL GUARD

Ed's Army National Guard unit was deployed to Iraq in February 2004. Ed is very down-to-earth in describing what happened:

"In November 2004, we were on a regular patrol in a Bradley Fighting Vehicle, looking for bad guys. We found them when they initiated contact with two rocket-propelled grenades (RPGs). I was standing in the turret at the time, and one of the RPGs found its way into the Bradley, exploding and taking off my leg and the leg of one of my men."

Though Ed's unit got the insurgents who had injured him and the other soldier and finished off the battle that ensued, it was the end of the war for Ed and the other man, who found themselves at Walter Reed Army Medical Center two days later.

Recuperation: Ed remained at Walter Reed Army Medical Center until he was medically retired on April 2, 2005. He underwent several surgeries and did physical rehabilitation every day, and takes the stoic attitude toward the ordeal that one might expect of a fully indoctrinated member of the armed forces: "Oh, I guess there were hard days and easy days. I learned to walk again. That's what matters."

Involvement with Wounded Warrior Project: Ed found a Wounded Warrior Project backpack in his room one day when he returned from surgery; and that, he said, "was very necessary at the time."

Like many injured soldiers coming home from the wars in Iraq and Afghanistan, Ed arrived in a hospital gown. He had no other clothing, and his family didn't know to bring any along when they rushed to Walter Reed to see him. So the shorts and T-shirts in the WWP backpack were a big plus. But the first thing he mentioned—with gratitude—was the razor and shaving cream. Apparently, after being shifted around for a few days, he was darn good and ready for a nice shave!

His next WWP contacts were with representatives of the organization who dropped by to say hello, bring a friendly word from one wounded warrior to another, and answer questions. But the impact of the Wounded Warrior Project became truly significant in Ed's life when he went on a skiing trip with the organization.

"That was huge," Ed exclaimed. "I used to run for fun. I loved going fast, but all that suddenly stopped when I was injured. Then, just five or six weeks after I was wounded, I was on the side of a mountain, skiing. I was going fast again, and it got my brain to realize something very important: I wasn't as disabled as I thought I was.

"It's pretty amazing as I look back on it; I actually learned how to ski before I got my prosthetic leg. I recently got certification to teach adaptive skiing, so I can teach other amputees and people with physical limitations how to do this. That's how important I think this is to recovery."

Employment Narrative: After Ed left Walter Reed, his old civilian job was waiting for him; but, after his experiences in Iraq, a certain restlessness set in. For one thing, he wanted to get more involved with the Wounded Warrior Project and asked Executive Director John Melia about volunteer opportunities. Ed said he was surprised when John explained that the organization was expanding its staff to meet the needs of growing numbers of injured veterans from Iraq and Afghanistan, and asked if Ed would like to work for WWP. Ed took up that offer and hasn't looked back.

Pointing out that he had an MBA and a job waiting for him when he returned to civilian life, he said, "These 19-year-old kids, they don't have everything all set up for them. They need everything when they get out—absolutely everything. And I need to be there helping to make sure they get it.

"This work with the Wounded Warrior Project allows me to do just that. I'm in the right place, doing just the right work."

Feelings about Helping Other Vets through WWP: Ed uses the Wounded Warrior Project logo to explain his feelings:

"Our logo shows a soldier carrying a wounded guy who can no longer carry himself. I was once that wounded guy. Now, I'm doing the carrying. That's the way it is with all of us in the Wounded Warrior Project. Here you see people who were paralyzed in combat teaching other wounded troops how to ski. Think about how powerful that is."

Speaking of the WWP mission, he added, "I'll tell you, we aren't looking for a handout or for pity. We're strong people, we don't need that. What we want is the opportunity to help each other as we move forward into the main-

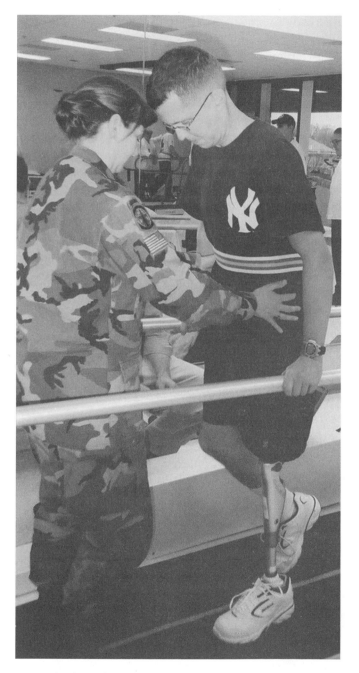

*Ed Salau, who was injured in Iraq while serving in the
National Guard, is now helping others through the
Wounded Warrior Project.*

stream of life as fully productive citizens." Ed is aware that the equipment and rehabilitation he received as a war-wounded veteran are superior to what many civilians get following amputations. He therefore looks for opportunities to work with professionals in the prosthetics field as they seek to apply the lessons of war-related prosthetic technology and rehabilitation to civilian amputees. He encourages other amputee veterans to do the same.

Feelings about Military Service: "What I did was valuable and necessary. I'm proud of what I did for America, and I'd do it all again if I had to."

LT. COL. ANDREW LOURAKE

Air Force Lt. Col. Andrew Lourake, an amputee who remained on active duty as a pilot, demonstrates how he switches modes on his computerized prosthesis that allows him to fly. His current prosthetic leg has two modes, one for walking and one for flying. The improved prosthesis being developed will have up to 10 modes and allow for remote-controlled switching.

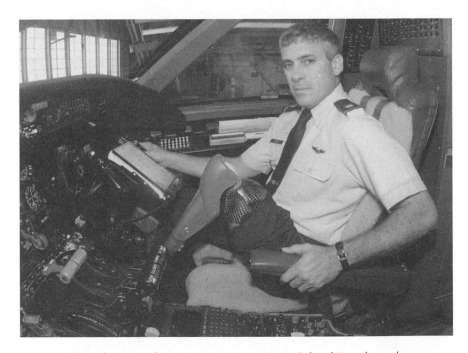

Lt. Col. Andrew Lourake sits in an Air Force C-20. Colonel Lourake underwent an above-the-knee amputation in June 2002. He was medically cleared to return to flying status and attended formal training to get requalified to fly.
(U.S. Air Force photo by Bobby Jones)

ARMY SGT. DENNIS CLINE

Army Sgt. Dennis Cline never was the kind of child who put together plastic models. More of an outdoor kid, he preferred doing anything outside—biking, hiking, hunting, fishing—to putting together a model.

Still, here he sat one recent day, as an adult, with his instructions and wheels and gears and rubber belts scattered about, putting together a racecar model. And he considers himself lucky to be doing it. Cline's left hand was claimed by a rocket-propelled grenade while on a patrol "outside the wire" in Afghanistan in 2006.

"I know I'm lucky," he said. "That RPG penetrated through the truck, through my hand, through the backpack with three 60 mm HE [high explosive] rounds and into a can of 40 mm HE rounds and didn't detonate any of it.

"That truck could have easily been a pink mess," he said.

Pulled up to a table in the bustling occupational therapy room of Walter Reed Army Medical Center here, Cline put the model together piece by piece, working on his fine motor skills with his prosthetic hand.

The room is white, square, filled with small weights, ropes and puzzles. Off to one side is a room set up like an apartment with a kitchen.

Amputees work individually and with therapists to regain skills they had before their injuries. Tasks as simple as brushing their teeth can be frustrating and cumbersome.

"We take it for granted, our fine motor coordination—to be able to grab a tooth brush and squeeze the tube of toothpaste just hard enough to get enough toothpaste on your brush. Or to have your arms and be able to pick up a shirt and be able to stick your arms through, . . . to be able to put it over your head," said Harvey Naranjo, a certified occupational therapy assistant at the center.

"Those are all tasks that we take for granted. . . . For someone who has been injured, it can be extremely trying," he said.

Naranjo said he works with amputees to get them to the point that they can reintegrate as much as possible back into normal life. He teaches them to use their prostheses in simple daily tasks. They learn to cook, clean, make their beds, tie their shoes, dress, and function as they did before their injuries.

"When you've been doing it the same way your whole life, and all of the sudden you have your dominant hand gone, . . . it is sometimes very difficult to relearn," he said.

Cline has three prosthetic hands, each having different functions, from normal wear to carrying heavy objects. He said it has taken months of hard work to learn to use them without breaking things in his grip.

"It takes a lot of practice and a lot of work to be able to use these," Cline said. "When you push down on something, it can easily break what you're trying to hold. It took a lot of time learning how much force to use. I would sit there and use my finger and practice how much muscle to use to grab my finger without smashing it.

"I'm to the point now where I can shake somebody's hand with it and not hurt them," he said. "It's got to the point now where it's pretty much second nature."

Cline said his love for the outdoors and strong desire for independence drove his recovery.

"To me, I love being outdoors. I love doing stuff. It was very important to me to regain my independence by being able to use my hand. A lot of things I like to do you can't do with one hand," he said.

"I made it my goal to try and use this as best as possible to give me back my independence . . . so I can get around and do things. There are very few things [now] that I can't do," he said.

One of the highlights of his recovery was learning to shoot a weapon again. The Fire Arms Training System at the center is a computer-generated weapons-training lab that helped him learn to fire using his prosthetic hand. For an outdoorsman like Cline, the therapy helped restore some normalcy to his life.

"As soon as I was able to get around a little more freely they had me down here shooting," he said. "As your recovery progresses, it allows you to know that you are a little more independent and you can do things that you used to do before.

"Originally I felt out of my comfort zone. I wasn't able to hold the weapon. I wasn't able to feel the weapon responding to the trigger squeeze," he said. "Now I can do it, and it feels as normal as it's going to get. It's a second nature again. It's more comfortable. I'm confident; I know I can hit the target."

The longtime outdoorsman already is hunting again, he said. Since his recovery, Cline has taken three deer, five ducks and three geese. He's practicing tying flies with plans to learn fly-fishing. Cline also recently skied for the first time since his injury.

"It just takes time. You've got to learn how to do things differently, . . . so you learn to adapt and overcome," he said.

Cline said he plans to go to college when he leaves the military. He has served in the Army for seven years and has been away from his wife and three children for nearly half of that time.

He also plans to organize a group of injured combat vets who regularly meet and travel for outdoor activities, he said.

Cline said getting away from the hospital is key in the recovery process. "The biggest thing I've noticed is that when I'm able to get out and do something that I like to do, it helps relieve a lot of the stressors that you have on your life," he said.

Cline offered simple advice for those beginning their recovery.

"If there is something you want to do, don't give up. There will be a way to do it," he said. "Yeah, life sucks now; . . . don't give up. Never give up. It doesn't matter what you do in life, you never give up. Once you give up, you're done."

SGT. ANDREW BUTTERWORTH

"Normal" is a relative term, and for one former North Carolina Army National Guard sergeant, it's distinctly different today from what it was in 2004.

On November 15 of that year, Army Sgt. Andrew Butterworth was serving in Iraq. After patrolling in the northeastern part of the country, he and members of his unit were heading home.

"They were waiting for us," he said. "[We] had an RPG, a rocket-propelled grenade, hit our Bradley [fighting vehicle]. It went right through the turret."

While the grenade caused some severe injuries, it could have been worse. Of the nine soldiers in the vehicle, Butterworth and his lieutenant were the only two seriously injured.

"I lost my right leg, and my lieutenant lost his left leg," he said. "Nobody was killed, except [the insurgents]."

Both Butterworth and his lieutenant got to Walter Reed Army Medical Center shortly after their injuries occurred. Their stays were short-lived, though.

"As far as I know, and unless somebody tells me different, I think we got out of there the fastest of all the amputees there," he said. "They were telling my family that I'd probably be there for six to eight months to a year or more."

But after only three and a half months, with the help of a cane, Butterworth walked out of Walter Reed on his good leg and a new prosthetic. The amazing progress was the result of friendly competition between Butterworth, also known as "Butter," and his lieutenant.

"It was who could do what first," he said. "That really helped both of us out."

On April 1, 2006, Butterworth was officially medically retired and began to embrace his new version of normal by attending a winter sports clinic in Aspen, Colorado. During that trip he decided that life may be different, but he wouldn't let his injury shape the future.

"I threw the cane away and started walking without it," he said. "I knew if I didn't start walking without it, I never would, so I just got rid of it."

With that act, Butterworth began to make good on a promise he made. When he first saw his family after the injury, he told them he wasn't going to let it slow him down.

"I guess it's just the way I was raised," he said. "It was just something else for me to learn how to do.

"I just kind of took it in stride, no pun intended," he chuckled.

Butterworth, who used to do electrical work for a living, now works as the Wounded Warrior Project's benefits liaison for the southeast region of the country. The job means a lot of time on the road and away from Bonzo, the orange tabby cat he said helps him keep his sanity, but he calls it his dream job.

The former soldier has a couple other dreams as well: a family and a college education.

He's already learned some important lessons not taught in a classroom, including the fact that there are two types of amputees: "those that have fallen and those that are about to."

And he's taught a few along the way.

"(Wounded warriors) aren't done. There's nothing that they can't do," Butterworth said. "You just have to meet it head-on and take it for what it is and see it as a new challenge."

This shouldn't be anything new for service members, he said.

"We've always got hard things to do, physically and mentally, emotionally," he said. "There's no reason to complain. We all have our days."

Some of those days leave him feeling like a 70-year-old man, he said. Some days that feeling wins out, and he can stay in bed. More often than not, though, he feels pretty good and enjoys some of his favorite activities, including hiking, camping, skiing and riding his motorcycle.

"People are like, 'You still ride a motorcycle? You're missing a leg,'" he said. "So what? Physically, I guess you would think I'm somewhat normal, besides the fact that I'm missing a leg.

"At some point you're going to be just as 'normal' as anybody else," he added.

MATT WATTERS

When Matt Watters deployed to war as a U.S. Army Ranger for the second time in 2003, he never expected the life-changing experience that would occur. Now a patrol officer in Tacoma, Washington, he serves his community and nation with a similar purpose—but a different mission.

Watters recently attended the Managing Civil Actions in Threat Incidents Basic course at the Center for Domestic Preparedness in Anniston, Alabama. At first look you may notice something that sets this officer apart from his classmates—or you may not. Saving American lives, regardless of the situation, is a responsibility that Watters takes pride in, as a citizen. In 2003, as his unit fought to root terrorists from hiding in western Iraq, he was severely injured.

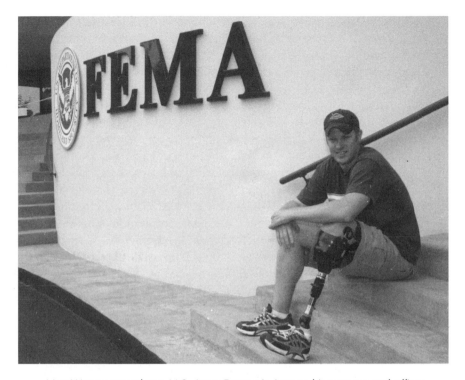

Matt Watters served as a U.S. Army Ranger in Iraq and is now a patrol officer in Tacoma, WA.

"We were raiding a settlement of enemy fighters camped near the Syrian border," said Watters. "They were pretty well emplaced despite our aerial support's efforts to disrupt them and aid our advance."

As gunships destroyed much of the camp, a section from the 2nd Ranger Battalion was preparing to join the fight using troop transport helicopters. When the special operations unit reached ground, they quickly formed an offensive line and began returning enemy fire. No longer covered by darkness due to burning structures, Watters' unit approached a well-entrenched enemy.

Within minutes of returning enemy fire and destroying many fighters, a terrorist fighter fired a Rocket Propelled Grenade—an RPG. The grenade first hit the earth, and bounced directly to Watters, resulting in severe injuries to his left leg, as well as other parts of his body. Ultimately, his lower left leg was completely blown away by the impact.

"I was injured on June 11, 2003, and received my final surgery in July," said Watters. "I also lost the top of my right thumb, and received shrapnel wounds that caused severe nerve damage near my left elbow and right calf muscle."

After extensive recovery time and rehabilitation Watters was medically retired as a sergeant in October 2004. He received the Purple Heart Medal for his injuries and the Bronze Star for Valor for his actions under fire. Remarkably, only two other Rangers were injured by AK-47 rifle fire, and no U.S. soldiers were killed.

Watters' love for the Army and serving his country as a soldier made leaving the military a tough decision. He says that despite his injuries, he had planned to leave military service at the end of his contract and explore other opportunities.

"I wanted to be with my family more," said the husband and father of two. "But if they had made Europe an option, I might have stayed," he said laughing.

"When I first noticed Matt Watters and learned about his circumstances, the thoughts that ran through my mind were pure admiration of his discipline, determination, and dedication to the force," said Gary Pippin, assistant course manager for law enforcement protective measures and other CDP courses. "His focus and mission are still the same—to protect and serve. He's a great young man with a positive attitude about life."

Watters added, "I was looking at either firefighting or law enforcement." "I was first looking to apply at the fire department, but in the end I was drawn to serving as a cop—like my father."

No stranger to challenges, Watters made two attempts at the police academy before completing his training in January 2005. During his first attempt, he experienced a large abscess to his injured leg that resulted in emergency surgery.

"It seems like I'm continually drawn to run after people with guns," he smiled. "[As a police officer] I haven't been fired upon, but I have arrested armed suspects." Watters maintains two different prosthetics and says he doesn't let his disability interfere with his duties.

"I walked into the mall one day to take care of some juvenile shoplifters and I got a lot of looks," he said. I was in uniform and wearing the leg that doesn't require a shoe, and is similar to a spring you may see amputee runners wear. I'm walking down the main corridor, and I sounded like a pirate. An employee from another store said, 'you are going to scare those kids.' I said, 'that's the point.'"

Watters added that the law enforcement course at the CDP is knowledge he needed. He indicated it isn't first-hand information that comes naturally, and is glad he attended the training.

"The course is good and all police officers should attend it," he said. "When it comes to dealing with large crowds, this course demands attention and tells the crowd, 'we're here now, and we're in charge.' The course stresses teamwork and working together as one."

Watters emphasized his surprise at the diverse training programs. He said he arrived at the CDP for one course, and found many other courses from which he and other emergency responders would benefit.

"Whether they are medical professionals, firefighters, or ambulance carriers, the training here is worthwhile," he stressed. "If you have an emergency or major disaster and the responders have this training, you're going to save time and you're going to save lives."

With his desire to serve his country or community—whether in the military abroad or stateside as a law enforcement officer—Watters serves as an example of citizenship and an inspiration to all Americans. When facing a possible debilitating injury, Watters recovered and returned to work serving his nation—just in a different uniform, and wearing one boot.

"A person who leaves a position of serving his country during war after an injury like that and takes on a job in law enforcement is brave and courageous," said Pippin. "This is a person who loves himself, his family, and his country. There aren't many that are made like this young man."

"I couldn't stop serving. Serving is in my blood and it's not in me to give up," Watters pointed out. "Everyone can't be in the military, but all Americans can serve in some way. We should all give something back."

SGT. ERIC EDMUNDSON

In November 2007 a former Army sergeant and his family settled into a brand new house in New Bern, NC, custom-built to ensure his war injuries will not keep him from independent living.

"Well, we need the house because Eric is in a wheelchair all the time, so we need it so he can get around the house by himself," said Stephanie Edmundson, wife of Eric Edmundson. The former soldier was wounded by a roadside bomb while riding in a Stryker armored vehicle on October 2, 2005, in Iraq, according to Homes for Our Troops officials, which took on the project for the family. The explosion left Edmundson unable to talk, walk, eat or drink, though he does have the ability to move his legs.

The home features wide doorways, an open architecture without hallways, lower counters, sturdy hand rails and other hardware for accessibility.

"He can move his chair with his feet," Stephanie said. "So he can help himself. . . . Quality of life is important in having Eric home, being able to be a husband and dad."

More than a dozen businesses in the New Bern area donated building materials, engineering services and labor for the project. In the end, the total cost for Homes for Our Troops was $5,000. Since the project came in so far under

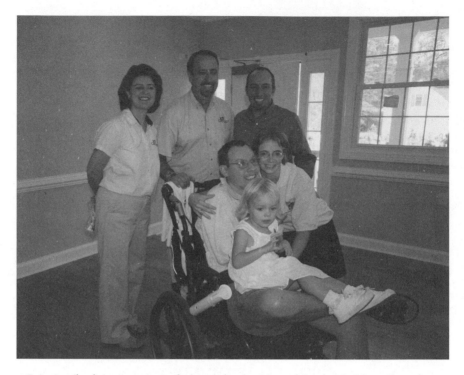

Enjoying the first moments in their new home, Eric and Stephanie Edmundson, front, are joined by Donna and Bill Russell of Kit Corp., left, and John Gonsalves, president and founder of Homes for Our Troops, far right.

budget, another home will be built for another wounded warrior, said John Gonsalves, president of the group.

It was one of nine homes built by the end of 2007.

"They are just an awesome family, the three of them together . . . their gratitude," said Donna Russell, who with her husband Bill Russell, owns the Kit Corp., which acted as lead contractor for the project. "He just brought things home . . . for us, so that we understand the sacrifices that they make every day."

"One of the things I always say about our projects is that they end up being a reflection of the community," said Kirt Rebello, chief project officer at Homes for Our Troops. "And if you look at this house, the community really stepped up."

Donating their resources was not a difficult decision for the local business people, according to Donna Russell.

"It just makes us proud to be able to do something so small to touch their lives to make it a little better," she said.

MORE SUPPORT

The new $3.5 million Warrior and Family Support Center in Fort Sam Houston, Texas, is 10 times the size of the previous facility. It provides a nurturing and comfortable environment where returning soldiers and their families can rest and recover.

Since opening its doors in December 2003, the Warrior and Family Support Center, formerly the Soldier and Family Assistance Center, has accommodated more than 180,000 visits from wounded warriors and their families—family members who have left their jobs and homes to come to Fort Sam Houston to help with the rehabilitation of their loved ones.

The old center had outgrown its space, due to the length of the war and an increase in wounded warriors, officials said. The additional influx required a permanent facility to meet all of the Warrior and Family Support Center operations.

The new building provides a "living room" environment, a place for social interaction and recreation between wounded warriors and their families. It was designed with wounded warriors' requirements in mind—fully wheelchair-accessible, with an atmosphere that will encourage healing. The facility has a computer classroom, kitchen, dining room, conference room, adequate bathrooms, and storage and social-gathering areas. It also provides opportunities in training for new job skills.

Spc. Francesca Duke, who was injured by a car bomb in Ramadi, Iraq, was an outpatient receiving treatment at Brooke Army Medical Center. She recalled her first encounter with the center.

"The Warrior and Family Support Center is where my mother and I found solace; it is one of the beginning steps in aiding in the recovery process for all heroes injured in support of operations Enduring [Freedom] and Iraqi Freedom. This is your home away from home," Spc. Duke said.

WOUNDED WARRIOR WIVES

Operation Homefront and its online community, CinCHouse.com, launched Wounded Warrior Wives, a project to provide comprehensive support to caregivers of wounded warriors. Operation Homefront's mission is to provide emergency services and morale to troops, the families they leave behind during deployments, and wounded warriors when they return home. Its popular online magazine and community, CinCHouse.com, attracts hundreds of thousands of military wives each month looking for information and advice. Wounded Warrior Wives combines the best of both to wounded warriors and their families from the crisis phase to their return to "normal" life.

"As we reach peak levels of wounded warriors returning from Iraq and Afghanistan, Operation Homefront and the military wives on CinCHouse.com are increasingly concerned about the family support system that will help these warriors return to normal—in particular, the spouses who make key health and logistical decisions while also providing emotional support," said Meredith Leyva, founder of Operation Homefront.

"Once military health care providers have done their magic, family support is key to warriors' physical and mental recuperation, yet the wives who lead the family effort have almost no resources or emotional support themselves," Leyva continued. "Wounded Warrior Wives is designed to unite and serve a new generation of veterans' families."

Operation Homefront understands the critical role played by spouses in caring for wounded warriors. While the military sees to their physical health, the key to the short- and long-term stability and full restoration of our wounded warriors lies in support of their spouses. Moreover, it is the spouses—not the wounded warriors—who are most responsible for key family issues such as financial viability and seeking assistance, so reaching out to spouses makes more sense than directly targeting wounded warriors, many of whom are recuperating from traumatic brain injuries and PTSD.

Note: In April 2010 Congress approved the Caregivers and Veterans Omnibus Health Services Act. Title 1 provides caregivers with assistance and support services, medical care for family caregivers, counseling and mental health services and lodging and subsistence for attendants.

The law includes provisions that help provide support for the caregivers of seriously injured Iraq and Afghanistan veterans, helps improve services for our nation's 1.8 million women veterans, and helps expand the availability of health care for veterans and services preventing veterans from becoming homeless. These measures and others honor the sacrifices of our men and women who have served this country proudly, the commitment and dedication of those who care for our wounded service members every day, and our nation's sacred responsibility to stand by our troops, our veterans, and their families.

Here's a quick look at what the Caregivers and Veterans Omnibus Health Services Act of 2010 does:

- Provides veterans' caregivers with training, counseling, supportive services, and a living stipend; provides health care to the family caregivers of injured veterans under the Civilian Health and Medical Program of the Department of Veterans Affairs (CHAMPVA); requires independent oversight of the caregiver program;
- Requires the VA to report to Congress on its comprehensive assessment of the barriers in providing health care to the 1.8 million women veterans cur-

rently receiving VA health care, and it requires the VA to train its mental health providers in the treatment of military sexual trauma. It also mandates that the VA implement pilot programs to provide child care to women veterans receiving medical care and provide readjustment services to women veterans;

- Expands the VA's authority to provide incentives so that the VA can recruit and retain high-quality health care providers; provides travel reimbursements for veterans receiving treatment at VA facilities and grants for veterans service organizations transporting veterans residing in highly rural areas;
- Authorizes the Secretary to utilize non-VA facilities for the care and treatment of veterans suffering from TBI when the Secretary: (1) is unable to provide such treatment or services at the frequency or for the duration necessary; or (2) determines that it is optimal to the veteran's recovery and rehabilitation;
- Establishes and increases eligibility for Iraq and Afghanistan service members, including National Guard and reserve members, to receive readjustment counseling; requires the VA to conduct a study on veteran suicides;
- Emphasizes the VA's commitment to provide medical care for certain Vietnam-era veterans exposed to herbicide and Gulf War-era veterans who have insufficient medical evidence to establish a service-connected disability; and
- Eliminates copayments for veterans who are catastrophically disabled.

For more information, go to www.govtrack.us/congress/billsearch.xpd.

9

Handling Bereavement

Nothing can prepare you for the loss of a loved one, yet when the unthinkable does happen, it may be of some comfort to know that you are not alone. There are support groups to help you through your grief, counselors to give advice on the many decisions that have to be made at this very difficult time, and a wide range of government and non-government benefits and assistance available in recognition of the sacrifice made by your service member.

GRIEF SUPPORT

VA Bereavement Counseling

VA Vet Centers provide bereavement counseling to all family members including spouses, children, parents and siblings of service members who die while on active duty. This includes federally activated members of the National Guard and Reserve Components.

Phone: 202-461-6530
Website: www.va.gov

Civilian Grief Support Resources

AARP Grief and Loss Programs

Offers a wide range of resources and information on grief and loss issues to bereaved adults and their families. Programs include one-to-one outreach support, a grief course, support groups, interactive online support groups, and informational booklets and brochures.

Phone: 202-434-2260
Website: www.aarp.org/griefandloss
Email: griefandloss@aarp.org

The Dougy Center

Offers an extensive list of books about children and grief, and addresses of child grief treatment providers state-by-state. Support information is offered for an audience of children, as well as for caring adults wanting to help a grieving child.

Phone: 503-775-5683
Website: www.dougy.org

Gold Star Moms

Provides support for mothers who have lost sons or daughters in the war. The name comes from the custom of families of servicemen hanging a banner called a Service Flag in the window of their homes. The Service Flag had a star for each family member in the military. Living servicemen were represented by a blue star, and those who had lost their lives were represented by a gold star. Membership is open to any American woman whose child has died in the line of duty of the United States Armed Forces. Stepmothers and adoptive mothers are eligible for membership under certain circumstances. Husbands of Gold Star Mothers may become Associate Members, who do not vote or pay dues. Gold Star Mothers is made up of local chapters, which are organized into departments.

Website: www.goldstarmoms.com

Gold Star Wives

An organization of military widows and widowers whose spouse died while on active duty or from service connected disabilities.

Website: www.goldstarwives.org

Grief Recovery Helpline

The Grief Recovery Helpline is a toll-free service provided by the Grief Recovery Institute, an organization that trains professionals and nonprofessionals on dealing with grief.

Phone: 800-445-4808
Websites: www.grief-recovery.com; www.fallenheroesfund.org

GriefShare

Provides a national network of support groups to assist any person suffering from grief over the loss of a loved one. Offers information, referrals, and literature.

Phone: 919-562-2112
Website: www.griefshare.org
Email: info@griefshare.org

Hope for the Warriors

A national not for profit whose mission is to enhance quality of life for U.S. service members and their families nationwide who have been adversely affected by injuries or death in the line of duty. Hope for the Warriors actively seeks to ensure that the sacrifices of wounded and fallen warriors and their families are never forgotten nor their needs unmet, particularly with regard to the short- and long-term care of the severely injured. It assists families of deceased through its immediate needs, spouse scholarships and A Warrior Wish programs.

Website: www.hopeforthewarriors.org

Rainbows

Establishes peer support groups in churches, schools or social agencies for children and adults.

Phone: 800-266-3206
Website: www.rainbows.org
Email: info@rainbows.org

Segs4Vets

The Segs4Vets program, with a goal of providing Segways to the men and women of the United States military who while serving our country in Operation Iraqi Freedom and Operation Enduring Freedom sustained injuries which resulted in permanent disability and difficulty walking, was conceived by Disability Rights Advocates For Technology (DRAFT) with the assistance of General Ralph "Ed" Eberhart.

Website: www.draft.org

OTHER ORGANIZATIONS OFFERING TRAGEDY ASSISTANCE

Air Compassion for Veterans www.aircompassionforveterans.org
American Legion Auxiliary www.legion.org
Angels 'n Camouflage www.angelsncamouflage.org
Angels of Mercy www.mcleanpost270.org
Armed Forces Foundation www.armedforcesfoundation.org
Blue Star Mothers of America, Inc. www.bluestarmothers.org
Caring for Troops www.caringfortroops.com
Children of Fallen Soldiers Relief Fund www.childrenoffallensoldiersrelief
    fund.org
Coming Home Project www.cominghomeproject.net
Eagle's Watch Foundation www.eagleswatchfoundation.org
Freedom Is Not Free www.freedomisnotfree.com
Hope Coming Ministries www.hopecoming.com/military.html
Local Heroes, Inc. mass-localheroes.org
Marine Parents www.marineparents.com
Military Child Education Coalition www.militarychild.org
National Homeland Defense Foundation www.nhdf.org
National Next of Kin Registry www.nokr.org
Operation Ensuring Christmas www.opchristmas.org
Operation Family Fund www.operationfamilyfund.org
Operation First Response www.operationfirstresponse.org
Operation Homefront www.operationhomefront.net
Operation Remembrance www.operationremembrance.org
Our Fallen Soldier www.ourfallensoldier.com
PFC Geoffrey Morris Memorial Foundation http://heroesoffreedommemorial
    .org
Project Compassion www.heropaintings.com
Project Prayer Flag www.projectprayerflag.org
Sew Much Comfort www.sewmuchcomfort.org
SOFAR: Strategic Outreach to Families of All Reservists www.sofarusa.org
Soldiers' Angels www.soldiersangels.com
Summit Supports Our Troops www.ssot.org
Tragedy Assistance Program for Survivors (TAPS) www.taps.org
U.S. Troop Support Foundation www.ustroopsupport.org
United We Serve www.unitedweservemil.org
USA Cares www.usacares.org
Veteran Love and Appreciation Fund www.veteranlove.com
Veterans of Foreign Wars (VFW) www.vfw.org
Veterans Outreach Center, Inc. www.veteransoutreachcenter.org
Warrior Foundation www.warriorfoundation.com

Society of Military Widows

Offers support and assistance for widows of members of all U.S. uniformed services.

Phone: 800-842-3451
Website: www.militarywidows.org
Email: benefits@militarywidows.org

Tragedy Assistance Program for Survivors (TAPS)

Provides support for surviving family members of deceased service members —including crisis information, problem-solving assistance and liaison with military agencies.

Phone: 800-959-8277
Website: www.taps.org

Young Widows

Provides an online support group for young widows and widowers. Also provides a listing of local face-to-face support groups, links to other related online email discussion groups and websites for young widows and widowers.

Website: www.youngwidow.org

Youth Grief Support Resources

Tragedy Assistance Program for Survivors (TAPS)

TAPS offers programs and information for parents of grieving children, literature recommendations, as well as specific programs geared towards kids, including TAPS Good Grief Youth Camp for surviving family members between 2 to 20 years of age.

Phone: 800-959-8277
Website: www.taps.org

Death Certificate

The military will assign a Casualty Assistance Officer (CAO) who should provide a copy of the death certificate within ten working days. You may need multiple copies of the death certificate as proof of death in order to settle the estate.

Burial

The CAO will work with the Military Medical Support Office to coordinate the delivery of the remains. Surviving family members should notify their CAO of the location of any burial and funeral services. Remains will be transported to that location at government expense generally within 7 to 10 days in the case of a death overseas. However, transportation could take longer depending on the circumstances of the conflict.

Under certain circumstances, the military will conduct an investigation into the casualty incident, but the military does not conduct an investigation in all instances. If there is an investigation, family members may request copies of any investigation or accident report by contacting their CAO.

All service members who die while on active duty and former service members who have received a discharge under conditions other than dishonorable may be buried in any Department of Veterans Affairs (VA) national cemetery if there is space available. National cemeteries offer a variety of gravesite options, although not all are available at every cemetery. The surviving family members may either directly, or through a funeral director, select and contact the national cemetery to make the arrangements. Eligible spouses and dependents may be buried with the service member in a national cemetery, including Arlington National Cemetery, at no cost to the family.

The deceased service member does not need to be buried in a veterans cemetery in order for surviving family members to receive funeral benefits from the military.

A military funeral is not necessary, but if requested includes an honor guard, the presentation of the United States burial flag and the playing of "Taps."

The VA provides a flag, at no cost, to drape the casket or accompany the urn of a deceased veteran. The CAO, the National Cemetery Administration or a funeral director should be able to assist in obtaining a burial flag.

Burial and Memorial Benefits

Veterans discharged from active duty under conditions other than dishonorable and service members who die while on active duty, as well as spouses and dependent children of veterans and active duty service members, may be eligible for VA burial and memorial benefits. The veteran does not have to pre-decease a spouse or dependent child for them to be eligible.

With certain exceptions, active duty service beginning after September 7, 1980, as an enlisted person, and after October 16, 1981, as an officer, must be for a minimum of 24 consecutive months or the full period of active duty (as in the case of reservists or National Guard members called to active duty for a limited duration). Eligibility is not established by active duty for training in the reserves or National Guard. Reservists and National Guard members, as well as their spouses and dependent children, are eligible if they were entitled to retired pay at the time of death, or would have been if over age 60.

VA national cemetery directors verify eligibility for burial in their cemeteries. A copy of the veteran's discharge document that specifies the period(s) of active duty and character of discharge, along with the deceased's death certificate and proof of relationship to the veteran (for eligible family members) are all that are usually needed to determine eligibility.

Under Section 2411 of Title 38 of the United States Code, certain otherwise eligible individuals found to have committed federal or state capital crimes are barred from burial or memorialization in a VA national cemetery, and from receipt of government-furnished headstones, markers, burial flags, and Presidential Memorial Certificates. For more information contact the nearest national cemetery, listed by state in the VA facilities section at the end of this book, or visit the website at www.cem.va.gov.

Burial in VA National Cemeteries

Burial in a VA national cemetery is available for eligible veterans, their spouses and dependents at no cost to the family and includes the gravesite, graveliner, opening and closing of the grave, a headstone or marker, and perpetual care as part of a national shrine. For veterans, benefits also include a burial flag (with case for active duty) and military funeral honors. Family members and other loved ones of deceased veterans may request Presidential Memorial Certificates.

The VA operates 131 national cemeteries in 39 states, of which 71 are open for new casketed interments and 21 are open to accept only cremated remains. Burial options are limited to those available at a specific cemetery but may include in-ground casket, or interment of cremated remains in a columbarium, in ground or in a scatter garden. Contact the nearest national cemetery to determine if it is open for new burials and which options are available.

Six national cemeteries opened in 2008 near Bakersfield, CA; Birmingham, AL; Greenville, SC; Jacksonville, FL; Philadelphia, PA; and Sarasota, FL. The funeral director or the next of kin makes interment arrangements by contacting the national cemetery in which burial is desired. The VA normally does not conduct burials on weekends. Gravesites cannot be reserved; however, the VA will honor reservations made under previous programs.

Surviving spouses of veterans who died on or after January 1, 2000, do not lose eligibility for burial in a national cemetery if they remarry. Burial of dependent children is limited to unmarried children under 21 years of age, or under 23 years of age if a full-time student at an approved educational institution. Unmarried adult children who become physically or mentally disabled and incapable of self-support before age 21, or age 23 if a full-time student, also are eligible for burial.

Headstones and Markers

Veterans, active duty service members, retired reservists, and National Guard service members are eligible for an inscribed headstone or marker for their grave at any cemetery—national, state veterans, or private. VA will deliver a headstone or marker at no cost, anywhere in the world. For certain veterans whose deaths occurred on or after November 1, 1990, VA may provide a government headstone or marker even if the grave is already marked with a private one.

Spouses and dependent children are eligible for a government headstone or marker only if they are buried in a national or state veterans cemetery.

Flat markers are available in bronze, granite or marble. Upright headstones come in granite or marble. In national cemeteries, the style chosen must be consistent with existing monuments at the place of burial. Niche markers are available to mark columbaria used for inurnment of cremated remains.

Headstones and markers previously provided by the government may be replaced at the government's expense if badly deteriorated, illegible, vandalized or stolen. To check the status of an application for a headstone or marker for a national or state veterans cemetery, call the cemetery. To check the status of one being placed in a private cemetery, call 800-697-6947.

Inscription: Headstones and markers must be inscribed with the name of the deceased, branch of service, and year of birth and death. They also may be inscribed with other markings, including an authorized emblem of belief and, space permitting, additional text including military rank; war service such as "World War II"; complete dates of birth and death; military awards; military organizations; civilian or veteran affiliations; and words of endearment.

Private Cemeteries: To apply for a headstone or marker for a private cemetery, mail a completed VA Form 40-1330 (available at www.va.gov/vaforms/va/pdf/40-1330.pdf), Application for Standard Government Headstone or Marker, and a copy of the veteran's military discharge document to Memorial Programs Service (41A1), Department of Veterans Affairs, 5109 Russell Rd., Quantico, VA 22134-3903. The application and supporting documents may also be faxed toll-free at 800-455-7143.

Before ordering, check with the cemetery to ensure that the additional headstone or marker will be accepted. Any placement fee will not be reimbursed by VA.

"In Memory Of" Markers: The VA provides memorial headstones and markers, bearing the inscription "In Memory Of" as the first line, to memorialize those whose remains were not recovered or identified, were buried at sea, donated to science or cremated and scattered. Eligibility is the same for regular headstones and markers. There is no fee when the "In Memory Of" marker is placed in a national cemetery. Any fees associated with placement in another cemetery will not be reimbursed by the VA.

Presidential Memorial Certificates

Certificates are issued upon request to recognize the military service of honorably discharged deceased veterans. Next of kin, relatives and friends may apply for a certificate by mailing a completed VA Form 40-0247 (available at www.va.gov/vaforms/va/pdf/VA40-0247.pdf), Presidential Memorial Certificate Request Form, and a copy of the veteran's military discharge document to Presidential Memorial Certificates (41A1C), Department of Veterans Affairs, 5109 Russell Rd., Quantico, VA 22134-3903. The request form and supporting documents may also be faxed toll-free at 800-455-7143.

Burial Flags

VA will furnish a U.S. burial flag for memorialization of:

1. Veterans who served during wartime or after January 31, 1955.
2. Veterans who were entitled to retired pay for service in the reserve or National Guard, or would have been entitled if over age 60.
3. Members or former members of the Selected Reserve who served their initial obligation, or were discharged for a disability incurred or aggravated in line of duty, or died while a member of the Selected Reserve.

Reimbursement of Burial Expenses

The VA will pay a burial allowance up to $2,000 if the veteran's death is service-connected. In such cases, the person who bore the veteran's burial expenses may claim reimbursement from the VA.

In some cases, the VA will pay the cost of transporting the remains of a service-connected veteran to the nearest national cemetery with available gravesites. There is no time limit for filing reimbursement claims in service-connected death cases.

Burial Allowance: The VA will pay a $300 burial and funeral allowance for veterans who, at time of death, were entitled to receive pension or compensation or would have been entitled if they weren't receiving military retirement pay. Eligibility also may be established when death occurs in a VA facility, a VA-contracted nursing home or a state veterans nursing home. In non-service-connected death cases, claims must be filed within two years after burial or cremation.

Plot Allowance: The VA will pay a $300 plot allowance when a veteran is buried in a cemetery not under U.S. government jurisdiction if: the veteran was discharged from active duty because of disability incurred or aggravated in the line of duty; the veteran was receiving compensation or pension or would have been if the veteran was not receiving military retired pay; or the veteran died in a VA facility. The $300 plot allowance may be paid to the state for the cost of a plot or interment in a state-owned cemetery reserved solely for veteran burials if the veteran is buried without charge. Burial expenses paid by the deceased's employer or a state agency will not be reimbursed.

Military Funeral Honors

Upon request, the DoD will provide military funeral honors consisting of folding and presentation of the United States flag and the playing of "Taps." A funeral honors detail consists of two or more uniformed members of the armed forces, with at least one member from the deceased's branch of service.

Family members should inform their funeral directors if they want military funeral honors. The DoD maintains a toll-free number (877-MILHONR) for use by funeral directors only to request honors. The VA can help arrange honors for burials at VA national cemeteries. Veterans' service organizations or volunteer groups may help provide honors. For more information, visit www.militaryfuneralhonors.osd.mil.

Veterans Cemeteries Administered by Other Agencies

Arlington National Cemetery: Administered by the Department of the Army. Eligibility is more restrictive than at VA national cemeteries. For information, call 703-607-8000, write Superintendent, Arlington National Cemetery, Arlington, VA 22211, or visit www.arlingtoncemetery.org.

Department of the Interior: Administers two active national cemeteries— Andersonville National Cemetery in Georgia and Andrew Johnson National Cemetery in Tennessee. Eligibility is similar to VA national cemeteries.

State Veterans Cemeteries: Sixty-nine state veterans cemeteries offer burial options for veterans and their families. These cemeteries have similar eligibility requirements but usually require some residence. Some services, particularly for family members, may require a fee. Contact the state cemetery or state veterans affairs office for information. To locate a state veterans cemetery, visit www.cem.va.gov/cem/scg/lsvc.asp.

Death Gratuity

The death gratuity is a one-time non-taxable payment to help surviving family members deal with the financial hardships that accompany the loss of a service member. It is a payment of $100,000 for survivors of those whose deaths occurred under the following conditions:

- A member of an armed force under his jurisdiction who dies while on active duty or while performing authorized travel to or from active duty;
- A reserve of an armed force who dies while on inactive duty training (with exceptions);
- Any reserve of an armed force who assumed an obligation to perform active duty for training, or inactive duty training (with exceptions) and who dies while traveling directly to or from that active duty for training or inactive duty training;
- Any member of a reserve officers' training corps who dies while performing annual training duty under orders for a period of more than 13 days, or while performing authorized travel to or from that annual training duty; or any applicant for membership in a reserve officers' training corps who dies while attending field training or a practice cruise or while performing authorized travel to or from the place where the training or cruise is conducted; or
- A person who dies while traveling to or from or while at a place for final acceptance, or for entry upon active duty (other than for training), in an armed force, who has been ordered or directed to go to that place, and who
- Has been provisionally accepted for that duty; or
- Has been selected for service in that armed force.

The death gratuity amount is made payable to survivors of the deceased in this order:

1. The member's lawful surviving spouse.
2. If there is no spouse—to the child or children of the member, regardless of age or marital status, in equal shares.
3. If none of the above—to the parents, or brothers and/or sisters, or any combination as designated by the deceased member.
4. Natural father or mother.
5. Father or mother through adoption, in equal shares.
6. Natural brothers and sisters.
7. Any person who acted as guardian for not less than one year at any time before the deceased member's entry into active service.

8. Brothers and sisters of half-blood and those through adoption.
9. Surviving parents, in equal shares.
10. Surviving brothers and sisters, in equal shares.

The death gratuity is not paid to any other person when there are no survivors as listed above. If an eligible beneficiary dies before receiving the amount to which entitled, such amount is paid to the then living survivor(s) first listed above.

The claim form required to apply for this benefit is DD Form 397, Claim Certification and Voucher for Death Gratuity Payment.

Retiree Within 120 Days of Separation from Active Duty

A lump-sum gratuitous $12,420 payment is made to eligible beneficiaries when death occurs within 120 days after retiring. There is no death gratuity payment for retiree's family when the retiree dies past 120 days of active duty service. The Defense Finance and Accounting Service issues this payment only if the Veterans' Administration (VA) determines death was caused by an illness or injury incurred while the retiree was on active duty. The term "active duty" encompasses full-time active reserve personnel traveling directly en route to or from or participating in annual training (AT), active duty training (ADT), initial active duty training (IADT), active duty for special work (ADSW), special active duty training (SADT) or inactive duty training (IDT) and Guard personnel traveling directly en route to or from or participating in AT, ADT, full time national guard duty (FTNGD), temporary tour of active duty (TTAD), IADT or IDT. This amount is excludable from gross income for tax purposes. The death gratuity payment is made to survivors of the deceased in this order:

1. The deceased member's surviving spouse.
2. If there is no spouse, to the child or children of the member, regardless of age or marital status, in equal shares (state laws guide payment to minor children).
3. If none of the above, to the parents, or brothers and/or sisters, or any combination as designated by the deceased member.

The death gratuity is not paid to any other person when there are no survivors as listed above. If an eligible beneficiary dies before receiving the amount to which entitled, such amount is paid to the then living survivor(s) first listed above.

Death Pension

The VA provides pensions to low-income surviving spouses and unmarried children of deceased veterans with wartime service.

Table 9.1. Death Pension Rates

Recipient of Pension	Maximum Annual Rate
Surviving spouse	$7,933
(with dependent child)	$10,385
Permanently housebound	$9,696
(with dependent child)	$12,144
Needs regular aid and attendance	$12,681
(with dependent child)	$15,128
Each additional dependent child	$2,020

Eligibility: To be eligible, spouses must not have remarried and children must be under age 18, or under age 23 if attending a VA-approved school, or have become permanently incapable of self-support because of disability before age 18.

The veteran must have been discharged under conditions other than dishonorable and must have had 90 days or more of active military service, at least one day of which was during a period of war, or a service-connected disability justifying discharge. Longer periods of service may be required for veterans who entered active duty on or after September 8, 1980, or October 16, 1981, if an officer. If the veteran died in service but not in the line of duty, the death pension may be payable if the veteran completed at least two years of honorable service.

Children who become incapable of self-support because of a disability before age 18 may be eligible for the death pension as long as the condition exists, unless the child marries or the child's income exceeds the applicable limit.

A surviving spouse may be entitled to a higher income limit if living in a nursing home, in need of the aid and attendance of another person or is permanently housebound.

Payment: The death pension provides a monthly payment to bring an eligible person's income to a level established by law. The payment is reduced by the annual income from other sources such as Social Security. The payment may be increased if the recipient has unreimbursed medical expenses that can be deducted from countable income.

Dependency and Indemnity Compensation

Dependency and Indemnity Compensation (DIC) is a monthly benefit paid to eligible survivors of certain deceased veterans.

DIC is a monthly benefit paid to eligible survivors of the following:

- Military service member who died while on active duty, OR
- Veteran whose death resulted from a service-related injury or disease, OR

- Veteran whose death resulted from a non-service-related injury or disease, and who was receiving, or was entitled to receive, VA compensation for service-connected disability that was rated as totally disabling
  - for at least 10 years immediately before death, OR
  - since the veteran's release from active duty and for at least five years immediately preceding death, OR
  - for at least one year before death if the veteran was a former prisoner of war who died after September 30, 1999.

The surviving spouse is eligible if he or she:

- validly married the veteran before January 1, 1957, OR
- was married to a service member who died on active duty, OR
- married the veteran within 15 years of discharge from the period of military service in which the disease or injury that caused the veteran's death began or was aggravated, OR
- was married to the veteran for at least one year, OR
- had a child with the veteran, AND
- cohabited with the veteran continuously until the veteran's death or, if separated, was not at fault for the separation, AND
- is not currently remarried.

Note: A surviving spouse who remarries on or after December 16, 2003, and on or after attaining age 57, is entitled to continue to receive DIC.

The surviving child(ren) if he or she is:

- unmarried AND
- under age 18, or between the ages of 18 and 23 and attending school.

Note: Certain helpless adult children are entitled to DIC. Call the toll-free number (800-827-1000) for the eligibility requirements for those survivors. The surviving parents may be eligible for an income-based benefit.

Monthly Rate (for 2011)

Dependency and indemnity compensation is paid to a surviving spouse at the monthly rate of **$1,154**.

Additional Allowances

- Add **$246** if at the time of the veteran's death, the veteran was in receipt of or entitled to receive compensation for a service-connected disability rated totally disabling (including a rating based on individual unemployability) for a continuous period of at least 8 years immediately preceding death AND the surviving spouse was married to the veteran for those same 8 years.

- Add **$286** per child for each dependent child under age 18
- If the surviving spouse is entitled to A&A, add **$286.**
- If the surviving spouse is entitled to Housebound, add **$135.**

Note: DIC apportionment rates approved by the Under Secretary for Benefits will be the additional allowance received for each child.

Whenever there is no surviving spouse of a deceased veteran entitled to dependency and indemnity compensation, dependency and indemnity compensation shall be paid in equal shares to the children of the deceased veteran at the following monthly rates divided by the number of children:

1. one child, $488;
2. two children, $701;
3. three children, $915; and
4. more than three children, $1,099, plus $174 for each child in excess of three.

The Application Process

You can apply by filling out VA Form 21-534 (Application for Dependency and Indemnity Compensation, Death Pension and Accrued Benefits by a Surviving Spouse or Child), and submitting it to the VA regional office that serves your area.

GI Bill

If the deceased service member contributed to the Montgomery GI Bill education program, the designated life insurance beneficiary or surviving spouse is entitled to a refund of any money collected through payroll deductions but not used in education benefits during the service member's lifetime.

Estate Matters

The manner in which an estate is settled is governed principally by the laws of the state of the deceased service member's legal residence.

Some assets, including bank and brokerage accounts and real property (i.e., houses and condominiums), are held by two or more persons, such as a husband and wife. In many cases these jointly held assets, such as joint bank accounts or jointly owned homes, provide for the surviving joint owner to become the sole owner automatically upon the death of the service member. This type of ownership is called "joint ownership with rights of survivorship." Ownership of these items passes automatically to the surviving joint owner, so they are not governed by a will.

When the deceased service member signed up for many military-sponsored programs, the forms gave the service member the option of designating a person, known as the beneficiary, to receive those assets in the event of death. These programs include military-sponsored life insurance and benefit plan programs like the death gratuity, Survivor Benefit Plan (SBP) and Thrift Savings Plan (TSP). Additionally, a service member usually designates a beneficiary to receive any final pay, unpaid leave and unpaid installments of a reenlistment bonus. The Casualty Assistance Officer (CAO) should have access to the forms the service member used to designate beneficiaries of military-sponsored assets. These items are distributed automatically to the designated beneficiaries, so they are not considered part of the decedent's estate and a will has no effect on their distribution.

If the service member died with a valid will in place, the distribution of the remaining assets will be made according to the instructions in the will. If the will was prepared with the assistance of a military Legal Assistance Officer, the Legal Assistance Office will assist in the settlement of the estate or will refer surviving family members to a civilian lawyer.

The will should name an executor, who has the responsibility of safeguarding and collecting the decedent's assets for distribution according to the will. The executor pays the decedent's debts and taxes first and then distributes the remaining assets according to the will.

The executor must "probate" the will by filing it, along with supporting evidence of its authenticity and a death certificate, in the local court with jurisdiction over wills and estates. Once the court reviews the will and any other necessary documentation, the court grants the executor the official power to collect the assets and to make the distributions under the will.

A person who does not have a valid will at the time of death is said to have died "intestate." That person's personal property is divided according to the intestacy laws of the state where the decedent resided, while real property (i.e., real estate) is distributed according to the intestacy laws of the state where the property is located. Generally, the intestacy laws provide for a surviving spouse, children, or parents to receive the assets.

Federal Taxes

A final income tax return must be filed on behalf of the deceased spouse or family member regardless of the timing or circumstances of death. Under most circumstances a surviving spouse is eligible to file a joint income tax return with the deceased service member for the year the death occurred, provided that the surviving spouse did not remarry before the end of the year.

In addition, under most circumstances the surviving spouse may file a joint return for the next two years after the service member's death if the surviving spouse remains unmarried throughout the year and maintains a household which is the principal place of residence of a child (including a stepchild) for whom the surviving spouse is entitled to take a dependency deduction.

The income tax return for the year in which the service member died is generally due by April 15 of the following year. However, extensions are generally available upon a timely request. Also, an automatic extension may be available because of the military service of the deceased service member. (See also Tax Matters in chapter 6 for more information about extensions, refunds and exclusions.)

If estate tax returns are required, the returns should be filed by the court-appointed executor or administrator of the estate. Federal returns and any estate taxes for the estate of a deceased person generally are due nine months after the date of death. If the deceased service member died while serving in a combat zone or died from wounds, disease or other injury received in a combat zone, special reduced estate tax rates will apply. Generally, no federal estate tax will be due with respect to any property received by a surviving spouse, whether outright or in certain types of trusts, from the deceased service member's estate, regardless of the size of the estate. The surviving family member (or the court-appointed executor or administrator, if there is such a person) should consult a tax professional regarding the filing requirements, estate tax rates, available credits and deductions and applicable deadlines.

Generally, any life insurance proceeds received as a result of the death of a service member will not be subject to income tax. However, the life insurance policy itself may be includible in the estate of the deceased service member and therefore may be subject to estate tax.

All DIC payments are exempt from tax.

Life Insurance

All members of the uniformed services are eligible for a life insurance policy under the Service Members' Group Life Insurance (SGLI) program. Coverage is available in increments up the maximum of $400,000. However, service members can, and often do, choose a lesser amount of coverage or decline coverage altogether because they do not wish to pay the full premium amount.

Service members may also obtain additional coverage from private insurance companies through individual policies or, for some reservists, an employer-sponsored group plan. Persons listed as beneficiaries on the SGLI Election & Certificate (Form SGLV 8286), a form completed by the service member, are entitled to the SGLI proceeds. A service member's records, including this form, are maintained by the branch of the service member's armed services.

If the service member did not designate a beneficiary on the form, the proceeds will automatically be paid in the following order:

1. the surviving spouse;
2. the child or, if more than one child, to the children in equal shares, with the share attributable to any deceased child to be distributed among the descendants, if any, of that child;
3. the parents in equal shares or all to the surviving parent;
4. a duly appointed executor or administrator of the insured's estate; or
5. other next of kin.

The CAO should assist surviving beneficiaries in filing a claim using Claim for Death Benefits (SGLV Form 8283). The beneficiary of a private life insurance policy starts the claim process by notifying the insurance company of the service member's death. Many insurance companies offer toll-free hotlines and websites to help beneficiaries file claims.

Social Security Administration Includes Survivor Benefits

Death Benefit

A one-time payment of $255 may be made to a surviving spouse of the deceased service member if the service member earned enough work credits to qualify for Social Security benefits. The surviving spouse is entitled to the payment if the spouse is eligible to receive the survivor benefits described below or if the spouse was living with the deceased service member at the time of death. If there is no surviving spouse, or the surviving spouse is not eligible, then a child of a deceased service member may be eligible to receive the death benefit.

Survivor Benefits

Surviving family members of a deceased service member may be entitled to receive any Social Security benefits that would have been paid to the service member. The following surviving family members are eligible:

1. A spouse or divorced spouse age 60 or older;
2. A disabled spouse or disabled divorced spouse age 50 or older;
3. Unmarried children under age 18, or under age 19 if they are still attending high school full-time. Under some circumstances, benefits may be paid to

stepchildren, grandchildren, or adopted children who can establish their prior financial dependency on the deceased service member.

4. Children of any age who were disabled before age 22 and remain disabled;
5. A spouse or divorced spouse, regardless of age, who is responsible for the care of the children of the deceased service member who are under age 16, as long as the spouse meets Social Security income requirements; and
6. Parents of the deceased service member beginning at age 62 if they can establish that they were more than 50% financially dependent on the deceased service member.

An expedited claims procedure is available to the surviving family members of service members who died during Operation Iraqi Freedom or other military operations. The Military Casualty Expedited Service Hotline will accept claims for survivor benefits over the telephone at 866-777-7887.

The Social Security office will immediately process the application upon receipt. Surviving family members may also file for Social Security benefits by calling the Social Security Administration's general information telephone number (800-772-1213) or by visiting a local Social Security office.

You will need the name, Social Security number, date of birth, and date of death of the deceased service member; and the names, Social Security numbers and dates of birth of the surviving family members making the claim, including the same information for any children.

In most cases, the claim for benefits under the expedited claims procedure will be processed for payment within 48 hours.

It is possible to receive Social Security benefits and work at the same time. However, depending on the surviving family member's age, the Social Security benefits to which the surviving family member is entitled could be reduced if the surviving family member earns more than a specified minimum. In general, a surviving spouse will become ineligible for benefits if he or she remarries before the age of 60, unless the later marriage ends by death, divorce or annulment. A surviving spouse who remarries after age 60 (age 50 if disabled) can still collect benefits.

Other Benefits for Survivorship

Relocation Travel Expenses

Depending on the location of travel, surviving family members may be eligible for reimbursement of travel costs incurred in connection with relocation following the service member's death. Reimbursement may be available for travel either to the service member's home of record, the residence of the service member's dependents or another authorized location. In order to be reimbursed, travel generally must take place within one year of the service member's death.

Shipment of Personal Effects and Household Goods

The military generally will pay for the movement of the personal effects and household goods of the deceased service member to one of the following locations: the member's last permanent duty station; the member's home of record; the home of the member's dependents; the home of the next of kin; or to other persons legally entitled to receive custody of the service member's personal effects or household goods.

Both temporary and non-temporary storage may be available in connection with a shipment of personal effects and household goods. Temporary storage may be available for up to 90 days from the date of the service member's death. Non-temporary storage may be available for up to a year from the date of the service member's death.

Assistance

Basic Allowance for Housing

Surviving family members can continue to live in military housing for six months from the date of death of the service member. If surviving family members leave military housing before the expiration of this six-month period, they will be paid the Basic Allowance for Housing (BAH) for the remaining time.

If surviving family members do not live in military housing, they may receive the BAH or, if applicable, overseas housing allowance for six months from the date of death of the service member.

VA Home Loan Guarantee

Surviving family members concerned about their ability to make mortgage payments while the deceased service member's estate is being settled should contact the financial institution which holds the mortgage to discuss the situation.

A surviving spouse may also be eligible for assistance with the mortgage through the VA home loan program. Having a VA-guaranteed home loan means that the VA Regional Loan Centers can offer financial counseling to help avoid foreclosure.

Surviving spouses of service members who died on active duty or as a result of a service-connected disability may be eligible to receive a VA-guaranteed home loan. In order to be eligible for the home loan guarantee, the surviving spouse must not have remarried. A regional VA office can provide more details on the amount of guarantee.

State Benefits

Many states have passed laws providing certain rights, benefits and privileges to the surviving spouses and children of deceased service members. These benefits include educational assistance, employment opportunities and tax relief. Information on the laws pertaining to a particular state may be obtained from local government officials, the nearest VA office, and local veterans' organizations such as the American Legion, Veterans of Foreign Wars and Disabled American Veterans.

Education

The Department of Veterans Affairs (VA) administers the Survivors' and Dependents' Educational Assistance Program (DEA), which provides education and training opportunities for eligible dependents of a service member. The program offers up to 45 months of education benefits that may be used for a high school diploma or GED, college, graduate school, business, technical or vocational courses, certificate programs, apprenticeships and on-the-job training. Benefits vary depending on the type of educational facility attended and whether the attendee is enrolled full-time or otherwise.

Checks are normally sent at the beginning of each month for the previous month's activity. Payments for on-the-job or apprenticeship training are not released until after a monthly report of hours worked is processed. If fewer than 120 hours are worked in a month, less than a full benefit payment is made. Payments for correspondence courses are made each calendar quarter after a certification of lessons completed is processed.

Sons and daughters of deceased service members are generally eligible for education benefits from age 18 to age 26. Surviving spouses generally must use any available DEA benefits within 20 years from the first date of eligibility.

Those who wish to enroll in the program must obtain VA Form 22-5490, Application for Survivors' and Dependents' Educational Assistance. The school or training program must certify to the VA an applicant's enrollment in the educational program before DEA benefits will be paid.

For surviving spouses, DEA benefits do not affect Dependency and Indemnity Compensation.

Other Benefits

• Financial reimbursement for tutors and work-study benefits are also available. The application for tutorial assistance should be made on VA Form 22-1990t, Application and Enrollment Certification for Individualized Tutorial Assistance.

- Any student receiving VA education benefits who attends school at least three-quarters of the time may be eligible for work-study benefits, including employment at the school veterans' office, VA Regional Office, VA medical facilities or approved state employment offices. Work-study students are paid at the state or federal minimum wage, whichever is greater. The application for work-study benefits should be made on VA Form 22-8691, Application for Work-Study Allowance.
- Many states offer free tuition to state-sponsored institutions of higher learning, such as state universities, to eligible applicants, while other states offer subsidized, rather than free, tuition. Surviving family members should contact the state's veterans affairs office, which will often oversee military service-related education benefits for the state.
- There are many scholarships available for dependents of service members, and a scholarship specifically designed for the surviving family members of deceased veterans. Each scholarship has its own set of criteria to determine eligibility.

Medical

Generally, surviving spouses and children of deceased service members continue to be eligible for TRICARE health benefits. The service's personnel department determines eligibility for health care coverage. Please visit www .tricare-osd.mil for more information. Surviving spouses remain eligible for TRICARE unless and until they remarry. However, under certain circumstances, if the marriage is later annulled, the spouse may regain eligibility for TRICARE.

Children of the deceased service member are also eligible for TRICARE. This includes children (1) born within marriage, (2) adopted children and (3) children born outside of marriage to a male service member whose paternity has been established in court, or who resided with the service member and received more than 50% of his or her financial support from the service member.

Children may retain their health care coverage benefits until they marry or reach their 21st birthday, whichever comes first. Children enrolled as full-time students in accredited schools can extend care coverage until their 23rd birthday. Severely disabled children may be covered by TRICARE indefinitely in some circumstances.

Surviving spouses and children of reservists and guardsmen called to active duty service for a period of more than 30 consecutive days are eligible for TRICARE.

To receive TRICARE, surviving family members must register with the Defense Enrollment Eligibility Reporting System (DEERS). DEERS is a worldwide computerized database of uniformed service members and their family members and is the key to receiving health care benefits. In order to ensure continuation of benefits under TRICARE, surviving family members must update their enrollment through DEERS each year.

Surviving family members who are 65 years of age or older must enroll in Medicare (Part B) to remain eligible for TRICARE. In addition, if a surviving spouse or child is eligible for Medicare (Part A) as a result of a disability or certain types of kidney diseases, the person who is eligible must also be enrolled in Medicare (Part B) to remain eligible for TRICARE.

Surviving family members remain eligible for TRICARE benefits at the active duty dependent rates for three years after the service member's death. At the end of the three-year period, TRICARE eligibility continues but at the retiree dependent rates, which are higher.

Conversion to the retiree dependent rates should occur automatically; however, surviving family members receiving TRICARE coverage should verify their continued enrollment at the time of conversion.

Surviving family members who are not eligible for TRICARE may be eligible for the Civilian Health and Medical Program of the Department of Veterans Affairs (VA), or CHAMPVA, a health benefits program run by the VA. CHAMPVA is a "fee for service" program, meaning it provides partial reimbursement for most medical expenses. Surviving spouses remain eligible for CHAMPVA unless they remarry before the age of 55. However, if the marriage later ends in divorce, is annulled or the subsequent spouse dies, the surviving spouse may regain eligibility for CHAMPVA.

Children may retain their CHAMPVA benefits until they marry or they reach their 18th birthday, whichever comes first. Children enrolled in accredited schools as full-time students can extend coverage to their 23rd birthday. If a full-time student incurs a disabling illness or injury and is no longer enrolled as a full-time student, eligibility for reinstatement of benefits may continue for six months after the disability ceases, for two years after the onset of the disability, or until the student's 23rd birthday, whichever comes first.

For a more complete description of CHAMPVA's benefits and costs, visit their website at www.va.gov/hac/champva/handbook/chandbook.pdf.

Dental

Generally, surviving spouses and children of deceased service members are eligible for TRICARE's dental programs. The eligibility requirements for TRICARE's dental programs (TDP) are the same as those for the health benefits.

Retirement

Military retirement benefits may include the following:

Survivor Benefit Plan

The Survivor Benefit Plan (SBP) is a monthly annuity, or regular cash payment, paid to a surviving spouse, and in some cases to the eligible children, of a service member who is retirement-eligible at the time of Dependency and Indemnity Compensation (DIC) payments and death, and who dies while on active duty. The SBP is intended to supplement Social Security benefits.

The SBP payment is equal to 55% of the retirement pay to which the service member would have been entitled if the member had retired on the date of death. This is based upon the service member's years of active service. The amount of the cash payment is reduced by the amount of the monthly DIC payment that a surviving spouse receives from the Department of Veterans Affairs. When a surviving spouse reaches age 62, the annuity is reduced to 35% because a surviving spouse becomes eligible for individual Social Security benefits. The SBP annuity is paid until the surviving spouse dies. If a surviving spouse remarries before age 55, payment will be suspended. If a surviving spouse remarries at age 55 or older, however, the spouse will continue to receive the monthly annuity for life.

If the service member elected coverage for both a spouse and for children, the full amount of the annuity is payable to the surviving spouse as long as the spouse remains eligible. If the spouse loses eligibility because of remarriage before age 55 or death, the children of the service member are entitled to the full SBP annuity. The annuity is then paid in equal shares to eligible children under age 18, or under age 22 if the children are full-time students. The coverage stops when the children either reach age 22, leave school, become part-time students or marry.

A child who is disabled before age 18, or before age 22 if the child is a full-time student when the disability occurs, is an eligible beneficiary for life so long as the disability continues and the child remains incapable of self-support. The monthly annuity for children is 55%, is payable for life for permanently disabled children, and is not reduced by DIC payments or when a disabled child attains age 62 and the child becomes eligible for individual Social Security retirement benefits.

Supplemental Survivor Benefit Plan

The Supplemental Survivor Benefit Plan (SSBP) is an additional benefit that the deceased service member might have elected for the service member's designated beneficiaries. Under the SSBP, a surviving spouse continues to receive higher benefits once the spouse reaches age 62, which is when the SBP annuity would otherwise be reduced to 35%. If the service member elected the SSBP, the total payment received by surviving family members could be anywhere between 40% to 55% of the eligible retirement pay, depending on the amount of supplemental benefits the member elected.

Reserve Component Survivor Benefit Plan

The Reserve Component Survivor Benefit Plan (RCSBP) is a monthly annuity paid to the surviving spouse or, in some cases, eligible children, of a Reserve Component member. Members become eligible only after accruing twenty "qualifying" years of service, which should be reported to the member in a twenty-year eligibility letter. In order to participate in this program, the member must have made an election within 90 days of receiving notice of eligibility. The same restrictions that affect the SBP also affect the RCSBP. If a service member is eligible for both SBP and RCSBP benefits, the beneficiary must choose to receive benefits under only one of the plans.

Thrift Savings Plan

The Thrift Savings Plan (TSP) is a federal government-sponsored retirement savings and investment plan. In October 2000, the TSP was extended to members of the military. The TSP is a defined contribution plan and is similar to a 401(k) plan. If a service member dies while on active duty, the entire account balance in the TSP is distributed to the beneficiary designated by the service member on the Designation of Beneficiary Form. Under certain circumstances, payments may be subject to tax. Surviving spouses may be able to roll over the payment to another qualified retirement plan or traditional Individual Retirement Account (IRA) without incurring federal income taxes. Payments to beneficiaries other than surviving spouses are not eligible for tax-free rollovers. Designated beneficiaries are strongly encouraged to consult a tax professional concerning the tax consequences of receiving any TSP distributions.

VA Death Pension

If the service member's death was determined to be outside of the line of duty by the VA, surviving family members still may be eligible for benefits from a VA Death Pension. Benefits would be payable if the service member completed at least two years of active honorable service.

Contact the nearest VA Regional Office for more information.

Private Retirement Benefits

Entitlement to private benefits depends on the plan and its eligibility and vesting rules, which are usually based on years of service with the employer or membership with the union. All private plans have standards that must be met in order to qualify for benefits. Only those benefits that the employee has earned and is eligible to take from the plan—the so-called vested benefits—are paid. Under many circumstances, receipt of private retirement benefits is subject to tax. Beneficiaries are strongly encouraged to consult a tax professional before making any decisions related to retirement benefits.

10

Resources

This section contains a comprehensive list of organizations, agencies, and websites offering advice, information, and support.

General Information

American Red Cross

While providing services to 1.4 million active duty personnel and their families, the Red Cross also reaches out to more than 1.2 million members of the National Guard and the reserves and their families who reside in nearly every community in America. Red Cross workers in hundreds of chapters and on military installations brief departing service members and their families regarding available support services and explain how the Red Cross may assist them during the deployment.

Both active duty and community-based military can count on the Red Cross to provide emergency communications that link them with their families back home, access to financial assistance, counseling and assistance to veterans. Red Cross Service to the Armed Forces personnel work in 756 chapters in the United States, on 58 military installations around the world, and with our troops in Kuwait, Afghanistan and Iraq.

www.redcross.org

Angels 'n Camouflage

A cooperative initiative with various organizations across the country, Angels 'n Camouflage, Inc. reinforces the importance and advantages of supporting our veterans and deployed service members. Since its inception in 2002, Angels 'n Camouflage, Inc. has helped thousands of veterans and troops through "Mail Call," and emergency assistance for those veterans homeless or injured from combat.

www.angelsncamouflage.org

Deployment Health Clinical Center

Health Clinical Center of the Department of Defense: Health information for clinicians, veterans, family members and friends.

www.pdhealth.mil

Marine Corps League

The Marine Corps League was founded by Maj. Gen. Commandant John A. Lejeune in 1923 and chartered by an Act of Congress on August 4, 1937. Its membership of 51,500 is comprised of honorably discharged, active-duty and reserve Marines with 90 days of service or more, and retired Marines. Contact the Marine Corps League at 800-625-1775, 703-207-9588, or fax at 703-207-0047.

www.mcleague.com

Military OneSource

Military OneSource is a "one stop shop" for information on all aspects of military life. From information about financial concerns, parenting, relocation, emotional well-being, work, and health, to many other topics, Military OneSource can provide a wealth of information. There are many informative topics on the website specific to wounded service members and families. For example, by clicking on Personal & Family Readiness and selecting Severely Injured Service Members, you can access topics such as "Coping with Compassion Fatigue," "Finding Temporary Work During a Loved One's Extended Hospitalization," and "Re-establishing Intimacy After a Severe Injury."

In addition to the comprehensive information available online, there are 24 hour a day, seven day a week (24/7) representatives available at the 800 number provided below.

Calling will provide you with personalized service specific to your needs. You can call the same representative back for continuity of service, as each person has their own extension. Military OneSource is closely aligned with the Military Severely Injured Center. You can call Military OneSource as a parent, spouse or service member. The information you need is a phone call away (800-342-9647).

www.militaryonesource.com

The Military Order of the Purple Heart

The Military Order of the Purple Heart provides support and services to all veterans and their families. This website includes information on VA benefits assistance, issues affecting veterans today, and links to other key websites for veterans.

www.purpleheart.org

National Resource Directory
Packed with information about employment, transition assistance, vocational rehabilitation and transitioning from military to civilian employment.
www.nationalresourcedirectory.gov

Noncommissioned Officers Association (NCOA)
NCOA was established in 1960 to enhance and maintain the quality of life for noncommissioned and petty officers in all branches of the Armed Forces, National Guard and reserves. The association offers its members a wide range of benefits and services designed especially for current and former enlisted service members and their families. Those benefits fall into these categories: Social Improvement Programs to help ensure your well-being during your active military career, your transition to civilian life and throughout your retirement; Legislative Representation to serve as your legislative advocate on issues that affect you and your family, through our National Capital Office in Alexandria, VA; Today's Services to help save you money through merchant program discounts. Contact NCOA at 800-662-2620.
www.ncoausa.org

Returning Veterans Resource Project NW
Provides free counseling for veterans and families in Oregon
www.returningveterans.com

Transition Assistance Online
The largest source of transition assistance information, jobs and tools for today's separating military.
www.taonline.com

Veterans Health Information
A list of links to civilian and military health care information.
www.va.gov/health

Veterans of Foreign Wars (VFW)
The Veterans of Foreign Wars has a rich tradition of enhancing the lives of millions through its legislative advocacy program that speaks out on Capitol Hill in support of service members, veterans and their families, and through community service programs and special projects. From assisting service members in procuring entitlements, to providing free phone cards to the nation's active-duty military personnel, to supporting numerous community-based projects, the VFW is committed to honoring our fallen comrades by helping the living. Contact the VFW at 202-453-5230, or fax at 202-547-3196.
www.vfw.org

Veterans Outreach Center
The Veterans Outreach Center proactively seeks out veterans in need who continue to suffer in silence—battling personal wars that can be won, with our

help. VOC's collaborative approach to treatment cares for the whole person; veterans receive the breadth of services needed to regain their mental, physical and economic health, reconnect with themselves and the community, and resume productive lives.

www.veteransoutreachcenter.org

Vets 4 Vets
Outreach support groups run by vets for Iraq-era vets
www.vets4vets.com

Women Veterans Health Program
Provides full range of medical and mental health services for women veterans.
www.womenshealth.va.gov

Army Reserve Websites

U.S. Army Reserves
www.usar.army.mil

Army Reserve Family Programs Online
Army Reserve Family and Readiness Program
www.arfp.org

Army National Guard Websites

Army National Guard
www.nationalguard.com

Guard Family Program
One stop to find information on programs, benefits, and resources on National Guard family programs.
www.jointservicessupport.org

Employment Support for the Guard and Reserve (ESGR)
www.esgr.org

Documents

Army: For everything you want to know about the free AARTS transcript (Army/American Council on Education Registry Transcript System), go to aarts.army.mil. This free transcript includes your military training, your Military Occupational Specialty (MOS), and college-level examination scores with the college credit recommended for those experiences. It is a valuable asset that you should provide to your college or your employer and it is available for active Army, National Guard and reserve soldiers.

Save Time and Money: Unless you know for sure that you need to take a particular course, wait until the school gets all your transcripts before you sign up for classes. Otherwise you may end up taking courses you don't need.

Navy and Marine Corps: Information on how to obtain the Sailor/Marine American Council on Education Registry Transcript (SMART) is available at https://www.navycollege.navy.mil. SMART is now available to document the American Council on Education (ACE) recommended college credit for military training and occupational experience. SMART is an academically accepted record that is validated by ACE. The primary purpose of SMART is to assist service members in obtaining college credit for their military experience. Additional information on SMART can also be obtained from your nearest Navy College Office or Marine Corps Education Center, or contact the Navy College Center.

Air Force: The Community College of the Air Force (CCAF) automatically captures your training, experience and standardized test scores. Transcript information may be viewed at the CCAF website: www.au.af.mil/au/ccaf.

Coast Guard: The Coast Guard Institute (CGI) requires each service member to submit documentation of all training (except correspondence course records), along with an enrollment form, to receive a transcript. Transcript information can be found at the Coast Guard Institute website: www.uscg .mil/hq/cg1/cgi/active_duty/go_to_college/official_transcript.asp.

Advocacy General

The American Legion
Since its founding in 1919, the American Legion has been an advocate for America's veterans, a friend of the U.S. military, a sponsor of community-based youth programs and a spokesman for patriotic values. It is the nation's largest veterans' organization, with nearly 2.7 million members and about 15,000 local "posts" in most communities and 6 foreign countries. The Legion provides free, professional assistance—for any veteran and any veteran's survivor—in filing and pursuing claims before the VA; it helps deployed service members' families with things ranging from errands to household chores to providing someone to talk to; and offers temporary financial assistance to help families of troops meet their children's needs. Contact the American Legion at 202-861-2700, ext. 1403, or fax at 202-833-4452.

www.legion.org

American Bar Association
The mission of the ABA Standing Committee on Legal Assistance for Military Personnel is to help the military and the Department of Defense improve the effectiveness of legal assistance provided on civil matters to an estimated nine million military personnel and their dependents.

www.americanbar.org/groups/legal_assistance_military_personnel.html

American Legion Auxiliary
The women of the American Legion Auxiliary educate children, organize community events and help our nation's veterans through legislative action and volunteerism. It is the world's largest women's patriotic service organization with nearly 1 million members in 10,100 communities.

www.alaforveterans.org

AMVETS
As one of America's foremost veterans' service organizations, AMVETS (or American Veterans) assists veterans and their families. A nationwide cadre of AMVETS national service officers (NSOs) offers information, counseling and claims service to all honorably discharged veterans and their dependents concerning disability compensation, VA benefits, hospitalization, rehabilitation, pension, education, employment, and other benefits. Call toll-free: 877-726-8387 or 301-459-9600.

www.amvets.org

Hope for the Warriors
The mission of Hope for the Warriors™ is to enhance quality of life for U.S. service members and their families nationwide who have been adversely affected by injuries or death in the line of duty. Hope for the Warriors™ actively seeks to ensure that the sacrifices of wounded and fallen warriors and their families are never forgotten nor their needs unmet, particularly with regard to the short- and long-term care of the severely injured.

On their own, our service members and their families are awe-inspiring in the face of their disabilities and hardships—courageous and resolute. But it is with the support of a grateful nation that they remain unfaltering in their determination and find hope and purpose beyond recovery. As a united support network, all individuals, whether of great or small means, can find an opportunity to honor those who have willingly sacrificed to defend and protect our freedom. They have designed special projects and programs that allow and encourage community involvement.

www.hopeforthewarriors.org

Military Order of the Purple Heart of the USA (MOPH)
The Military Order of the Purple Heart represents combat wounded veterans in the nation's capital. This means that the voice of the combat-wounded veteran is heard in Congress, at the Department of Defense and at the Veterans Administration. The MOPH is constantly alert to any legislation which affects its members. The MOPH also works on combat-wounded veterans' behalf. Contact MOPH at 703-642-5360.

www.purpleheart.org

National Veterans Foundation
Serves the crisis management, information and referral needs of all U.S. veterans and their families through management and operation of the nation's only toll-free helpline for all veterans and their families; public awareness programs that shine a consistent spotlight on the needs of America's veterans, and outreach services that provide veterans and families in need with food, clothing, transportation, employment, and other essential resources. Call toll-free: 888-777-4443.
www.nvf.org

Patients

Defense Centers of Excellence for Psychological Health and Traumatic Brain Injury
DCoE serves warriors and their families who need help with psychological health and traumatic brain injury issues, promoting resilience, recovery and reintegration.
www.dcoe.health.mil

Helping Our Heroes Foundation
HOHF provides funding, services, and volunteers to complement the support of our military injured in either Operation Enduring Freedom or Operation Iraqi Freedom. We provide mentors and patient advocates, identify and fund educational opportunities for the service member, coordinate specialty counseling (financial assistance, career, housing, etc.), and assist with emergency funding needs. We ask that service members approach official resources and channels for assistance before requesting support from the foundation, as we are a volunteer organization with limited financial resources. This special fund is to help service members and their families on a case by case basis. The Army Wounded Warrior Program makes referrals to this foundation.
www.helpingourheroes.org

Coalition to Salute America's Heroes
Our mission is to help provide the support needed to overcome the many challenges our returning wounded heroes face so that they may regain a rewarding and productive life.
www.saluteheroes.org

Wounded Warrior Project
The WWP seeks to assist those men and women of our Armed Forces who have been severely injured during the conflicts in Iraq, Afghanistan, and other locations around the world. At the Wounded Warrior Project we provide

programs and services designed to ease the burdens of the wounded and their families, aid in the recovery process, and smooth their transition back to civilian life. Our work begins at the bedside of the severely wounded, where we provide comfort items and necessities, counseling, and support for families. We help to speed rehabilitation and recovery through adaptive sports and recreation programs, raising patients' morale, and exposing them to the endless possibilities of life after an injury. Finally, we provide a support mechanism for those who have returned home by providing outreach and advocacy on issues like debt and disability payments that will affect their family's future. Call: 540-342-0032 or email: info@woundedwarriorproject.org.

www.woundedwarriorproject.org

Disability/Benefits

Disabled American Veterans (DAV)

The DAV is dedicated to one single purpose: building better lives for all of our nation's disabled veterans and their families. DAV provides a variety of free services to America's veterans and service members, which include reviewing Medical Evaluation Board (MEB) results, representation before a Personnel Evaluation Board (PEB), and submission of claims before the VA for disability compensation, rehabilitation and other benefit programs. Contact DAV toll-free at 877-426-2838 or call 202-554-3501 or fax at 202-554-3581.

www.dav.org

Military Severely Injured Center (MSI Center)

The Military Severely Injured Center is dedicated to providing seamless, centralized support—for as long as it may take—to make sure that injured service members and their families achieve the highest level of functioning and quality of life. If you are a severely injured service member or the family member of a severely injured service member, the MSI Center can help you cut red tape; understand what benefits are available to you; identify resources; and obtain counseling, information, and support.

Injured service members and their families can call us 24 hours a day, 7 days a week, at 888-774-1361 for this free service. A care manager will give you personal, ongoing assistance related to:

- financial resources
- education, training, and job placement
- information on VA benefits and other entitlements
- home, transportation, and workplace accommodations
- personal, couple, and family issues counseling
- personal mobility and functioning

MSI Center coordinates closely with AW2. There is a MSI Center representative at the MTF. The MSI Center also provides educational materials that can help you understand and tackle issues related to concerns that injured service members often have. This can be anything from helping children and spouses with the challenges they face, to concerns about making homes and vehicles accessible, to building new relationships.

The MSI Center also provides a Career Center that supplements the services related to career planning, including employment and benefits information for both injured service members and their spouses.

The MSI Center differs from other resources in that it has representatives from other government agencies available to them as part of the center. It also works with nongovernment (non-profits) organizations. You do not need a physician referral to use this resource. You can use this service regardless of other agencies you may be dealing with.

www.military.com/support

Veterans of Foreign Wars
The VFW has more than 100 trained service officers to assist any veteran, or their dependents, obtain federal or state entitlements. Annually, VFW service officers process thousands of veterans' claims, which have resulted in the recovery of hundreds of millions dollars in disability compensation claims for veterans. Service officers, who must pass rigorous testing and annual certification, also assist veterans in discharge upgrades, record corrections, education benefits and pension eligibility. In addition, service officers regularly inspect VA health care facilities and national cemeteries, and employment specialists monitor laws concerning veterans' preference in federal employment. The VFW also monitors medical and health issues affecting veterans as well as providing veterans with up-to-date information on diabetes, post-traumatic stress, Agent Orange exposure and Persian Gulf syndrome. To help veterans, the VFW Tactical Assessment Center is a 24-hour help line for veterans with questions or concerns about VA entitlements. Call toll-free 800-VFW-1899 or call 202-453-5230.

www.vfw.org

Other Disability Websites

Allsup Inc.—Disabilty Coordination Services
www.allsupinc.com

American Association of People with Disabilities (AAPD)
www.aapd.com

American Disabled for Attendant Programs Today
www.adapt.org

American Disability Association (ADAnet)
www.adanet.org

Consortium for Citizens with Disabilities (CCD)
www.c-c-d.org

Disability Advocacy Work With Networking
home.earthlink.net/~dawwn

Disability Rights Advocates
www.dralegal.org

Disability Rights California
www.disabilityrightsca.org

Disability Rights Education and Defense Fund
www.dredf.org

Invisible Disabilities Advocate
Helping people understand chronic, debilitating illness.
www.invisibledisabilities.com

Mays Mission
Dedicated to assisting the disabled and promoting public awareness on disabilities.
www.maysmission.org

National Alliance of the Disabled (NAOTD)
naotd.wheelboat.com

National Disability Rights Network (NDRN)
www.ndrn.org

National Patient Advocate Foundation
www.npaf.org

National Organization on Disability
www.nod.org

Road Access for Disabled Americans
www.digitalthreads.com/rada

The Disability Advocacy Council
www.disabilityadvocacycouncil.org

Victims of Crime With Disabilities Resource Guide
www.uwyo.edu/wind

Families

National Military Family Association (NMFA)

Serving the families of those who serve, the National Military Family Association—"The Voice for Military Families"—is dedicated to serving the families and survivors of the seven uniformed services through education, information, and advocacy. NMFA is the only national organization dedicated to identifying and resolving issues of concern to military families. Contact NMFA at 800-260-0218, 703-931-6632, or fax at 703-931-4600.

www.militaryfamily.org

Legal Resources

ABA Commission on Mental and Physical Disability Law

www.americanbar.org/groups/public_services/mental_physical_disability.html

DisabilityClaims.com

The resource for disability legal issues.

www.disabilityclaims.com

DiscriminationAttorney.com

Civil rights law guide.

www.discriminationattorney.com

FindLaw

Internet legal resources.

www.findlaw.com

National Disability Rights Network (NDRN)

www.ndrn.org

Neurotrauma Law Nexus

www.neurolaw.com

Disability—General

Benefits.gov

Find out which government benefits you may be eligible for.

www.benefits.gov

DisabilityInfo.gov

Official benefits website of the U.S. government. Information and benefits on over one thousand benefits and assistance programs.

www.disability.gov

Disability Information and Resources
This information-packed site is maintained solely by Jim Lubin, a C2 quadriplegic who is dependent on a ventilator to breathe.
   www.makoa.org

VA Polytrauma System of Care
Polytrauma care is for veterans and returning service members with injuries to more than one physical region or organ system, one of which may be life threatening, and which results in physical, cognitive, psychological, or psychosocial impairments and functional disability.
   www.polytrauma.va.gov

Brain Injury

Brain Injury Association of America
Leading national organization serving and representing individuals, families, and professionals who are touched by a life-altering, often devastating, traumatic brain injury. Call the family help line toll-free at 800-444-6443.
   www.biausa.org

Brain Injury Information Network
Started by caregivers who had loved ones with various types of brain injuries.
   www.tbinet.org

Traumatic Brain Injury Survival Guide
Online book regarding traumatic brain injury.
   www.tbiguide.com

PTSD

National Center for Post-traumatic Stress Disorder
The National Center for PTSD aims to advance the clinical care and social welfare of U.S. veterans through research, education and training on PTSD and stress-related disorders.
   www.ptsd.va.gov

Rehabilitation

Association for Service Disabled Vets
Rehabilitation programs serving military veterans who sacrificed their wellbeing for the freedom of the world.
   www.asdv.org

Intrepid Fallen Heroes Fund

The Intrepid Fallen Heroes Fund is a leader in supporting the men and women of the Armed Forces and their families. Begun in 2000 under the auspices of the Intrepid Museum Foundation, and established as an independent not-for-profit organization in 2003, the Fund has provided close to $60 million in support for the families of military personnel lost in service to our nation, and for severely wounded military personnel and veterans. These efforts are funded entirely with donations from the public, and hundreds of thousands of individuals have contributed to the Fund. 100% of contributions raised by the Intrepid Fallen Heroes Fund go towards these programs; all administrative expenses are underwritten by the Fund's Trustees.

From 2000 to 2005 the Fund provided close to $20 million to families of United States military personnel lost in performance of their duty, mostly in service in Iraq and Afghanistan. The Fund provided unrestricted grants of $11,000 to each spouse and $5,000 to each dependent child; and $1,000 to parents of unmarried service members. The payments were coordinated with the casualty offices of the Armed Forces, to ensure all families received these benefits. In 2005 a new law substantially increased the benefits granted to these families. With that mission therefore accomplished, the Fund redirected its support toward the severely injured.

In January 2007, the Fund completed construction of a $40 million world-class state-of-the-art physical rehabilitation center at Brooke Army Medical Center in San Antonio, Texas. The "Center for the Intrepid" serves military personnel who have been catastrophically disabled in operations in Iraq and Afghanistan, and veterans severely injured in other operations and in the normal performance of their duties. The 60,000 square foot center provides ample space and facilities for the rehabilitation needs of the patients and their caregivers. It includes state-of-the-art physical rehabilitation equipment and extensive indoor and outdoor facilities. The center is co-located with two 21-room Fisher Houses that house the families of patients.

Although sufficient funding has been received for the center's construction costs, the Fund is accepting donations to provide additional services for our wounded military and veteran heroes and their families. The Fund's Board of Trustees is currently determining, in consultation with the Armed Forces and the Department of Veterans Affairs, the next area of need for our wounded military personnel and veterans that the Fund will address.

www.fallenheroesfund.org

Amputees

Amputee Coalition of America
Aims to reach out to people with limb loss and empower them through education support and advocacy.
   www.amputee-coalition.org

Amputee Resource Foundation of America
Performs charitable services and conducts research to enhance productivity and quality of life for amputees in America.
   www.amputeeresource.org

The National Amputation Foundation
The National Amputation Foundation has programs and services geared to help the amputee and other disabled people. The AMP to AMP Program provides a home, hospital, or nursing home visit for peer counseling and support to any person who has had or will be having a major limb amputation. If the person does not live within a drivable distance, we will call them to offer the same support. The Medical Equipment Give-Away Program offers to any person in need, donated medical equipment. This includes wheelchairs, walkers, commodes, canes and crutches. Other services include information on recreational activities for amputees; booklets and pamphlets providing information specific to the needs of above-the-knee, below-the-knee, and arm amputees; hospital visits and running bingo games; contact information for veterans benefits; and referral service to other amputee organizations. Call 516-887-3600 or email: amps@aol.com.
   www.nationalamputation.org

Spinal Injury/Paralysis

National Spinal Cord Injury Association
Leading the way in maximizing the quality of life and opportunities for people with spinal cord injuries and diseases since 1948.
   www.spinalcord.org

Neurotrauma Registry (for brain and spine injuries)
Provides an inclusive resource list for those with acquired brain injury, spinal cord injury or other complex neurotrauma.
   www.neure.org

Paralyzed Veterans of America (PVA)
The PVA has a wide range of expertise in representing veterans with severe injuries, especially spinal cord dysfunction. Assistance is provided in all areas of benefits and health care issues, including: compensation, prosthetics, spe-

cially adapted housing, education and employment services, automobile adaptive equipment, health care advocacy, and other areas to assist in the transition to civilian life. Email: info@pva.org.

www.pva.org

United Spinal Association
United Spinal Association is dedicated to enhancing the lives of all individuals with spinal cord injury or disease by ensuring quality health care, promoting research, advocating for civil rights and independence, educating the public about these issues, and enlisting its help to achieve these fundamental goals. Programs include: counseling and referral, accessibility training and education, assistive technology resources, inclusion and integration advocacy, disability information and publications, educational outreach and training, wheelchair repair and parts, counseling and referral, accessibility training and education, individual and system advocacy, benefits advisement and assistance, Americans With Disabilities Act (ADA) technical assistance and advocacy, sports and recreation opportunities, and peer counseling. Call toll-free: 800-807-0192 or email: info@unitedspinal.org.

www.unitedspinal.org

Spinal Cord Injury and Disease—General Resources

American Association of Spinal Cord Injury Nurses
nurses.ascipro.org

American Association of Spinal Cord Injury Psychologists and Social Workers
psychologists-social-workers.ascipro.org

American Paralysis Association
www.apacure.com

American Paraplegia Society
physicians.ascipro.org

American Spine Injury Association (ASIA)
www.asia-spinalinjury.org

Apparelyzed
Spinal cord injury peer support
www.youtube.com/user/Apparelyzed

Canadian Paraplegic Association
www.canparaplegic.org

Christopher and Dana Reeve Paralysis Resource Center
A national clearinghouse for information, referral and educational materials on paralysis and spinal cord injury.
www.christopherreeve.org

Consortium for Spinal Cord Medicine
www.scicpg.org

The Healthy Gimp
Disability and spinal cord injury information.
www.rexdonald.com

InjuryBoard.com—Spinal Cord Injury Resource
wiki.injuryboard.com/help-center/spinal-cord-injuries/default.aspx

Paralyzed Veterans of America
www.pva.org

Push to Walk
www.pushtowalknj.org

Rick Hansen Institute
www.rickhansen.org

RVL S.C.O.R.E. International
A not-for-profit organization that assists paralyzed individuals.
www.rvlscore.org

Spinal Cord Injury Association—Greater Boston Chapter
www.sciboston.com

Spinal Cord Injury Association of Illinois
www.sci-illinois.org

Shake-a-Leg-Miami
www.shakealegmiami.org

Spinal Cord Injuries Australia
www.scia.org.au

SPINALCORD: Spinal Cord Injury Information Network
www.spinalcord.uab.edu

Spinal Cord Injury
jwright.best.vwh.net/scifyi

Spinal Cord Injury Manual for Patients and Families
calder.med.miami.edu/pointis/sciman.html

Spinal Cord Injury Resource Center
www.spinalinjury.net

Spinal Cord Society
www.spinalcordsociety.com

Syringomyelia Facts
www.syringo.org

The QUAD LINK
thequadlink.webs.com

The Spinal Cord Information Pages
Your one-stop site for all SCI information!
www.sci-info-pages.com

The Spinal Cord Injury Zone
www.spinalcordinjuryzone.com

The Steadward Centre for Personal & Physical Achievement
Formerly the Rick Hansen Center.
www.steadwardcentre.org

Treatment Centers/Rehabilitation

California Spine Institute
www.spinecenter.com

Kessler Rehabilitation Corporation
www.kessler-rehab.com

Madonna Rehabilitation Hospital
www.madonna.org

Magee Rehabilitation—Philadelphia
www.mageerehab.org

Mt. Sinai Medical Center Rehabilitation Medicine
www.mssm.edu/departments-and-institutes/rehabilitation-medicine

National Rehabilitation Information Center
www.naric.com

New England Regional Spinal Cord Injury Center
www.bmc.org/spinalcordinjurycenter.htm

NW Regional Spinal Cord Injury System
sci.washington.edu

Pushing Boundaries
Intensive exercise rehab for people with spinal cord injuries.
  www.pushingboundaries.org

Rehabilitation Institute of Chicago
  www.ric.org/conditions/spinal-injury-rehabilitation/index.aspx

Spine and Peripheral Nerve Surgery Center
  neurosurgery.mgh.harvard.edu/spine

The International Spinal Injuries & Rehabilitation Centre
  www.royalbucks.co.uk/rehabilitation.html

Thomas Land Publishers: Topics in Spinal Cord Injury Rehabilitation
  thomasland.metapress.com/content/300382

Research for Treatment/Cure

American Paralysis Association
  www.apacure.com

CenterWatch Clinical Trials Listing Service
  www.centerwatch.com

Christopher Reeve Paralysis Foundation
  www.christopherreeve.org

Claire E. Hulsebosch, PhD
Investigating the mechanisms of recovery after spinal cord injury.
  www.utmb.edu/ncb/faculty/Hulsebosch.asp

Cleveland FES Center
Restoring function through electrical stimulation.
  fescenter.org

Cure Paralysis Now
  www.cureparalysisnow.org

iCORD
International Collaboration on Repair Discoveries
  icord.org

Kessler Foundation
  www.kesslerfoundation.org

Project RESTORE
  www.hopkinsmedicine.org/neurology_neurosurgery/specialty_areas/
  project_restore

Restorative Therapies
  www.restorative-therapies.com

Reeve-Irvine Research Center
  www.reeve.uci.edu

Spinal Cord Research Centre
  www.scrc.umanitoba.ca

Spinal Cord Society
  www.spinalcordsociety.com

Spinal Research
A cure for paralysis from spinal cord injury
  www.spinal-research.org

The Miami Project to Cure Paralysis
  www.miamiproject.miami.edu

The Myelin Project
A non-profit organization engaged in research to find a way to repair myelin
as soon as possible.
  www.myelin.org

Translational Pain Research at the Brigham and Women's Hospital
  www.brighamandwomens.org/research/labs/paintrials/research

Bulletin Boards/Chat

Arizona Spinal Cord Injury Support Group
  health.groups.yahoo.com/group/azscisupportgroup/?tab=s

CareCure for the Spinal Cord Injury Community
  sci.rutgers.edu

Disability Chat Links
  www.makoa.org

MGH Neurology—Neurology Web-Forum
  neurosurgery.mgh.harvard.edu/webforum.htm

National Spinal Cord Injury Association
  www.spinalcord.org

Newsletters/Magazines

Electric Edge
  www.ragged-edge-mag.com

NSCIA Factsheets
www.sci-info-pages.com/factsheets.html

New Mobility Magazine
www.newmobility.com

Paralinks Electronic Magazine
www.paralinks.net

Spinal Cord Injury Update
sci.washington.edu/info/newsletters/update.asp

Articles/Pamphlets

Assist Cough in SCI
makoa.org/vent/assistcough.htm

Autonomic Dysreflexia
calder.med.miami.edu/pointis/automatic.html

Spinal Cord Injury Forum Reports
sci.washington.edu/info/forums/reports.asp

Segs4Vets
The Segs4Vets program provides Segways to military members who were injured while serving in Operation Iraqi Freedom and Operation Enduring Freedom resulting in permanent disability and difficulty walking.
www.segs4vets.com

Psychotherapy

Strategic Outreach to Families of All Reservists
Provides psychological services to families of reservists.
www.sofarusa.org

The Coming Home Project
The Coming Home Project is a non-profit organization devoted to providing compassionate care, support and stress management tools for Iraq and Afghanistan veterans and their families. It is a group of veterans, psychotherapists and interfaith leaders committed to helping transform the wounds of war. They help veterans and family members rebuild the connectivity of mind, heart, body and spirit that combat trauma can unravel; renew their relationships with loved ones; and create new support networks. They help build a safe space—a community—for veterans and their families to come together and share their stories, struggles and accomplishments. Single veterans are also most welcome.

The Coming Home Project offers a range of free services: workshops and retreats; psychological counseling; training for care providers; and community forums. Programs address the mental, emotional, spiritual and relationship challenges faced by veterans and families before, during and after deployment. All programs are free and confidential. Everyone is welcome.
www.cominghomeproject.net

The Soldiers Project
The Soldiers Project provides free psychotherapy for those looking for relief from PTSD or depression. The group received a large grant from the International Psychoanalytic Association to host the Hidden Wounds of War: Pathways to Healing Conference in May 2008. It was open to all therapists, veterans, current service members and their families. The Soldiers Project primarily covers all of Southern California, including San Diego, yet the network has expanded its care to Chicago, Seattle and New York. Anyone seeking help can call The Soldiers Project. Call 818-761-7438.
www.thesoldiersprojcct.org

Trauma Center of Los Angeles Institute and Society for Psychoanalytic Studies (LAISPS)
A group of licensed psychiatrists, psychologists, social workers and marriage and family therapists who volunteer part of their time to help military personnel and their loved ones prior to, during, and post-deployment from OEF or OIF.
www.laisps.org

Vision Loss

American Foundation for the Blind
Expanding possibilities for people with vision loss.
www.afb.org

Blinded Veterans Association
If you are a blind or visually impaired veteran; if you are a relative or a friend; or if you just want to get involved; write, email, or give BVA a call. The Blinded Veterans Association (BVA) is an organization specifically established to promote the welfare of blinded veterans. BVA is here to help veterans and their families meet the challenges of blindness. The BVA promotes access to technology and guidance about the practical use of the latest research. The BVA will also advocate for the blinded veteran and their families in both the private and public sectors. Call toll-free 800-669-7079.
www.bva.org

Guide Dogs

The Guide Dog Foundation for the Blind provides dogs for the blind and visually impaired.

www.guidedog.org

Learning Ally

Our vision is for all people to have equal access to the printed word.

www.learningally.org

Braille

Ai Squared

ZoomText screen magnification software.

www.aisquared.com

Braille Planet, Inc.

www.brailleplanet.org

Duxbury Systems

Braille translation software.

www.duxburysystems.com

Braille Printers and More

Key2Speak

Software that reads aloud what you type.

www.softpedia.com/get/Others/Miscellaneous/Key2Speak.shtml

Tack-tiles®

Braille learning blocks.

www.tack-tiles.com

Telesensory Blindness/Low Vision Products

The Internet Braille Wizard Access 20/20

Braille translator.

www.tbase.com

Hearing Loss

Center for Hearing and Communication

The world's leading not-for-profit hearing rehabilitation and human service agency for infants, children, and adults who are hard-of-hearing, deaf and blind.

www.chchearing.org

Hearing Loss Association of America
The Hearing Loss Association of America exists to open the world of communication for people with hearing loss through information, education, advocacy, and support.
www.shhh.org

Advanced Hearing Aid Center
www.advancedhearing.com

Nextalk
Video remote interpreting.
nextalk.com

SoundBytes
The hearing enhancement resource company.
www.soundbytes.com

Wheelchairs—Power Wheelchairs

1800Wheelchair.com
Manual and electric wheelchairs, power mobility scooters, and walkers.
www.1800wheelchair.com

21st Century Scientific
Power wheelchair manufacturer.
www.wheelchairs.com

AllegroMedical
Wheelchairs and power scooters.
www.allegromedical.com

Bruno Independent Living Aids
www.bruno.com

Durable Medical
Durable medical equipment, power and electric wheelchairs.
www.durablemedical.com

Invacare
Power and manual wheelchairs.
www.invacare.com

MobilityPro
Power wheelchairs, scooters, lift chairs and accessories.
www.mobilitypro.com

Sunrise Medical
Quickie electric wheelchairs.
  www.sunrisemedical.com

Rolltalk
Electric wheelchairs.
  www.rolltalk.com

TheMedSupplyGuide
Electric wheelchairs.
  www.themedsupplyguide.com

Wheelchairs at SpinLife.com
From walkers to power wheelchairs.
  www.spinlife.com

Manual/Sports Wheelchairs

Mobility Sports
Provider of custom wheelchairs and custom sleds for sled hockey.
  www.mobilitysports.com

Melrose Kiwi Concept Chairs
  www.wheelchairs.co.nz

MobilityPro
Wheelchairs and accessories.
  www.mobilitypro.com

SportAid-MedAid
Sports wheelchairs.
  www.sportaid.com

TheMedSupplyGuide
Manual wheelchairs.
  www.themedsupplyguide.com

All-Terrain Wheelchairs

Achievable Concepts
Adapted recreation and sporting equipment.
  www.achievableconcepts.com.au

Beach Wheelchairs
Handicapped recreational surf chair.
  www.beachwheelchair.com

Hotshot Products
www.hotshotproducts.org

Magic Mobility
Four-wheel-drive power wheelchair.
www.magicmobility.com.au

TracAbout.com
tracabout.com

Wheelchair Accessories

Aquila Corp.
Wheelchair cushion manufacturer.
www.aquilacorp.com

AllegroMedical
Wheelchairs and power scooters.
www.allegromedical.com

BXL International Sales
"K-Special Back," wheelchair seating components.
www.bxlintl.com

Diestco Manufacturing Co.
Products for wheelchairs and scooters.
www.diestco.com

Frog Legs Inc.
Shock-absorbing devices which replace the front forks.
www.froglegsinc.com

Greentyre Airless Wheelchair Tire
www.greentyre.com

Grover Gear Wheelchair Equipment
www.grovergear.com

Haseltine Systems Corporation
Containers to protect wheelchairs during air travel.
www.haseltine.com

Magic Wheels 2
Speed wheelchair drive.
www.magicwheels.com

MBL A/S Denmark
Wheelchair components manufacturer.
   www.mbl.dk

NPC Robotics
Wheelchair motor repair.
   www.npcrobotics.com

EaseCushion
Active massage wheelchair cushion.
   www.easecushion.com

WestCanProducts
Wheelchair supplies.
   www.westcanproducts.com

Scooters

Bruno Independent Living Aids
   www.bruno.com

MobilityPro
Scooters and accessories.
   www.mobilitypro.com

Scoot-Around North America
Electric scooter rentals.
   www.scootaround.com

TravelScoot
Lightweight mobility travel scooters.
   www.travelscoot.com

Other

Bodypoint Designs
Wheelchair seating accessories.
   www.bodypoint.com

Dana Douglas Inc.
Supporting all your needs, specialized models of wheeled walkers.
   www.danadouglas.com

Mobility-Advisor.com
Serves as an educational guide on wheelchair options, mobility resources and recreational outlets.
www.mobility-advisor.com

SoloRider Industries, Inc.
Multifunctional golf cart can be used for the disabled golfer.
www.solorider.com

Wheelchair
An online resource for the disabled community. It features informative articles about wheelchairs, wheelchair accessories and wheelchair sports.
www.newdisability.com

The Wheelchair Site
Independent consumer's guide to wheelchairs, scooters and accessories.
www.thewheelchairsite.com

Wheelchair Buying Guide
www.wheelchair-guide.com

Wheelchair Buying Guide
www.1800wheelchair.com

World Wide Wheelchairs
www.usedwheelchairs.com

Speech Recognition/Voice Controlled Systems

Dragon Speech Recognition Software
nuance.com/dragon/index.htm

e-Speaking
Free voice command and control program for Windows computers.
www.e-speaking.com

IBM
Embedded ViaVoice
www-01.ibm.com/software/pervasive/embedded_viavoice

Kempf Katalavox Voice Control Systems
www.katalavox.com

Continuous Speech

IBM
ViaVoice
  www-01.ibm.com/software/pervasive/embedded_viavoice

Nuance (formerly Dragon Systems)
  www.nuance.com

Synapse
TAP Universal and UNIX voice recognition.
  www.synapse-ada.com

Computer Vision and Voice

Synapse
Speech recognition systems.
  www.synapsestore.com

Augmentative Communication Devices

Prentke Romich Company
Communication without limitations.
  www.prentrom.com

RehabTool.com
Adaptive and assistive technology.
  www.rehabtool.com

ZYGO Industries
Augmentative communication systems.
  www.zygo-usa.com

Medical Supplies/Equipment

AllegroMedical
  www.allegromedical.com

ConvaQuip
Obese and bariatric patient aids
  www.convaquip.com

Elite Medical
Crutches, forearm crutches, guardian crutches, walk easy crutches.
  www.elitemedical.com

HDIS
Medical supplies.
www.hdis.com

Medical Plus Supplies
www.medicalplussupplies.com

MedLogic SuperSkin
Helps prevent skin breakdown.
www.medlogic.com

Ocelco Medical Supply
Patient aid equipment and parts.
www.ocelco.com

Posey Company
Health care products.
www.posey.com

TheMedSupplyGuide
www.themedsupplyguide.com

WHYP Inc.
Medical supplies for persons with disabilities.
www.whyp.com

Assistive Devices

Able-Phone
Hands-free phone.
www.ablephone.com

Access with Ease
Independent living products.
www.accesswithease.com

Access to Recreation
Independent living products.
www.accesstr.com

Concepts
Adapted recreation and sporting equipment.
www.achievableconcepts.com.au

Adaptive Technologies & Research
The Adapt-A-Grip System.
www.adapt-technologies.com

AllegroMedical
www.allegromedical.com

Comfort House
Products that make life easier, arthritis and independent living aids.
www.comforthouse.com

Contact Assistive Technology
Assistive listening, low vision products, accessibility, mobility and self-help aids.
www.contactassist.com

Dining with Dignity
Utensils for the disabled.
www.diningwithdignity.com

Dragonfly Toys
www.dragonflytoys.com

Dynamic Living
Solutions for easier living.
www.dynamic-living.com

Extensions for Independence
Mouthstick devices.
mouthstick.net

Flip Lacer
The belt buckle for shoe laces.
www.sheltonproducts.com/fliplacer.html

Independent For Life
www.independentforlife.com

North Coast Medical
Functional solutions for independent living.
www.ncmedical.com

Patterson Medical (formerly Sammons Preston)
Products for personal independence.
www.pattersonmedical.com

Petite Baubles Boutique
Custom medical ID alert bracelets for babies, kids, teens and adults.
www.petitebaublesboutique.com

R.D. Equipment, Inc.
Tub slide shower chair, electric leg bag emptier.
www.rdequipment.com

Seeing with Sound—The vOICe
Seeing with your ears.
 www.seeingwithsound.com

Technical Solutions Australia
 www.tecsol.com.au

The High Tech Store
 www.hightech-store.com

WestCanProducts
Aids to daily living products.
 www.westcanproducts.com

WisEnt
Products for personal independence.
 www.wisent.com

Transfer/Lift Devices

ADI Rides
Anti-slip transfer boards and more.
 www.accessibledesigns.com

Liftran Mobility
Lifts and transfers.
 www.liftran.com

Liko
Patient lifts, overhead lift systems.
 www.liko.com/na/north-america

Med-Lift & Mobility
Power lift/power recline chairs.
 www.medlift.com

MobilityPro
Power wheelchairs, scooters, lift chairs and accessories.
 www.mobilitypro.com

RAND-SCOT
EasyPivot Patient Lif
 www.randscot.com/lifts

SureHands
 www.surehands.com

Uplift Seat Assist
www.up-lift.com

Exercise

Access to Recreation
Cycles, exercisers.
www.accesstr.com

Endorphin Corporation
Fitness and rehabilitation products.
www.endorphin.net

Therapeutic Alliances Inc.
www.musclepower.com

Uppertone Unassisted
Muscle strengthening system for quads.
www.quadriplegia.com

Hygiene

AEROLET
Promotes independent and safe toilet use.
www.clos-o-mat.com/ad_aerolet_toilet_lift.html

Freedom Industries
Unique line of leg bag release systems.
www.freedomprod.com

GEBERIT
ShowerToilet
www.plumbum.com/geberit.htm

Hy-Gina Care
Portable personal showering system.
www.wheelsunlimited.com/hygina.html

PIE Medical
Pulsing water therapy for the bowel.
www.piemed.com

R.D. Equipment, Inc.
Electric leg bag emptier.
www.rdequipment.com

SelfWipe
Bathroom toilet aid.
 www.selfwipe.com

Urological

180 Medical
Disposable medical supply company specializing in intermittent catheters.
 www.180medical.com

BioDerm
Manufacturer of the external continence device for men (ECD)
 www.bioderm-inc.com/index.html

Comforthouse
Incontinence products.
 www.comforthouse.com

Grandview Wholesale Medical Supply
Incontinence supplies and medical supplies.
 store.grandviewmedical.com

Home Care Delivered
Incontinence supplies.
 www.homecaredelivered.com

LL Medico.com
Incontinence products.
 www.llmedico.com

SecurePersonalCare.com
Adult briefs and incontinence products.
 www.securepersonalcare.com

Clothing

Sew Much Comfort
Their mission is to design, create and deliver specialized clothing to recovering service members. Sew Much Comfort is an all-volunteer organization that provides free underwear, pants, shorts and shirts. The adaptive clothing uses Velcro seams enabling you to dress with ease and access your wounds for treatment. This free clothing is available to you at most MTFs. Please ask for a sample and give it a try.
 www.sewmuchcomfort.org

AbleApparel
Adaptive clothing, bibs.
www.ableapparel.com

Adaptations by Adrian
Adaptive clothing for disabilities, wheelchair users, g-tubes and orthopedic limitations.
www.adaptationsbyadrian.com

Adaptive Clothing Showroom
Large, affordable selection of special needs clothing and accessories for the disabled or handicapped.
www.adaptiveclothingshowroom.com

Buck and Buck Designs
Adaptive clothing for home health care and nursing home residents.
www.buckandbuck.com

Care Apparel Industries, Inc.
Adaptive apparel and footwear for men and women with specialty products for the geriatric and wheelchair community.
www.careapparel.com

Clothing Solutions
Adaptive Clothing for easy and enhanced dressing dignity in nursing home facilities and home health care.
www.clothingsolutions.com

Comfort Clothing
Adaptive clothing for nursing home and home health care residents.
www.comfortclothing.com

Easy Access Clothing
www.easyaccessclothing.com

Easy Does It
Special adaptive clothing featuring front closure Velcro-brand fasteners.
www.myeasydoesit.com

Farabloc Pain Management Clothing and Products
www.farabloc.com

Innovative Plums
Cosy Toes Blanket
http://www.stay-put-blankets.com/cosy-toes.html

Janska
Clothing that comforts.
 www.janska.com

Liftvest
 www.liftvest.com

Mini-Miracles
Special needs clothing for children.
 www.minimiracles.ca

MJ Designs
Adaptive and everyday wear.
 www.mjdesignsinc.com

The Odd Shoe Exchange
For amputees and people with odd shoe sizes.
 www.angelfire.com/in2/oddshoes

Personal Care Wear
Maker of the Honor Guard personal care garment and the Shower Shield.
 www.personalcarewear.com

Pip Squeakers
Fun shoes for your baby and toddler.
 www.pipsqueakers.com

Professional Fit Clothing
Stylish, affordable clothing for adults and children with disabilities.
 www.professionalfit.com

Rolli-Moden
Designer clothing for wheelchair users.
 www.rollimoden.de

Shop on the Net
Adaptive clothing, nursing home clothing, clothing for special needs.
 www.shop-onthenet.com

Simplantex
Stylish weather wear and casual wear for the wheelchair user.
 www.simplantex.co.uk

Silvert's
Special needs clothing, elderly care, physically challenged disabled clothes, fashions.
 www.silverts.com

Specially For You
Clothing for the physically challenged.
  www.speciallyforyou.net

Spec-L
Clothing needs of residents in convalescent and nursing facilities.
  www.spec-l.com

USA Jeans
Wheelchair clothing and pants designed for sitting.
  www.wheelchairjeans.com

Wardrobe Wagon
Special needs clothing store.
  www.wardrobewagon.com

Disabilities/Health-Related Magazines/Newsletters

ABILITY Magazine
  www.abilitymagazine.com

Closing The Gap
  www.closingthegap.com

Deaf Digest
  deafdigest.org

DisabledPerson.Com
  www.disabledperson.com

Electric Edge
  www.ragged-edge-mag.com

Inclusion Daily Express
Daily email news service on disability rights, community inclusion and integration.
  www.inclusiondaily.com

Mainstream
Magazine of the able-disabled.
  www.mainstream-mag.com

New Mobility Magazine
  www.newmobility.com

Palaestra
Forum of sport, physical education & recreation for those with disabilities.
  www.palaestra.com

Reach Out Magazine
Bringing people with disabilities together.
www.reachoutmag.com

Spinal Cord Injury Update Newsletter
sci.washington.edu/info/newsletters/update.asp

Family and Support

General

Army Morale Welfare and Recreation
Army recreation programs.
www.armymwr.com

Army OneSource
Website of choice for Army families providing accurate, updated articles and information on various topics.
www.myarmyonesource.com

Azalea Charities
Provides comfort and relief items for soldiers, sailors, airmen and Marines sick, injured or wounded from service in Iraq and Afghanistan. It purchases specific items requested by Military Medical Centers, VA Medical Centers and Fisher House rehabilitation facilities each week. It also provides financial support to CrisisLink, a hotline for wounded soldiers and their families, and Hope for the Warriors, special projects for wounded soldiers.
www.azaleacharities.com

Blue Star Mothers of America
A non-profit organization of mothers who now have, or have had, children honorably serving in the military. Their mission is "supporting each other and our children while promoting patriotism."
www.bluestarmothers.org

Heroes4Heroes
Heroes4Heroes supports injured military members and their families, and the Armed Services YMCA, at the Naval Medical Center San Diego and Camp Pendleton.
www.heroes4heroes.org

The Military Family Network
One nation, one community, making the world a home for military families.
www.emilitary.org

Military Connection
Comprehensive military directory providing information on job postings, job fairs, and listings.
www.militaryconnection.com

Military Homefront
Website for reliable quality of life information designed to help troops, families, and service providers.
www.militaryhomefront.dod.mil

National Military Family Association
NMFA's primary goals are to educate military families concerning their rights, and benefits and services available to them; to inform them regarding the issues that affect their lives; and to promote and protect the interests of military families by influencing the development and implementation of legislation and policies affecting them. Great publications online such as "Resources for Wounded and Injured Service Members and Their Families" and "Your Service Member Your Army—A Parent's Guide."
www.militaryfamily.org

The National Remember Our Troops Campaign
The National Remember Our Troops Campaign works to recognize military service members and their families by providing an official U.S. Blue or Gold Star Service Banner. The Star Service Banner displayed in the window of a home is a tradition dating back to World War I.
www.nrotc.org

Strategic Outreach to Families of All Reservists
Strategic Outreach to Families helps reservist families reduce their stress and prepare for the possibility that their reservist or Guard member may exhibit symptoms of trauma from serving in a combat zone. The goal of SOFAR is to provide a flexible and diverse range of psychological services that fosters stabilization, aids in formulating prevention plans to avoid crises, and helps families to manage acute problems effectively when they occur.
www.sofarusa.org

Visiting

Fisher House Foundation is a not-for-profit organization that provides free or low-cost housing at Fisher Houses run by the organization for families of patients receiving medical care at many major military and Veterans Administration (VA) medical centers. Family members must meet certain requirements to be eligible to stay at a Fisher House. The eligibility requirements generally differ from those of an ITO and they are set by the local medical treatment facility and/or installation commander. The availability of space is not guaranteed.

Through its Hero Miles Program, the Fisher House Foundation makes airline tickets available to military personnel undergoing treatment at a military medical center or VA medical center incident to their service in Iraq, Afghanistan and the surrounding area.

Qualifying servicemen and servicewomen may be given free round-trip tickets on a number of major airlines to enable their family or close friends to visit them while they are in treatment.

A Fisher House is "a home away from home" for families of patients receiving medical care at many major military and VA medical centers. A Fisher House is a temporary residence for family members and is not a treatment facility, hospice or counseling center. The homes are normally located within walking distance of the treatment facility or provide transportation alternatives to the treatment facility. There are 35 Fisher Houses located on 18 military installations and eight VA medical centers.

Typically, the houses are 5,000 to 16,000 square-foot homes donated by the Fisher family and Fisher House Foundation. Each house is designed to provide eight to 21 suites. All are professionally furnished and decorated in the tone and style of the local region. The houses can accommodate 16 to 42 family members. They feature a common kitchen, laundry facilities, spacious dining room and an inviting living room with library, and toys for children.

Local medical treatment facilities and/or installation commanders establish eligibility criteria for each Fisher House. For a referral, the service member's family should contact the service member's physician, nurse, social worker, chaplain, or other medical treatment facility staff worker. Depending on the turnover rate and waiting list, availability might be limited to families of inpatients with life-threatening illnesses. A family's income and distance from home might also be considered.

Families of casualties from Operation Iraqi Freedom and Operation Enduring Freedom do not pay for lodging. Otherwise, the cost to stay at each Fisher House varies by location. However, the cost per family per day is typically nominal (approximately $10), and many of the Fisher Houses are free of charge.

www.fisherhouse.org

Transport/Travel

Air Compassion for Veterans
The mission of Air Compassion for Veterans is to provide medically related air transport to service members, veterans and their families affected by military

deployment in Operations Iraqi Freedom and Enduring Freedom. For more information, visit the website or call 888-662-6794.

www.aircompassionforveterans.org

Caregivers

National Family Caregivers Association
NFCA educates, supports, empowers and speaks up for the more than 50 million Americans who care for loved ones with a chronic illness.

www.nfcacares.org

Health Care Websites

TRICARE
www.tricare.mil

Post-Traumatic Stress Disorder (PTSD) Resources

DoD Mental Health Self-Assessment Program
www.militarymentalhealth.org

National Center for Post-Traumatic Stress Disorder (PTSD)
www.ptsd.va.gov

Ameriforce Deployment Guide
www.ameriforce.net/deployment

Courage to Care
www.usuhs.mil/psy/courage.html

Returning Reservists Resources
www.usuhs.mil/psy/GuardReserveReentryWorkplace.pdf

Continued Health Care Benefit Program (CHCBP
www.humana-military.com/chcbp/main.htm

VA Home Page
www.va.gov

VA Health Care Enrollment Resources
https://www.1010ez.med.va.gov/sec/vha/1010ez

VA Eligibility
www.va.gov/healtheligibility

TRICARE Dental Program
www.tricaredentalprogram.com

TRICARE Retiree Dental Program
www.trdp.org

Insurance

VA Office of Service Members' Group Life Insurance (OSGLI)
www.insurance.va.gov

OSGLI Contact Information
www.insurance.va.gov/sgliSite/miscellaneous/contact.htm

Form SGLV 8286, "Service Members' Group Life Insurance Election & Certificate"
www.insurance.va.gov/sgliSite/forms/8286.htm

Form SGLV 8286A, "Family Coverage Election (FSGLI)"
www.insurance.va.gov/sgliSite/forms/8286a.htm

Form SGLV 8714, "Application for Veterans' Group Life Insurance"
www.insurance.va.gov/sgliSite/forms/8714.htm

SGLI Conversion Policy
www.insurance.va.gov/sgliSite/SGLI/SGLI.htm

VA OSGLI Frequently Asked Questions
www.insurance.va.gov/sgliSite/SGLI/deployFAQ.htm

Veterans Benefits

Department of Veterans Affairs
www.va.gov

Vet Center Directory
www2.va.gov/directory

State Veterans Benefits Directory
www.military.com/benefits/content/veteran-state-benefits

Health Care Benefits
www.va.gov/health

Health Care Enrollment—Priority Groups
www.va.gov/healtheligibility

Education Benefits
www.gibill.va.gov

Compensation and Pension
www.vba.va.gov/bln/21/index.htm

Home Loan Guaranty
  www.benefits.va.gov/homeloans

Vocational Rehabilitation and Employment (VR&E)
  www.vba.va.gov/bln/vre/index.htm

DVA Life Insurance Programs
  www.insurance.va.gov

Finance

Military One Source
  www.militaryonesource.com

Annual Credit Report
  www.annualcreditreport.com

Experian National Consumer Assistance
  www.experian.com

Equifax Credit Information Service
  www.equifax.com

TransUnion
  www.transunion.com

VA Home Loan Resources
  www.benefits.va.gov/homeloans

Get Your W-2 from myPay
  https://mypay.dfas.mil/mypay.aspx

Relocation Websites

Relocation Assistance Office Locator
  www.militaryinstallations.dod.mil

Chamber of Commerce Locator
  www.chamberofcommerce.com

Military Personnel Portals

Army Knowledge Online (AKO)
  ako.ahp.us.army.mil

Navy Knowledge Online (NKO)
  https://wwwa.nko.navy.mil

Air Force Portal
www.my.af.mil

USA Travel Source
www.usa.com

Travel and Per Diem Information
www.defensetravel.dod.mil

"Special Needs" Resources
www.militaryhomefront.dod.mil

R&R

Wounded Warriors
The Wounded Warriors organization supports families of soldiers wounded, injured or killed in combat by offering the free use of two family-friendly resorts—the Bahama Bay Resort, minutes from Disney World, in Orlando, Florida, and the Victorian Resort and Conference Center in Galveston, Texas.
www.woundedwarriors.org

Sun Valley Adaptive Sports
Sun Valley Adaptive Sports is a nonprofit organization located in Ketchum, Idaho. Since the first days of helping people learn to ski SVAS has developed a national reputation of adaptive sports excellence. SVAS is recognized as one of the country's ski programs that provide adaptive ski lessons and equipment to disabled veterans who've served in Iraq and Afghanistan.
www.svasp.org

Transition

Sentinels of Freedom
Sentinels of Freedom's mission is to provide life-changing opportunities for service members who have suffered severe injuries and need the support of grateful communities to realize their dreams. Unlike any other time in history many more severely wounded are coming home faced with the challenges of putting their lives back together. Sentinels of Freedom provides "life scholarships" to help vets become self-sufficient. Sentinels succeeds because whole communities help. Local businesses and individuals not only give money, but also time, goods and services, housing and transportation.
www.sentinelsoffreedom.org

Veterans and Families Coming Home
Provides resources for vets to ease their transition from military to civilian life.
www.veteransandfamilies.org

General Transition-Related Websites

A Summary of Veterans' Benefits
www.vba.va.gov/bln/21/index.htm

Army Career and Alumni Program (ACAP)
www.acap.army.mil

Civilian Assistance and Re-Employment (CARE)
www.cpms.osd.mil/care

Department of Veterans Affairs (DVA)
www.va.gov

Department of Veterans Affairs Locations
www2.va.gov/directory

Department of Labor
www.dol.gov

Military Home Front
www.militaryhomefront.dod.mil

Military OneSource
www.militaryonesource.com

Operation Transition
https://www.dmdc.osd.mil/ot

Temporary Early Retirement Authority (TERA) Program
www.dmdc.osd.mil/tera

National Guard Transitional Assistance Advisors
www.jointservicessupport.org

Air Force Airman and Family Readiness Center
www.militaryinstallations.dod.mil

Navy Fleet and Family Support Center
www.cnic.navy.mil

Marines Career Resource Management Center (CRMC)/Transition & Employment Assistance Program Center
www.usmc-mccs.org/tamp/index.cfm

Marine for Life
www.marineforlife.org

Military Family Network
www.emilitary.org

Housing and the Home—General

Homes for Our Troops

Homes for Our Troops assists severely injured military members and their families by raising money and providing building materials and professional labor to build a new home or adapting an existing home for handicapped accessibility. For more information call 866-7-TROOPS.

www.homesforourtroops.org

Building Homes for Heroes

www.buildinghomesforheroes.com

Home Modification Resources

The following two agencies can help answer questions in all areas, including home modification and can direct you to other resources as well. Some of these other resources are found below:

The MSI Center (Department of Defense joint resources)

888-774-1361, 24 hours a day, 7 days a week

U.S. Army Wounded Warrior Program (AW2) (formerly DS3)

wtc.army.mil/aw2

Department of Veterans Affairs (VA)

Depending on your service-connected disability, you may be eligible for assistance under one or more of the following programs administered by the Department of Veterans Affairs.

www.va.gov (access specific information on the programs at this website)

- Specially Adapted Housing (SAH) grants
- Special Home Adaptations (SHA) grants
- Loan Guaranty Service: VA Home Loans
- Vocational Rehabilitation and Employment (VR&E): Independent Living Services
- Veterans Health Administration (VHA) Home Improvement and Structural Alterations (HISA) grants

U.S. Department of Housing and Urban Development 203(k) Rehab Program

www.hud.gov

ABLEDATA

ABLEDATA is a comprehensive, federally funded project that provides information on assistive technology and rehabilitative equipment available from sources worldwide. Offers fact sheets and consumer guides through the website or by mail. Call 800-227-0216.

www.abledata.com

Adaptive Environments Center, Inc.

The center provides consultation, workshops, courses, conferences, and other forums on accessible and adaptable design. Also offers publications through the website and by mail, including *A Consumer's Guide to Home Adaptation.*

www.adaptiveenvironments.org

Army Emergency Relief (AER)

This private nonprofit service organization provides interest-free emergency loans and grants to eligible recipients. Call 866-878-6378.

www.aerhq.org

Center for Universal Design

This website is a listing of helpful advice and links, including state-by-state information. Call 800-647-6777.

www.design.ncsu.edu/cud

Salute America's Heroes

Provides financial assistance for wheelchair-bound or blind veterans to purchase homes that will accommodate their disabilities.

www.saluteheroes.org

State and Local Government

Thousands of state agencies and city and county governments.

Home Automation

Adaptivation

Technology for people with mild to severe disabilities.

www.adaptivation.com

Applied Future Technologies, Inc.

www.appliedfuture.com

Home Automation Inc.

www.homeauto.com

Home Controls, Inc.

Home Automation Products

www.homecontrols.com

Home Automation Systems, Inc.

Home Automation Products

www.smarthome.com

HomeVision Home Automation Controller
www.csi3.com/homevis2.htm

IntellaVoice
Giving Every X-10 Automated Home a Voice
www.intellahome.com

JDS Technologies
Home Automation and Environmental Control
www.jdstechnologies.com

Leviton Mfg
Home automation, lighting controls
www.leviton.com

Omnipotence Software
ECS (Event Control System) Home Automation Software
omnipotencesoftware.com

PacificCable.com
X-10 home automation.
www.pacificcable.com

Personal Assistance Systems
smarthome.com

Rolltalk (Norway)
Electric wheelchairs with ECU.
www.rolltalk.com

SmartHome Discounts
www.smarthomediscounts.com

SMARTworld (Australia)
Home automation.
www.smart.com.au

X-10 Pro
Home automation products.
www.x10pro.com

X-10 USA
Home automation products.
www.x10.com

Telephones

Able-Phone
Adaptive telephones (switch or voice activated).
  www.ablephone.com

Accessible Cell Phones
Accessible cell phones for people with physical disabilities, the blind and visually impaired, the deaf and hard of hearing, people with cognitive disabilities and the elderly.
  www.etoengineering.com

Ameriphone
Assistive telephones (switch activated, TTY, big button, amplified).
  www.clarityproducts.com

ASL Product
Wireless remote telephone.
  www.asl-inc.com

GEWA Jupiter Speaker-Telephone
Hands-free telephone access.
  www.zygo-usa.com

Liberty Bell Communication System
Hands-free, 24-volt system, and TDMA, CDMA, or GSM phone (complete system) for wheelchair.
  www.planetmobility.com/store/phones

Vocalize
Voice-controlled Bluetooth cell phone system.
  www.broadenedhorizons.com/vocalize.htm

Microphones

Andrea Electronics
  www.andreaelectronics.com

Labtec
  www.labtec.com

Koss Corporation
  www.koss.com

Telex Computer Audio
Microphones and headsets for speech dictation, voice recognition, telephony, and cellular.
  www.telex.com

Shure TCHS Computer Wireless System
www.shure.com/wireless/default.asp

Switches

Artificial Language Laboratory Switches
www.msu.edu/~artlang/Switches.html

ASL Product
Wireless infrared transmitters/receivers and mouse emulators.
www.asl-inc.com

SCATIR Switch Page
www.msu.edu/~artlang/SCATIR.html

TAS Switch
www.msu.edu/~artlang/TAS.html

Enabling Devices
Toys for special children and enabling devices.
enablingdevices.com/catalog

Bed and Comfort Products

Air Support Therapies
users.erols.com/airsuprt

Aquila Corp
Wheelchair cushion manufacturer.
www.aquilacorp.com

FloCare Flotation
Health care water mattresses and waterbeds.
www.flobeds.com

Invacare Standard Products Group
www.invacare.com

Tempest International
Therapeutic Support Surfaces
www.tempestinternatrional.com/products

Turnsoft
Automatic turning mattress heals "decubitus."
www.turnsoft.com/tssystem.html

The EASE
Active Massage Wheelchair Cushion
www.easecushion.com

Environmental Control

Angel ECU
www.angelecu.com

Automatic Door Openers & Environmental Control Units for Disabled
www.barrier-free.com

Break Boundaries
REACH (Remote Electronic Access & Control Hands-free) Candle Automation
—The Butler™ controls your home's lighting with your voice commands.
www.breakboundaries.com

NanoPac—CINTEX4
An environmental control system for use with voice recognition systems (such as DragonDictate, NaturallySpeaking) or any other keyboard replacement.
www.nanopac.com

Home Automated Living
HAL2000 Home Automation voice recognition technology.
www.automatedliving.com

InterAct Plus
Imperium® Environmental Control System
www.ablenetinc.com/Home/Products/TashProducts

KELVIN Talking Thermostat
A voice-interactive programmable thermostat for the visually impaired, disabled, elderly or anyone who has difficulty seeing and programming a standard thermostat.
www.independentliving.com/prodinfo.asp?number=756990

Mastervoice—BUTLER-IN-A-BOX™
Home Automation & Voice Recognition Systems
www.avsi.us

Minomech Enterprises
Providing interfaces for computers, telephones, light switches or power-switches.
www.minomech.com

Multimedia Designs Inc.
Multimedia Max—voice operated computer and environmental control.
www.multimediadesigns.com

Q Systems Engineering
HomeSaver
www.qsystemsengineering.com

Quartet Technologies
Simplicity Series EC using Voice and/or Switches
www.qtiusa.com

SRS Technology Ltd
Smart home technology.
www.srstechnology.co.uk

XTG
Activate—a software package designed to interface voice recognition capabilities of the desktop PC with integrated control systems.
www.xtg.com

ZYGO Industries
Environmental Control Systems
www.zygo-usa.com

Lifts and Ramps

Adaptive Engineering Ltd.
www.adaptivelifts.com

All-ways Accessible, Inc.
www.awalifts.com

Ascension Portable Wheelchair Lifts
ADA-compliant portable wheelchair lifts that do not require a ramp.
www.wheelchairlift.com

Comforthouse
www.comforthouse.com/comfort.wheelram.html

Savaria
Elevators, lifts, stairlifts, van conversions
www.savaria.com

Discount Ramps
Affordable wheelchair ramps, wheelchair lifts, and other accessories
www.discountramps.com/portable_ramps.htm

EZ-Access
ezaccess.com

Garaventa Accessiblity
Stair-Lifts, vertical residential lifts and an emergency evacuation device for the mobility-impaired.
www.garaventa.ca

LiteRamp
Portable Wheelchair Ramps and Scooter Ramps
www.literamp.com

Loading Ramps
www.loadingramps.com

movemanSKG
Designs, supplies and installs platform lifts for wheelchair users.
www.moveman.co.uk

Pollock Lifts
Through floor domestic lifts, stair lifts, step lifts, platform lifts and overhead hoists.
www.pollocklifts.co.uk

Premier Lift Products
Residential elevators, commercial & residential wheelchair lifts
www.premierliftproducts.com

Startracks Mobility
Affordable Accessible Lift and Mobility Products
www.startracksmobility.com

ThyssenKrupp
www.tkaccess.com/wheelchair-lifts/wheelchairLifts.aspx

Transportation

Absolute Mobility Center
Northwest's largest dealer and rental service for wheelchair accessible vans
www.absolutemobilitycenter.com

Adaptive Equipment & Vehicles
Modified for Persons with Disabilities (NHTSA)
www.nhtsa.dot.gov/cars/rules/adaptive

Access AMS
Wheelchair Accessible Vans and Adaptive Driving Aids
www.accessams.com

Access Industries
Accessible vans
www.access-ind.com

Access Unlimited
Adaptive Transportation And Mobility Technology
www.accessunlimited.com

Accessible Vans of America
www.accessiblevans.com

AMS Vans, Inc.
Nationwide provider of wheelchair-accessible transportation
www.amsvans.com

Associated Handicapable Vans
www.rollxvans.com

Automotive Innovations
www.ai1.com/index.html (that's a "one" in "ai1")

Bruno Independent Living Aids
www.bruno.com

Braun Ability
www.braunability.com

Braun Corporation
Leader in handicapped-accessible vehicles, wheelchair lifts
www.braunlift.com

Freedom Motors
www.fminow.com

MobilityWorks!
www.mobilityworks.com

Mobility Sales
Wheelchair vans, Handicapped Vans—Nationwide Sales & Rental
www.mobilitysales.com

Motion Automotive Specialty
Meeting the Transportation Needs of the Physically Challenged
www.motionautomotive.com

Transit Plus Inc.
www.transitplus.com

Wheelchair Getaways
Wheelchair-accessible van rentals
   www.blvd.com/Travel_and_Recreation

Wheelchair Vans of America
   www.wheelchairvansofamerica.com

Homelessness

U.S. VETS
U.S. VETS is dedicated to helping homeless veterans. More than 250,000
veterans will sleep on the streets of our nation tonight. Our vision is that one
day there will no longer be homeless veterans in America. Contact U.S.
VETS at 202-546-6994 or by fax at 202-546-6748.
   www.usvetsinc.org

Financial

Social Security
The Social Security Administration has information which can help you understand better its programs and services.
   www.ssa.gov/woundedwarriors

The Social Security Office of Disability Home Page
   www.ssa.gov/pgm/disability.htm

Social Security Disability Secrets
   www.disabilitysecrets.com

Information About the Social Security Disability Program
   www.ssa.gov/pubs/10029.html

Frequently Asked Questions & Answers
   ssa-custhelp.ssa.gov

Social Security publications available
   www.ssa.gov/pubs

A few of the disability-related publications available:
How Work Affects Your Benefits
   www.ssa.gov/pubs/10069.html

Medicare
   www.ssa.gov/pubs/10043.html

Disability Benefits
   www.ssa.gov/pubs/10029.html

How We Decide If You Are Still Disabled
www.ssa.gov/pubs/10053.html

Survivors Benefits
www.ssa.gov/pubs/10084.html

Supplemental Security Income (SSI)
www.ssa.gov/pubs/11000.html

The Appeals Process
www.ssa.gov/pubs/10041.html

What You Need to Know When You Get Disability Benefits
www.ssa.gov/pubs/10153.html

What You Need to Know When You Get Your Retirement or Survivors Benefits
www.ssa.gov/pubs/10077.html

Working While Disabled—How We Can Help
www.ssa.gov/pubs/10095.html
pdf: www.ssa.gov/pubs/10095.pdf

Social Security: Understanding the Benefits
www.ssa.gov/pubs/10024.html
pdf: www.ssa.gov/pubs/10095.pdf

Financial Aid

Army Emergency Relief
AER is the Army's own emergency financial assistance organization and is dedicated to "Helping the Army Take Care of Its Own." AER provides commanders a valuable asset in accomplishing their basic command responsibility for the morale and welfare of service members.
www.aerhq.org

Operation First Response
Operation First Response's mission is to assist the wounded military and their families with personal and financial needs who are serving our country during Operation Iraqi Freedom and forward. Website includes online application for assistance.
www.operationfirstresponse.org

Evan Ashcraft Memorial Foundation
Provides funds to veterans and dependents of OIF for education and health care needs.
www.evanashcraft.org

Unmet Needs
VFW-sponsored program to help military families with financial hardship. Apply online or download an application from this website.
   www.vfw.org/Assistance/National-Military-Services

USA Cares
USA Cares is dedicated to helping service members and their families with quality of life issues using grants, counseling and mentorship. Requests for financial assistance can be done online.
   www.usacares.org

The Coalition to Salute America's Heroes
The Coalition to Salute America's Heroes was created to provide a way for individuals, corporations and others to help severely wounded and disabled Operation Enduring Freedom and Operation Iraqi Freedom veterans and their families. Founded in 2004 the coalition works with corporate sponsors, individual contributors and volunteers to provide an easy way for individuals and corporations to help veterans and their families rebuild their lives. You can help through tax-deductible donations, participating in programs that raise money, giving your time and by corporate sponsorships. Ninety-one percent of all money contributed goes directly to service members and their families.
   www.saluteheroes.org

Wounded EOD Warrior Foundation
The Wounded EOD Warrior Foundation is a nonprofit organization that provides funds and support to Explosive Ordnance Disposal families caring for their loved ones at military medical facilities. The support can include plane fare, accommodations, food vouchers or other travel expenses. Eligible families can also use benefits for other needs such as child care, mortgage and rent relief while visiting service members. The foundation depends on fundraisers and donations. It's the generosity of others that allows us to offer "compassionate solutions" to our Wounded EOD Warriors and their families during difficult times.
   www.woundedeodwarrior.org

Possible Alternative Technology Funding Sources/Low Cost

Assistive Technology Funding and Systems Change Project (ATFSCP)
   www.icdri.org/Assistive%20Technology/atfs.htm

Non-Profit Refurbished Computers Available for Disabled
   www.makoa.org/psa/computer.htm

Financing Assistive Technology: Handbook for Funding
   trace.wisc.edu/archive/fintech/fintech.html

emachines
www.emachines.com

WebTV
watap.org/resources/index.php?cat=2

Education and Training

Education

Operation Life Transformed
Operation Life Transformed provides military spouses, war-wounded care-givers and wounded soldiers funding for training in careers that are portable and flexible; the types suited to the military lifestyle. OLT partners with colleges and corporations for training, certification and licensing programs that lead to appropriate jobs.
www.operationlifetransformed.org

Education/Training Websites

VA Education Services (GI Bill)
www.gibill.va.gov

VA Regional Office Finder
www2.va.gov/directory

The Defense Activity for Non-Traditional Education Support (DANTES)
www.dantes.doded.mil/DANTES_Homepage.html

Department of Defense Voluntary Education Program
www.voled.doded.mil

Army (AARTS) Transcript
aarts.army.mil

Navy and Marine Corps (SMART) Transcript
https://smart.navy.mil/smart/welcome.do

Air Force (CCAF) Transcript
www.au.af.mil/au/ccaf

Coast Guard Institute Transcript
www.uscg.mil/hr/cg

Federal Financial Student Aid
federalstudentaid.ed.gov

Application Pell Grants or Federal Stafford Loans (FAFSA)
www.fafsa.ed.gov

Veterans' Upward Bound
www.navub.org

Education Resources

Students Seeking Disability Related Information
www.abilityinfo.com

AHEAD: Association on Higher Education and Disability
www.ahead.org

American Council on Education
www.acenet.edu

National Center for Learning Disabilities
www.ncld.org

OSERS: National Institute on Disability & Rehabilitation Research (NIDRR)
www2.ed.gov/about/offices/list/osers/nidrr/index.html

University Resources

Centennial College Centre for Students with Disabilities (CSD)
www.centennialcollege.ca/csd

Coalition of Rehab Engineering Research Organizations
crero.org

Curry School of Education
curry.virginia.edu

George Washington University Rehabilitation Counselor Education Programs
www.gwu.edu/~chaos

Iowa State University Student Disability Resources
www.dso.iastate.edu/dr

Johns Hopkins University Physical Medicine and Rehabilitation
www.hopkinsmedicine.org/rehab

Nebraska Assistive Technology Project
www.atp.ne.gov

Northwestern University Rehab Engineering, Prosthetics and Orthotics
www.nupoc.northwestern.edu

Ohio State University Disability Services
ods.osu.edu

Oklahoma State University National Clearing House of Rehabilitation Training Material
ncrtm.org

Tarleton State University
www.tarleton.edu

Thomas Edison State College Distance Learning
www.tesc.edu

University of California Berkeley School of Psychology
gse.berkeley.edu/program/sp/sp.html

University of California Los Angeles Disabilities and Computing Program
dcp.ucla.edu

University of Delaware Office of Disabilities Support Services
www.udel.edu/DSS

University of Georgia Disability Services
drc.uga.edu

University of Illinois at Urbana-Champaign Disability Resources
www.disability.illinois.edu

University of Kansas Medical Center, School of Allied Health
www.alliedhealth.kumc.edu

University of Minnesota Disability Services
ds.umn.edu

University of New Hampshire Institute on Disability
www.iod.unh.edu

University of Washington Department of Rehab Medicine
rehab.washington.edu

Victorian University, TAFE Services
www.vu.edu.au/higher-ed-and-tafe

West Virginia University Rehabilitation Research and Training Center (WVRTC)
www.icdi.wvu.edu

Wright State University Rehabilitation Engineering Info & Training
www.wright.edu/~aja.ash

Assistive Technology Programs

Applied Assistive Technology
www.atole.com

Arizona Technology Access Program
www.nau.edu/ihd/aztap

Maryland Technology Assistance Program
www.mdod.maryland.gov/MTAP%20Home.aspx

Oklahoma ABLE Tech Home Page
www.ok.gov/abletech

Partnerships in Assistive Technology
www.pat.org

UCP/NYC—Assistive Technology
www.ucpnyc.org

Washington Assistive Technology Alliance
watap.org

Wyoming New Options in Technology (WYNOT)
www.uwyo.edu/wind/watr

Financial Aid

fastWEB!
Financial Aid Search Through the Web
www.fastweb.com

FinAid
The Financial Aid Information Page
www.finaid.org

Financial Aid for Disabled Students
www.finaid.org/otheraid/disabled.phtml

FreSch!
www.freschinfo.com

MIUSA Financial Aid & Scholarship Options for Disability and Exchange
www.miusa.org

Workplace Technology Foundation
Offers micro-grants and awards to people with disabilities seeking education
or employment.
www.workplacefoundation.org

Transition Resources

Recovery and Employment Lifelines
The program seeks to support the economic recovery and reemployment of transitioning wounded and injured service members and their families by identifying barriers to employment or reemployment and addressing those needs. The program facilitates collaboration of federal and state programs and services with follow-up and technical assistance to assure success of wounded and injured service members. Call 888-774-1361.
www.dol.gov/vets/programs/Real-life/main.htm

E-VETS Resource Advisor
The e-VETS Resource Advisor assists veterans preparing to enter the job market. It includes information on a broad range of topics, such as job search tools and tips, employment openings, career assessment, education and training, and benefits and special services available to veterans. The e-VETS Resource Advisor was created to help veterans and their family members sort through the vast amount of information available on the Internet. Based on your personal profile and/or the various services you select, the e-VETS Resource Advisor will provide a list of website links most relevant to your specific needs and interests. The e-VETS Resource Advisor is one of several elaws Advisors developed by the U.S. Department of Labor to help employees and employers understand their rights and responsibilities under numerous Federal employment laws. The e-VETS Resource Advisor has two sections: General Services and Personal Profile. You are encouraged to use both sections to achieve the best results.
www.dol.gov/elaws/evets.htm

Army Community Service Employment Readiness Program
The goal and focus of this program is to help the military spouse find employment. The program provides education, employment, and volunteer information as well as career counseling and coaching. Job search assistance is provided.
www.myarmyonesource.com

Transition Assistance Program (TAP)
Program is geared to soldiers separating from the service. Pre-separation counseling, veterans' benefits briefings, and pre-discharge program are offered.
www.turbotap.org

Heroes to Hometowns
Helping severely injured service members and their families connect with their hometowns or new communities. The recuperation time after hospitalization and rehabilitation is crucial to an individual's recovery. Knowing that they are welcome in their new community and that there is a new life ahead can be the most significant part of this process.

The purpose of the Heroes to Hometowns Program is to help communities:

- Recognize the severely injured and embrace them as part of the community
- Assist them in making a seamless transition into their new hometown
- Provide a support network they can access when needed
- This program will promote community growth and:
  - Bring in a "champion" to support your community, or reach out to assist another community in need
  - Rally the community to provide what is needed
  - Connect the community with nationwide efforts and nationally accessible resources
  - Keep the community informed of severely injured service members interested in becoming a member of the community
  - Comfort all active duty and reserve military and their families by knowing that their communities support them

Call the Military Severely Injured Center at 888-774-1361 for more information or Pentagon Severely Injured Center at 703-692-2052.
  www.legion.org/heroes

Seamless Transition Assistance Program
  www.oefoif.va.gov

Seamless Transition Benefits
- Compensation and Pension—VA website hosting benefits information for veterans with disabilities.
- Education—Information on VA education benefits available for veterans.
- Home Loan Guaranty—VA's Home Loan Guaranty eligibility website.
- Vocational Rehabilitation and Employment—Rehabilitation counseling and employment advice for veterans who are disabled and in need of help readjusting.
- Insurance—VA life insurance program for disabled veterans.
- Burial—Information on burial benefits for certain qualified veterans.
- Women Veteran Benefits and the Center for Women Veterans—Two separate websites where you will find benefits issues and other programs unique to women veterans.
- Health and Medical Services—VA website for complete health and medical services information.
- Medical Care for Combat Theater Veterans—VA website with specific information for veterans of combat theater of operations.
- Special Health Benefits Programs for Veterans of Operations Enduring Freedom / Iraqi Freedom—VA health information website for OEF/OIF veterans specific to environmental agents issues.

- HealtheVet Web Portal—VA's NEW health portal has been developed for the veteran and family—to provide information and tools to enable one to achieve the best health.
- CHAMPVA (Civilian Health and Medical Program of the Department of Veterans Affairs)—CHAMPVA is a federal health benefits program administered by the Department of Veterans Affairs. CHAMPVA is a Fee for Service (indemnity plan) program. CHAMPVA provides reimbursement for most medical expenses—inpatient, outpatient, mental health, prescription medication, skilled nursing care, and durable medical equipment (DME). There is a very limited adjunct dental benefit that requires pre-authorization. CHAMPVA is available to certain veterans' family members who are not eligible for TRICARE.
- Transitioning from War to Home—Go to the VA website of the Vet Center Readjustment Counseling Service. Provides war veterans and their family members quality readjustment services in a caring manner, assisting them toward a successful post-war adjustment in or near their respective communities.
- State Benefits—Many states offer benefits for veterans. You should contact the VA regional office that serves your area to find out what your state may offer. You will find the area(s) served in the right-hand column of the web page at the other end of the link.

Work and Employment

Army Career and Alumni Program (ACAP)
The ACAP serves transitioning soldiers, veterans, retirees, and their family members. Services include a wide range of transition and job assistance activities. The ACAP has 53 centers and satellite offices, in locations around the world, which provide on-site services. Additionally, the ACAP website provides contact information for each center and satellite office, as well as a wealth of information and tools for clients who are not located near an ACAP facility. ACAP is also dedicated to serving soldiers, retirees, and veterans with severe service-connected disabilities.

http://myarmybenefits.us.army.mil/Home/Benefit_Library/Federal_Benefits_Page.html

The Army AW2 Soldier Connection
This website provides employers and disabled soldiers the ability to connect. Participating employers make employment opportunities available and provide an AW2 point of contact, who can provide interested soldiers with more information about employment opportunities for disabled veterans. Contact ACAP at 571-226-5043.

www.acap.army.mil

Give a Vet a Chance
GAVAC was incorporated for the purpose of helping out our nation's honorably discharged veterans and disabled veterans. Men and women from all over this nation, after having served in our Armed Forces, today, own and operate their own small businesses, but they need our support. During deployments, these men and women left behind their families and their businesses, to defend our beliefs. While they were serving, their businesses suffered, their families suffered, and their communities suffered. Some came home disabled for life, some never made it back. GAVAC's goal is to help out these heroes. With free advertising for their businesses, support and training for them, and nationwide networking, we aim to help them rebuild their lives, and their families' lives.

www.giveavetachance.com

Operation Warfighter
The purpose of this program is to provide service members with meaningful activity outside the hospital environment, and to offer them a formal means of transition back into the workforce. This is a voluntary program and has orientation sessions at the MTF. Call the Military Severely Injured Center for details: 888-774-1361.

www.militaryhomefront.dod.mil/tf/operationwarfighter

Swords to Plowshares
Founded in 1974, Swords to Plowshares is a community-based, not-for-profit organization that provides counseling and case management, employment and training, housing, and legal assistance to more than 1,500 homeless and low-income veterans annually in the San Francisco Bay Area and beyond. We promote and protect the rights of veterans through advocacy, public education, and partnerships with local, state, and national entities.

www.swords-to-plowshares.org

Employment Assistance

Employer Support of the Guard and Reserve (ESGR)
www.esgr.org

Department of Labor Resources
www.careeronestop.org
www.doleta.gov/programs
www.doleta.gov/jobseekers

One-Stop Career Center
www.servicelocator.org

Federal Job Search
www.usajobs.gov

DoD Civilian Careers
www.godefense.com

DoD Job Search
www.dod.jobsearch.org

Fed World Job Resource
www.fedworld.gov

Federal Employment Portal
www.opm.gov

Army Civilian Personnel Online
www.cpol.army.mil

Troops to Cops
www.cops.usdoj.gov

Career InfoNet
www.acinet.org/acinet

Careers in Government
www.careersingovernment.com

Vocational Information Center
www.khake.com

The Riley Guide
www.rileyguide.com

Veterans Employment and Training Service (VETS)
www.dol.gov/vets

DoD Spouse Career Center
www.military.com/spouse

Helpful Career Related Resources
www.military.com/veteran-jobs

Army Credentialing Opportunities Online (COOL)
www.army.mil/info/armylife/careermanagement

Navy Credentialing Opportunities Online (COOL)
https://www.cool.navy.mil

Helmets to Hardhats (H2H)
helmetstohardhats.org

Occupational Information Network (O*NET)
online.onetcenter.org

The Encyclopedia of Associations
library.dialog.com/bluesheets/html/bl0114.html

The Occupational Outlook Handbook
www.bls.gov/oco/home.htm

Military and Veteran Service Organizations
www.military.com/benefits/resources/military-and-veteran-associations

Troops to Teachers (TTT)
www.proudtoserveagain.com

State Employment Office Locator
www.naswa.org

Entrepreneurship and Business

U.S. Small Business Administration (SBA)
www.sba.gov

HUBZone Empowerment Contracting Program
https://eweb1.sba.gov/hubzone/internet

Veterans Business Outreach Centers (VBOC)

The Research Foundation of SUNY
www.rfsuny.org

The University of West Florida in Pensacola
www.vboc.org

The University of Texas–Pan American
www.coserve.org/vboc

Vietnam Veterans of California
www.vboc-ca.org

SCORE: Counselors to America's Small Business
www.score.org

Office of Small and Disadvantaged Business Utilization
www.osdbu.dot.gov

Center for Veterans Enterprise (CVE)
www.vetbiz.gov

Association of Small Business Development Centers (ASBDC)
www.asbdc-us.org

International Franchise Association (IFA)
www.franchise.org

Computers and Technology

Communications Devices

Computer/Electronic Accommodations Program (CAP)
CAP is committed to providing assistive technology and support to returning wounded service members. Accommodations are available for wounded service members with vision or hearing loss, upper extremity amputees as well as persons with communication and other disabilities to access the computer and telecommunication environment. Call: 703-681-8813 (V/TTY).
www.tricare.osd.mil/cap

Computer Adaptive Technologies

AbilityHub
Assistive technology for computers and disability.
www.abilityhub.com

Abledata Computer Access
www.abledata.com

About One Hand Typing and Keyboarding
www.aboutonehandtyping.com

Assistive Devices for Use with Personal Computers
makoa.org

Compusult Jouse2
Joystick-based mouse and keyboard alternative with built-in Morse code capability.
www.jouse.com

Darci Institute
Darci Too Keyboard and Mouse Emulator
www.westest.com/darci/index.html

Trace Computer Access Program
www.trace.wisc.edu/world/computer_access

Computer Access Software

Academic Software, Inc.
www.acsw.com

Click-N-Type Virtual Keyboard (FREE!)
cnt.lakefolks.com

Innovation Management Group
Supplier of onscreen keyboards and pointing device enhancements
www.imgpresents.com

Judy Lynn Software
Software for children with limited motor skills.
www.judylynn.com

Simply Powerful Technologies
On-screen keyboard
www.simplypowerful.com

Microsoft Accessibility Support
www.microsoft.com/enable

Neil Squire Foundation
www.neilsquire.ca

Origin Instruments
www.orin.com

Prentke Romich Company
www.prentrom.com

RehabTool.com
Adaptive and assistive technology.
www.rehabtool.com

RJ Cooper's Special Needs
On-screen keyboard with WordComplete
rjcooper.com/onscreen/index.html

WiViK
On-screen keyboard (virtual keyboard)
www.wivik.com

Words+, Inc.
WSKE II, the E Z Keys (Morse code input)
www.words-plus.com

KeyStrokes
On-screen keyboard software for the Mac
www.assistiveware.com

Input Devices

AssisTECH, Inc.
www.assistech.com

Bilbo Innovations
Keyboard control pedals.
www.bilbo.com/index.html

Don Johnston Incorporated
Communication computer access
www.donjohnston.com

GiveTech
For the disabled who can't afford computer input technology & another head pointer.
www.givetech.org

IBM ARC
User System Ergonomics Research (USER)
www.almaden.ibm.com

Keyboards

Adesso
www.adesso.com

Big Keys Plus
www.bigkeys.com

Key Tronic Corporation
www.keytronic.com

Infogrip
The BAT Personal One-Handed Keyboard
www.infogrip.com

Keyboard Alternatives and Vision Solutions
www.lowvision.org

Keyboards with Left or Right Single-Handed Dvorak Layout
www.onehandedkeyboard.com/dvorak.html

Matias Corporation
Half-Qwerty One-Handed Keyboard Software
half-qwerty.com

P.I. Engineering
X-keys programmable auxiliary keyboards
   www.ymouse.com

TACTUS keyboard
Useful for people who are visually impaired
   www.tactuskeyboard.com

Zygo Flexiboard
Alternative keyboard
   www.zygo-usa.com

Pointing Devices (Mice and Alternatives)

Cirque GlidePoint
Touchpad controllers
   www.cirque.com

CameraMouse
Hands-free computer mouse; computer control without headgear.
   cameramouse.com

eFMer camera technologies
Track! Hands free camera mouse (freeware)
   www.efmer.eu

GPK QuadTrac
Trackball for People With Quadriplegia
   www.spinalcord.uab.edu/show.asp?durki=21640

Logitech
   www.logitech.com

Madentec Limited
Head pointing, click/dwell, on-screen, switch access
   www.madentec.com

NaturalPoint trackIR
Control of your computer by tracking your body motion
   www.naturalpoint.com

NoHands Mouse
Foot-controlled mouse
   www.footmouse.com

Origin Instruments
HeadMouse Head-Controlled Pointing Systems
  www.orin.com

Prentke Romich Company
  www.prentrom.com

RJ Cooper's Special Needs
  rjcooper.com/sam-trackball/index.html

SEMCO
QuadJoy mouse for quadriplegic
  www.quadjoy.com

TetraMouse
Low-cost alternative computer mouse for people who cannot use their hands.
  tetralite.com/mouse

Eye Control

Eye Tracking
  www.cs.sunysb.edu/~vislab/projects/eye/index.html

VisionKey Computer Controller
  www.eyecan.ca

Switches

Madentech
  www.madentec.com

TAS Switch
  www.msu.edu/~artlang/TAS.html

AssisTECH
  www.assistech.com

Enabling Devices
  www.enablingdevices.com

Switcheroo Switch Interface and Single Switch/Button
  rjcooper.com/switcheroo

SwitcherHopper Switch Interface
  rjcooper.com/switchhopper

Touch Screen

KEYTEC
Magic Touch Screen, Magic Touch Monitor (CRT & LCD), and other touch-screen products
   www.magictouch.com

Voice (microphones)

Andrea Electronics
   www.andreaelectronics.com

Koss Corporation
   www.koss.com

Shure TCHS Computer Wireless System
   www.shure.com

Telex Computer Audio
Microphones and headsets for speech dictation, voice recognition, telephony, and cellular.
   www.telex.com

Books

All the titles below are available from Amazon (www.amazon.com):

Adaptive Technology for the Internet: Making Electronic Resources Accessible to All
Assistive Technology for Children with Disabilities: A Guide for Providing Family-Centered Services
Assistive Technology: Essential Human Factors
Alternative Computer Access: A Guide to Selection
Adapting PCs for Disabilities
Adaptive Technologies for Learning & Work Environments
Computer Applications in Occupational Therapy
Computer and Web Resources for People with Disabilities: A Guide to Exploring Today's Assistive Technology
Enabling Technology: Disabled People, Work, and New Technology
Information Access and Adaptive Technology
Living in the State of Stuck: How Technology Impacts the Lives of Persons with Disabilities
Making an Exceptional Difference: Enhancing the Impact of Microcomputer Technology on Children with Disabilities

Modern Morse Code in Rehabilitation and Education—New Applications in Assistive Technology
One-Hand Typing and Keyboarding Manual: With Personal Motivational Messages from Others Who Have Overcome!
One-Handed in a Two-Handed World (Second Edition)
Solutions Access Technologies for People Who Are Blind

Other

Apple
www.apple.com/accessibility

AssisTECH
Assistive technology and ADA compliant furniture.
www.assistech.com

Attention Control Systems
Planning and execution software for assisting brain-injured people gain independence
www.brainaid.com

EASI Equal Access to Software and Information
people.rit.edu/easi

EnableMart
Accessibility solutions store.
www.enablemart.com

IBM Special Needs Solutions
www-03.ibm.com/able/access_ibm/disability.html

LAB Resources
Assistive technology for special needs.
www.labresources-assistivetechnology.com

Laptop Laidback
The bed table for laptop computers.
www.laptop-laidback.com

Microsoft Accessibility Support
www.microsoft.com/enable

Onsight Ergonomics
Ergonomic computer products
www.onsightergo.com

Proportional Reading
Instant computer-assisted reading of any text.
www.proportionalreading.com

Simtech Publications
Switch-accessible software for the Mac.
www.marblesoft.com

Technical Solutions
Electronics for people with disabilities.
www.tecsol.com.au

Unicorn Quest
The kids' typing tutor game for one or two hands.
www.esmerel.com

Zygo Optimist
Personal pen computer
www.zygo-usa.com

Appendix A

VA POLYTRAUMA CENTERS

The following four centers are Polytrauma Network Sites. There are an additional seventeen Network Sites in the Northeast, Southeast, Central and West Coast regions.

Hunter Holmes McGuire Richmond–VA Medical Center
1201 Broad Rock Blvd.
Richmond, VA 23249
804-675-5000
800-784-8381

James A. Haley Tampa–Veterans' Hospital
13000, Bruce B. Downs Blvd.
Tampa, FL 33612
813-972-2000
888-716-7787

Minneapolis Veterans Affairs Medical Center
1 Veterans Dr.
Minneapolis, MN 55417
612-725-2000
866-414-5058

VA Palo Alto Health Care System
3801 Miranda Ave.
Palo Alto, CA 94304
650-493-5000
800-999-5021

Northeast

VA Boston Healthcare System Jamaica Plain Campus
150 South Huntington Ave.
Jamaica Plain, MA 02130
617-232-9500

Washington, DC, VA Medical Center
50 Irving St., NW
Washington, DC 20422
202-745-8000
888-553-0242

Syracuse VA Medical Center
800 Irving Ave.
Syracuse, NY 13210
315-425-4400
800-792-4334

Louis Stokes Cleveland–VA Medical Center—Wade Park Division
10701 East Blvd.
Cleveland, OH 44106
216-791-3800

James J. Peters Bronx–VA Medical Center
130 West Kingsbridge Rd.
Bronx, NY 10468
718-584-9000
800-877-6976

Richard L. Roudebush Indianapolis–VA Medical Center
1481 W. 10th St.
Indianapolis, IN 46202
317-554-0000
888-878-6889

Philadelphia VA Medical Center
University & Woodland Aves.
Philadelphia, PA 19104
215-823-5800
800-949-1001

Edward Hines, Jr.
Veterans Hospital
5th and Roosevelt Rd.

PO Box 5000
Hines, IL 60141
708-202-8387

Southeast

Lexington VA Medical Center
1101 Veterans Dr.
Lexington, KY 40502-2236
859-233-4511

Michael E. DeBakey Houston–VA Medical Center
2002 Holcombe Blvd.
Houston, TX 77030-4211
713-791-1414
800-553-2278

North Texas Health Care System–Dallas VA Medical Center
4500 South Lancaster Rd.
Dallas, TX 75216
214-742-8387
800-849-3597

Augusta VA Medical Center
1 Freedom Way
Augusta, GA 30904-6285
706-733-0188
800-836-5561

Central

Southern Arizona VA Health Care System
3601 South 6th Ave.
Tucson, AZ 85723
520-792-1450
800-470-8262

VA Eastern Colorado Health Care System
1055 Clermont St.
Denver, CO 80220
303-399-8020
888-336-8262

St. Louis VA Medical Center—Jefferson Barracks Division
1 Jefferson Barracks Dr.
St. Louis, MO 63125-4101
614-652-4100
800-228-5459

West Coast

VA Puget Sound Health Care System—Seattle Division
1660 S. Columbian Way
Seattle, WA 98108-1597
206-762-1010
800-329-8387

West Los Angeles Healthcare Center
11301 Wilshire Blvd.
Los Angeles, CA 90073
310-478-3711
800-952-4852

OTHER VA FACILITIES

Patients should call the telephone numbers listed to obtain hours of clinic operation and services. The following symbols indicate additional programs are available at medical centers
    * nursing-home care units
    # domiciliaries
    The following acronyms are used to indicate the specific type of clinic or site:

DC—dental clinic
MHC—mental health clinic
OSAC—outpatient substance abuse clinic
OSP—opiate substitution program
PTSD—post-traumatic stress disorder residential rehabilitation program
TWS—therapeutic work site
    Under the National Cemeteries listings, the acronym "NC" is used after the name of the town to designate locations of national cemeteries.

Alabama

Medical Centers

Central AL Veterans Health Care System: 800-214-8387
   Birmingham 35233, 700 S. 19th St., 205-933-8101
   Montgomery 36109, 215 Perry Hill Rd., 334-272-4670
*Tuscaloosa 35404, 3701 Loop Rd. East, 205-554-2000
#*Tuskegee 36083, 2400 Hospital Rd., 334-727-0550

Clinics

Anniston/Oxford 36203, 96 Ali Way, Creekside South, Oxford, 256-832-4141
Decatur/Madison 35758, 8075 Madison Blvd., Suite 101, Madison, 256-772-6220
Dothan 36301, 2020 Alexander Dr., 334-673-4166
Dothan MHC 36301, 3753 Ross Clark Cir., Suite 4, 334-678-1903
Florence Shoals Area Clinic 35660, 422 DD Cox Blvd., 256-381-9055
Gadsden 35906, 206 Rescia Ave., 256-413-7154
Huntsville 35801, 301 Governor's Dr., SW, 256-535-3100
Jasper 35501, 3400 Hwy 78 East, Medical Towers Suite 215, 205-221-7384
Mobile 36604, 1504 Springhill Ave., 251-219-3900

Regional Office

Montgomery 36109, 345 Perry Hill Rd., statewide 800-827-1000

Vet Centers

Birmingham 35233, 1500 5th Ave. S., 205-731-0550
Mobile 36606, 2577 Government Blvd., 251-478-5906

National Cemeteries

Fort Mitchell NC 36856, 553 Hwy. 165, Seale, 334-855-4731
Mobile NC 36604, 1202 Virginia St., 850-453-4846

Alaska

Medical Center

Alaska VA Healthcare System and Regional Office: Anchorage 99508-2989, 2925 DeBarr Rd, 907-257-4700
#Homeless Veterans Service: Anchorage 99503, 3001 C St., 800-764-2995

Clinics

Fairbanks 99703, Ft. Wainwright, Bassett Army Hospital, Gaffney Rd., Bldg. 4065, Rm. 169/176, 907-353-6370
Kenai 99611, 805 Frontage Rd., Suite 130, 907-283-2231 or 877-797-8924

Regional Office

Anchorage 99508-2989, 2925 De Barr Rd., statewide 800-827-1000

Benefits Office

Juneau 99802, PO Box 20069, 907-586-7472

Vet Centers

Anchorage 99508, 4201 Tudor Centre Dr., Suite 115, 907-563-6966
Fairbanks 99701, 540 4th Ave., Suite 100, 907-456-4238
Kenai 99669, Red Diamond Ctr., Bldg. F, Suite 4, 43335, Kalifornsky Beach Rd., 907-260-7640
Wasilla 99654, 851 E. West Point Dr., Suite 111, 907-376-4318

National Cemeteries

Fort Richardson NC 99505-5498, Building 997, Davis Highway, 907-384-7075
Sitka NC 99835, 803 Sawmill Creek Rd., 907-384-7075

American Samoa

Benefits Office

Pago Pago 96799, PO Box 1005, 684-633-5073

Arizona

Medical Centers

*Phoenix 85012, 650 East Indian School Rd., 602-277-5551, enrollment, ext. 6508, or 888-214-7264
*#Prescott 86313, 500 Hwy. 89 North, 928-445-4860 or 800-949-1005
*Tucson 85723, 3601 S. 6th Ave., 520-792-1450 or 800-470-8262

Clinics

Anthem 85086, 3618 W. Anthem Way, Bldg. 120D, 928-445-4860, ext. 7200, or 623-551-6092

Bellemont 86015, Camp Navajo Army Depot, PO Box 16196, 928-445-4860, ext. 7820, or 928-226-1056

Buckeye 85326, 1209 N. Miller Rd., 623-386-5785

Casa Grande 85222, Plaza del Sol, 900 E. Florence Blvd., Suites H&I, 520-629-4900 or 800-470-8262

Cottonwood 86326, 203 Candy Ln., Suite 5B, 928-649-1532

Globe 85501, 707 S. Broad St., 928-425-0027

Green Valley 85615, 380 W. Vista Hermosa, Suite 140, 520-629-4900 or 800-470-8262

Kingman 86401, 1726 Beverly Ave., 928-445-4860, ext. 6830, or 928-692-0080

Lake Havasu City 86403, 2035 Mesquite Ave., Southeast, 928-445-4860, ext. 7300, or 928-680-0090

Mesa 85212, 6950 E. Williams Field Rd., 602-222-6568, ext. 3311

Mena 71953, 1706 Hwy. 71 N., 479-394-4800

Payson 85541, 1106 N. Beeline Hwy., 928-472-3148

Safford 85546, Bureau of Land Management, 711 S. 14th Ave., 520-629-4900 or 800-470-8262

Show Low 85901, 2450 Show Low Lake Rd., Suites 1 & 3, 928-532-1069

Sierra Vista 85613, Ft. Huachuca, Bliss Army Health Center, Bldg. 45001, 520-629-4900 or 800-470-8262

Sun City 85351, 10147 W Grand Ave., Suite C, 602-222-2630, ext. 3732

Yuma 85365, Bureau of Land Management, 2555 E. Gila Ridge Rd., 520-629-4900 or 800-470-8262

Regional Office

Phoenix 85012, 3333 N. Central Ave., statewide 800-827-1000

Vet Centers

Phoenix 85012, 77 E. Weldon Ave., Suite 100, 602-640-2981
Prescott 86303, 161 S. Granite St., Suite B, 928-778-3469
Tucson 85719, 3055 N. 1st Ave., 520-882-0333

National Cemeteries

Nat. Mem. Cem. of AZ 85024, 23029, N. Cave Creek Rd., Phoenix, 480-513-3600
Prescott NC 86301, 500 Hwy. 89 N., 480-513-3600

Arkansas

Medical Centers

#*Central Arkansas Veterans Healthcare System: North Little Rock 72114,
    2200 Fort Roots Dr., 501-257-1000
Fayetteville 72703, 1100 N. College Ave., 479-443-4301
Little Rock 72205, 4300 W. 7th St., 501-257-1000

Clinics

El Dorado 71730, 460 West Oak, 870-862-2489
Ft. Smith 72917, Sparks Medical Plaza, 1500 Dodson Ave., 479-709-6850
Harrison 72601, Main St. Clinic, 707 N. Main St., 870-741-3592
Hot Springs 71913, 1661 Airport Rd., Suite B, 501-760-1513
Jonesboro 72401, 223 East Jackson, 870-972-0063
Mountain Home 72653, 405 Buttercup Dr., 870-425-3030
Paragould 72450, 1101 West Morgan, Suite 9, 870-236-9756
Texarkana 71854, 910 Realtor Ave., 870-216-2242

Regional Office

North Little Rock 72114, 2200 Fort Roots Dr., Bldg. 65, statewide 800-827-1000

Vet Center

North Little Rock 72114, 201 W. Broadway, Suite A, 501-324-6395

National Cemeteries

Fayetteville NC 72701, 700 Government Ave., 479-444-5051
Fort Smith NC 72901, 522 Garland Ave., 479-783-5345
Little Rock NC 72206, 2523 Confederate Blvd., 501-324-6401

California

Medical Centers

*Fresno 93703, 2615 E. Clinton Ave., 559-225-6100
#*Greater Los Angeles Health Care System: West Los Angeles 90073, 11301
    Wilshire Blvd., 310-478-3711
*Loma Linda Health Care System: Loma Linda 92357, 11201 Benton St.,
    909-825-7084 or 800-741-8387
*Long Beach Health Care System: Long Beach 90822, 5901 E. 7th St., 562-
    826-8000

*Northern California Health Care System:
  Martinez 94553, 150 Muir Rd., 925-372-2000
  Sacramento 95655, 10535 Hospital Way, 916-843-7000
*Palo Alto Health Care System:
  Livermore 94550, 4951 Arroyo Rd., 925-373-4700
  #*Menlo Park 94025, 795 Willow Rd., 650-493-5000
  Palo Alto 94304, 3801 Miranda Ave., 650-493-5000
*San Diego Health Care System: San Diego 92161, 3350 La Jolla Village
  Dr., 858-552-8585
*San Francisco 94121, 4150 Clement St., 415-221-4810

Clinics

Anaheim 92801, 1801 W. Romneya Dr., Suite 303, 714-780-5400
Antelope Valley/Lancaster 93536, 547 W. Lancaster Blvd., 661-729-8655
Atwater 95301, 3605 Hospital Rd., Suite D, 209-381-0105
Auburn 95603, 11985, Heritage Oaks Pl., 888-227-5404
Bakersfield 93301, 1801 Westwind Dr., 661-632-1800
Cabrillo/Long Beach 90810, 2001 River Ave., Bldg. 28, Long Beach, 562-388-8000
Capitola 95010, At Santa Cruz Vet Center, 1350 N. 41st St., Suite 102, 831-464-5519
Chico 95926, 280 Cohasset Rd., Suite 101, 530-879-5000
Chula Vista 91910, 835 Third Ave., 619-409-1600
Corona 92879, 800 Magnolia Ave, Suite 101, 951-817-8820
East Los Angeles 90040, 5400 E. Olympic Blvd., Suite 150, City of Commerce, 323-725-7557
Escondido 92025, 815 East Pennsylvania Ave., 760-466-7020
Eureka 95501, 714 F St., 707-442-5335
Fairfield 94535, 103 Bodin Cir., Building 778, Travis AFB, 707-437-1800
Gardena 90247, 1251 Redondo Beach Blvd., 3rd Fl., 310-851-4705
Imperial Valley 92227, 528 G St., Brawley, 760-344-9085
Los Angeles 90012, 351 E. Temple St., 213-253-2677
Mare Island 94592, 201 Walnut Ave., 707-562-8200
*Martinez 94553, 150 Muir Rd., 925-372-2000
McClellan 95652, 5342 Dudley Blvd., 916-561-7400
McClellan 95652, 5401 Arnold Ave., 916-561-7800 or 800-382-8387
Mission Valley 92108, 8810 Rio San Diego Dr., 619-400-5000
Modesto 95350, 1524 McHenry, Suite 315, 209-557-6200
Monterey 93955, located at Fort Ord, 3401 Engineer Lane, Seaside, 831-883-3800
Oakland 94612, 2221 Martin Luther King Jr. Way, 510-267-7820

Oakland MHC 94607, Oakland Army Base, 2505 West 14th St., 510-587-3434

Oxnard 93030, 250 W. Citrus Grove Ave., Suite 150, 805-983-6384

Palm Desert 92211, 41865, Boardwalk, Suite 103, 760-341-5570

Pasadena 91776, 420 W. Las Tunas, San Gabriel, 626-289-5973

Redding 96002, 351 Hartnell Ave., 530-226-7555

Sacramento MHC 95655, 10633, Grissom Rd., 916-366-5420 or 800-382-8387

San Bruno 94066, 1011 Sneath Ln., Suite 300, 650-553-8000

San Francisco 94107, 401 3rd St., 415-551-7300

San Jose 95119, 80 Great Oaks Blvd., 408-363-3000

San Luis Obispo 93401, 1288 Morro St., 200, 805-543-1233

Santa Ana 92704, 2740 S. Bristol St., Suite 110, 714-825-3500

Santa Barbara 93110, 4440 Calle Real, 805-683-1491

Santa Rosa 95404, 3315 Chanate Rd., 707-570-3855

*Sepulveda 91343, 16111 Plummer St., 818-891-7711

Sonora 95370, 19747 Greenley Rd., 209-588-2600

South Los Angeles/Lynwood 90262, 3737 E. Martin Luther King Jr. Blvd.,
Suite 515, Lynwood, 310-537-6825

Stockton 95231, co-located with San Joaquin General Hospital, 500 W. Hospital Rd., 209-946-3400

Sun City 92586, 28125 Bradley Rd., 130, 951-672-1931

Tulare 93274, 1050 N. Cherry St., 559-684-8703

Ukiah 95482, 630 Kings Ct., 707-468-7700

Upland 91786, 1238 E. Arrow Hwy., Suite 100, 909-946-5348

Victorville 92392, 12138 Industrial Blvd., Suite 120, 760-951-2599 or 800-741-8387

Vista 92083, 1840 West Dr., 760-643-2000

Whittier/Santa Fe Springs 90670, 10210 Orr and Day Rd., Santa Fe Springs,
562-864-5565

Regional Offices

Los Angeles 90024, Federal Bldg., 11000 Wilshire Blvd., serving counties of
Inyo, Kern, Los Angeles, San Bernardino, San Luis Obispo, Santa Barbara
and Ventura, statewide 800-827-1000

Oakland 94612, 1301 Clay St., Rm. 1300 North, serving all counties not
served by the Los Angeles, San Diego, or Reno VA Regional Offices, 800-827-1000

ᶜan Diego 92108, 8810 Rio San Diego Dr., serving Imperial, Orange, Riverside and San Diego, statewide 800-827-1000. The counties of Alpine, Lassen, Modoc, and Mono are served by the Reno, NV, Regional Office.

Benefits Office

Sacramento 95827, 10365 Old Placerville Rd., 916-364-6500

Vet Centers

Anaheim 92805, 859 S. Harbor Blvd., 714-776-0161
Chico 95926, 280 Cohasset Rd., Suite 100, 530-899-8549
Concord 94520, 1899 Clayton Rd., Suite 140, 925-680-4526
Corona 92879, 800 Magnolia Ave., 110, 951-734-0525
East Los Angeles 90022, 5400 E. Olympic Blvd., 140, 323-728-9966
Eureka 95501, 2830 G St., Suite A, 707-444-8271
Fresno 93726, 3636 N. 1st St., Suite 112, 559-487-5660
Gardena 90247, 1045 W. Redondo Beach Blvd., Suite 150, 310-767-1221
Marina 93933, 455 Reservation Rd., Suite E, 408-384-1660
North Bay 94928, 6225 State Farm Dr., Suite 101, 707-586-3295
Oakland 94612, 1504 Franklin St., 200, 510-763-3904
Redwood City 94062, 2946 Broadway St., 650-299-0672
Sacramento 95825, 1111 Howe Ave., Suite 390, 916-566-7430
San Bernardino 92408, 155 West Hospitality Lane, Suite 140, 909-890-0797
San Diego 92103, 2900 6th Ave., 619-294-2040
San Francisco 94102, 505 Polk St., 415-441-5051
San Jose 95112, 278 N. 2nd St., 408-993-0729
Sepulveda 91343, 9737 Haskell Ave., 818-892-9227
Ventura 93001, 790 E. Santa Clara, Suite 100, 805-585-1860
Vista 92083, 1830 West Dr., Suite 103, 760-643-2070
West Los Angeles 90230, 5730 Uplander Way, Suite 100, Culver City, 310-641-0326

National Cemeteries

Fort Rosecrans NC 92106, PO Box 6237, Point Loma, San Diego, 619-553-2084
Golden Gate NC 94066, 1300 Sneath Ln., San Bruno, 650-589-7737
Los Angeles NC 90049, 950 South Sepulveda Blvd., 310-268-4675
Riverside NC 92518, 22495, Van Buren Blvd., 951-653-8417
Sacramento Valley VA NC 95620, 5810 Midway Rd., Dixon, 707-693-2460
San Francisco NC 94129, PO Box 29012, Presidio of San Francisco, 650-589-7737
San Joaquin Valley NC 95322, 32053, West McCabe Rd., Gustine, 209-854-1040

Colorado

Medical Centers

*Grand Junction 81501, 2121 North Ave., 970-242-0731 or 866-206-6415
VA Eastern Colorado Health Care System: Denver 80220, 1055 Clermont St.,
    303-399-8020 or 888-336-8262

Clinics

Alamosa, CO 81101, 622 Del Sol Dr., 719-587-6800 or 866-659-0930
Aurora 80045, 13001 East 17th Place, Bldg. 500, 2nd Floor, 303-724-0190
Colorado Springs 80905, 25 N. Spruce St., 719-327-5660 or 800-278-3883
Durango 81301, 400 S. Camino del Rio, 970-247-2214
Fort Collins 80524, 1100 Poudre River Dr., 970-224-1550
Greeley 80631, 2020 16th St., 970-313-0027
LaJunta 81050, 1100 Carson Ave., Suite 104, 719-383-5195 or 877-329-2625
Lakewood 80228, 155 Van Gordon St., Suite 395, 303-914-2680
Lamar 81052, 201 Kendall Dr., 719-336-5972 or 866-240-2279
Montrose 81401, 4 Hillcrest Plaza Way, 970-249-7791
Pueblo 81008, 4112 Outlook Blvd., 719-553-1000 or 800-369-6748

Regional Office

Denver 80225, Mailing Address: PO Box 25126. Physical Address: 155 Van
    Gordon St., Lakewood, 80228, statewide 800-827-1000

Vet Centers

Boulder 80302, 2336 Canyon Blvd., Suite 130, 303-440-7306
Colorado Springs 80903, 416 E. Colorado Ave., 719-471-9992
Denver 80230, 7465 E. First Ave., Suite B, 303-326-0645

National Cemeteries

Fort Logan NC 80235, 3698 S. Sheridan Blvd., Denver, 303-761-0117
Fort Lyon NC 81038, 303-761-0117

Connecticut

Medical Centers

Connecticut Health Care System:
    *West Haven Division 06516, 950 Campbell Ave., 203-932-5711
    Newington Division 06111, 555 Willard Ave., 860-666-6951

Clinics

Danbury 06810, 7 Germantown Rd., 203-798-8422
New London 06320, 15 Mohegan Ave., 860-437-3611
Stamford 06905, 1275 Summer St., Suite 102, 203-325-0649
Waterbury 06706, 133 Scovill St., Suite 203, 203-465-5292
Windham 06226, 96 Mansfield St., 860-450-7583
Winsted 06098, 115 Spencer St., 860-738-6985

Regional Office

Hartford Bldg 2E, RM 5137, 555 Willard Ave., Newington, 06111-2693, state-wide 800-827-1000

Vet Centers

Norwich 06360, 2 Cliff St., 860-887-1755
Wethersfield 06109, 30 Jordan Lane, 860-563-2320
West Haven 06516, 141 Captain Thomas Blvd., 203-932-9899

Delaware

Medical Center

*Wilmington 19805, 1601 Kirkwood Hwy., 302-994-2511 or 800-461-8262

Clinics

Millsboro 19966, 214 W. DuPont Hwy., 302-934-0195
Seaford 19973, 121 S. Front St., 302-628-8324

Regional Office

Wilmington 19805, 1601 Kirkwood Hwy., local, 302-994-2511

Vet Center

Wilmington 19805, 1601 Kirkwood Hwy., Bldg. 3, 302-994-1660

District of Columbia

Medical Center

*Washington, DC 20422, 50 Irving St., NW, 202-745-8000

Clinic

Southeast 20032, 820 Chesapeake St., SE, 202-745-8685

Regional Office

Washington, DC 20421, 1722 I St., NW, local, 800-827-1000

Vet Center

Washington, DC 20011, 1250 Taylor St., NW, 202-726-5212

Florida

Medical Centers

#*Bay Pines 33744, 10000 Bay Pines Blvd., 727-398-6661
North Florida/South Georgia Veterans Health System:
   *Gainesville 32608, 1601 Southwest Archer Rd., 352-376-1611
   *Lake City 32025, 619 S. Marion Ave., 386-755-3016
*Miami 33125, 1201 NW 16th St., 305-575-7000
*Tampa 33612, 13000, Bruce B. Downs Blvd., 813-972-2000
*West Palm Beach 33410, 7305 N. Military Trail, 561-422-8262

Clinics

Boca Raton 33433, 900 Glades Rd., 561-416-8995
Brevard 32940, 2900 Veterans Way, Viera, 321-637-3788
Brooksville 34613, 14540 Cortez Blvd., 352-597-8287
Coral Springs 33065, 9900 W. Sample Rd., Suite 100, 954-575-4940
Daytona Beach 32114, 551 National Health Care Dr., 386-323-7500
Deerfield Beach 33442, 2100 SW 10th St., 954-570-5572
Delray Beach 33445, 4800 Linton Blvd., 561-495-1973
Dunedin 34698, 1721 Main St., 727-734-5276
Ellenton 34222, 4333 U.S. Hwy 301 North, 941-721-0649
Fort Myers 33916, 3033 Winkler Extension, 239-939-3939
Ft. Pierce 34950, 727 North US 1, 772-595-5150
Hollywood 33021, 3702 Washington St., Hollywood Pav., Suite 201, 954-
   986-1811
Homestead 33030, 950 Krome Ave., Suite 401, 305-248-0874
Jacksonville 32206, 1833 Blvd. St., 904-232-2751
Key Largo 33037, 105662 Overseas Hwy., 305-451-0164
Key West 33040, 1300 Douglas Cir., 305-293-4609
Kissimmee 34741, 201 Hilda St., 407-518-5004

Lakeland 33803, 3240 S. Florida Ave., 863-701-2470
Lecanto 34461, 2804 Marc Knighton Ct., Suite A, 352-746-8000
Leesburg 34748, 711 West Main St., 352-435-4000
Miami OSAC 33135, 1492 West Flagler St., Suite 102, 305-541-8435
Naples 34101, 2685 Horseshoe Dr., Suite 101, 239-659-9188
New Port Richey 34654, 9912 Little Rd., 727-869-4100
Oakland Park 33334, 5599 N. Dixie Hwy., 954-771-2101
Ocala 34470, 1515 E. Silver Springs Blvd., 352-369-3320
Okeechobee 34972, 1201 N. Parrott Ave., 863-824-3232
#*Orlando 32803, 5201 Raymond St., 407-629-1599
Panama City 32407, 6703 West Hwy. 98, Bldg. 387, 850-636-7000
Pembroke Pines 33024, 7369 Sheridan St., Suite 102, 954-894-1668
Pensacola South 32503, 312 Kenmore Rd., 850-476-1100
Pensacola North 32506, 7895-C Pensacola Blvd., 850-476-1100
Port Charlotte 33952, 4161 Tamiami Trail, 941-235-2710
Sanford 32771, 1403 Medical Plaza Dr., 109, 407-323-5999
Sarasota 34233, 5682 Bee Ridge Rd., Suite 100, 941-371-3349
Sebring 33870, 3760 US Hwy. 27 South, 863-471-6227
St. Augustine 32086, 1955 US 1 South, Suite 200, 904-829-0814
St. Petersburg 33711, 3420 8th Ave. South, 727-322-1304
Stuart 34997, 3501 SE Willoughby Blvd., 772-288-0304
Tallahassee 32308, 1607 St. James Ct., 850-878-0191
The Villages 32162, 1950 Laurel Manor Dr., Bldg. 204, 352-205-8900
Vero Beach 32960, 372 17th St., 772-299-4623
Zephyrhills 33531, 6937 Medical View Ln., 813-780-2550

Regional Office

St. Petersburg 33708, mailing address: PO Box 1437; physical address: 9500
  Bay Pines Blvd., statewide 800-827-1000

Benefits Offices

Fort Lauderdale 33301, VR&E, 299 East Broward Blvd., Room 324, 800-
  827-1000
Jacksonville 32256, VR&E, 7825 Baymeadows Way, Suite 120-B, 800-827-
  1000
Orlando 32801, 1000 Legion Pl., VR&E-Suite 1500, C&P-Suite 1550, 800-
  827-1000
Pensacola 32503-7492, C&P, 312 Kenmore Rd., Rm. 1G250, 800-827-1000
West Palm Beach 33410, C&P, 7305 North Military Tr., Suite 1A-167, 800-
  827-1000

Vet Centers

Fort Lauderdale 33304, 713 NE 3rd Ave., 954-356-7926
Jacksonville 32202, 300 East State St., 904-232-3621
Miami 33122, 8280 NW 27th St., Suite 511, 305-859-8387
Orlando 32822, 5575 S. Semoran Blvd., Suite 36, 407-857-2800
Palm Beach 33461, 2311 10th Ave., North 13, 561-585-0441
Pensacola 32501, 4501 Twin Oaks Dr., 850-456-5886
Sarasota 34231, 4801 Swift Rd., 941-927-8285
St. Petersburg 33713, 2880 1st Ave., N., 727-893-3791
Tallahassee 32303, 548 Bradford Rd., 850-942-8810
Tampa 33604, 8900 N. Armenia Ave., Suite 312, 813-228-2621

National Cemeteries

Barrancas NC 32508-1099, 80 Hovey Rd., Naval Air Station, Pensacola, 850-453-4846
Bay Pines NC 33504-0477, 10000 Bay Pines Blvd., North Bay Pines, 727-398-9426
Florida NC 33513, 6502 SW 102nd Ave., Bushnell, 352-793-7740
Saint Augustine NC 32084, 104 Marine St., 352-793-7740
South Florida NC 33467, 6501 South State Rd. 7, 561-649-6489

Georgia

Medical Centers

*Augusta 30904, 1 Freedom Way, 706-733-0188
*Decatur 30033, 1670 Clairmont Rd., 404-321-6111
#*Dublin 31021, 1826 Veterans Blvd., 478-272-1210

Clinics

Albany 31701, 417 4th Ave., 229-446-9000 or 877-216-4495
Athens 30610, 9249 Hwy 29 North, 706-227-4534
Columbus 31906, 1310 13th Ave., 706-257-7200
East Point 30344, 1513 Cleveland Ave., 404-321-6111
Lawrenceville 30043, 1970 Riverside Pkwy., 404-417-1750
Macon 31220, 5398 Thomaston Rd., Suite B, 478-476-8868 or 800-552-7483
Oakwood 30566, 3931 Mundy Mill Rd., Suite C, 404-728-8210
Savannah 31406, 325 W. Montgomery Cross Rd., 912-920-0214
Smyrna 30082, 582 Concord Rd., 404-417-1760
Valdosta 31602, 2841 North Patterson, 229-293-0132

Regional Office

Decatur 30033, 1700 Clairmont Rd., statewide 800-827-1000

Vet Centers

Atlanta 30324, 1440 Dutch Valley Place, Suite G, 404-347-7264
Savannah 31406, 8110A White Bluff Rd., 912-652-4097

National Cemeteries

Georgia NC 30114, 2025 Mt. Carmel Church Lane, Canton, 866-236-8159
Marietta NC 30060, 500 Washington Ave., 866-236-8159

Guam

Clinic

Agana Heights 96919, US Naval Hospital, Bldg 1, E-200, Box 7608, 671-344-9200

Benefits Office/Vet Center

Hagatna 96910, 222 Chalan Santo Papa St., Suite 202, 671-472-7217

Hawaii

Medical Center

Honolulu 96819-1522, Pacific Islands Health Sys., 459 Patterson Rd., 808-433-0600

Clinics

Hilo 96720, 1285 Wainuenue Ave., Suite 211, 808-935-3781
Honolulu PTSD 96819, 3375 Koapaka St., 808-566-1546
Kauai: Lihue 96766, 3-3367 Kuhio Hwy., Suite 200, 808-246-0497
Kona: Kailua-Kona 96740, 75-5995 Kuakini Hwy., Suite 413, 808-329-0774
Maui: Kahului 96732, 203 Ho'ohana St., Suite 303, 808-871-2454

Regional Office

Honolulu 96819-1522, 459 Patterson Rd., E Wing. Mailing address: PO Box 29020, Honolulu, HI 96820 (800-827-1000 from Hawaii, Guam, Saipan, Rota and Tinian; 877-899-4400 from American Samoa)

Benefits Offices

Hilo 96720, VR&E, 891 Ululani St., 808-961-3413
Kahului 96732, VR&E, 203 Ho'ohana St., 808-873-9426

Vet Centers

Hilo 96720, 120 Keawe St., Suite 201, 808-969-3833
Honolulu 96814, 1680 Kapiolani Blvd., Suite F3, 808-973-8387
Kailua-Kona 96740, Pottery Terrace, Fern Bldg., 75-5995 Kuakini Hwy.,
  # 415, 808-329-0574
Lihue 96766, 3-3367 Kuhio Hwy., Suite 101, 808-246-1163
Wailuku 96793, 35 Lunalilo, Suite 101, 808-242-8557

National Cemetery

National Cemetery of the Pacific 96813-1729, 2177 Puowaina Dr., Honolulu,
  808-532-3720

Idaho

Medical Center

*Boise 83702, 500 West Fort St., 208-422-1000

Clinics

Pocatello 83201, 444 Hospital Way, Suite 801, 208-232-6214
Twin Falls 83301, 260 2nd Ave, E., 208-732-0947

Regional Office

Boise 83702, 805 W. Franklin St., statewide 800-827-1000

Vet Centers

Boise 83705, 5440 Franklin Rd., Suite 100, 208-342-3612
Pocatello 83201, 1800 Garrett Way, 208-232-0316

Illinois

Medical Centers

Chicago 60612, Jesse Brown VA, 820 S. Damen Ave., 312-569-8387
*VA Illiana Health Care System 61832, Danville Med. Ctr., 1900 E.
Main St., 217-554-3000 or 800-320-8387

*Hines 60141, Roosevelt Rd. & 5th Ave., 708-202-8387
*Marion 62959, 2401 W. Main St., 618-997-5311
#*North Chicago 60064, 3001 Green Bay Rd., 847-688-1900

Clinics

Aurora 60506, 1700 N. Landmark Rd., 630-859-2504
Belleville 62223, 6500 W. Main St., 618-398-2100
Chicago—Lakeside 60611, 333 E. Huron, 312-569-8387
Chicago 60643, 2038 W. 95th St., 773-239-7134
Chicago Heights 60411, 30 E. 15th St., Suite 207, 708-756-5454
Decatur 62526, 3035 E. Mound Rd., 217-875-2670
Effingham 62401, Lincolnland Bldg., 1901 S. 4th St., 217-347-7600
Elgin 60120, 450 Dundee Ave., Suite 100, 847-742-5920
Evanston 60202, 107-109 Clyde St., 847-869-6315
Freeport 61032, 1301 Kiwanis Dr., 608-280-7038
Galesburg 61401, 387 E. Grove St., 309-343-0311
Joliet 60435, 2000 Glenwood Ave., 815-744-0492
LaSalle 61301, 2970 Chartres St., 815-223-9678
Manteno 60950, One Veterans Dr., 815-468-1027
McHenry 60050, 620 S. Route 31, 815-759-2306
Mt. Vernon 62864, 1 Doctors Park Rd., 618-246-2910 or 2911
Oak Lawn 60453, 4700 W. 95th St., Suite 104, 708-499-3675
Oak Park 60302, 149 S. Oak Park Ave., 708-386-3008
Peoria 61605, 411 Martin Luther King Jr. Dr., 309-497-0790
Quincy 62301, 1707 North 12th St., 217-224-3366
Rockford 61108, 4940 East State St., 815-227-0081
Springfield 62702, 700 N. 7th St., Suite C, 217-522-9730

Regional Office

Chicago 60612, 2122 W. Taylor St., statewide 800-827-1000

Vet Centers

Chicago 60643, 2038 W. 95th St., Suite 200, 773-881-9900
Chicago Heights 60411, 1600 S. Halsted St., 708-754-0340
East St. Louis 62203, 1265 N. 89th St., Suite 5, 618-397-6602
Evanston 60202, 565 Howard St., 847-332-1019
Moline 61265, 1529 46th Ave., 6, 309-762-6954
Oak Park 60302, 155 S. Oak Park Blvd., 708-383-3225
Peoria 61603, 3310 N. Prospect Rd., 309-671-7300
Springfield 62702, 624 S. 4th St., 217-492-4955

National Cemeteries

Abraham Lincoln NC 60421, 27034, South Diagonal Rd., Elwood, 815-423-9958
Alton NC 62003, 600 Pearl St., 314-260-8720
Camp Butler NC 62707, 5063 Camp Butler Rd., Springfield, 217-492-4070
Danville NC 61832, 1900 East Main St., 217-554-4550
Mound City NC 62963, Junction Hwy., 37 & 51, 314-260-8720
Quincy NC 62301, 36th and Maine St., 309-782-2094
Rock Island NC 61299-7090, Rock Island Arsenal, Bldg. 118, 309-782-2094

Indiana

Medical Centers

Indianapolis 46202, 1481 W. 10th St., 317-554-0000
Northern Indiana Health Care System:
  *Fort Wayne 46805, 2121 Lake Ave., 260-426-5431
  *Marion 46953, 1700 E. 38th St., 765-674-3321

Clinics

Bloomington 47403, 455 S. Landmark Ave., 812-336-5723
Crown Point 46307, 9330 S. Broadway, 219-662-5000
Evansville 47713, 500 E. Walnut, 812-465-6202
Greendale 47025, 1600 Flossie Dr., 812-539-2313
Lawrenceburg 47025, 710 W. Eads Pkwy., 812-539-2313
Muncie/Anderson 47304, 3500 W. Purdue Ave., 765-284-6822
New Albany 47150, 811 Northgate Blvd., 502-287-4100
Richmond 47374, 4351 South A St., 765-973-6915
South Bend 46614, 55725 S. Ironwood Rd., 574-229-4847 or 866-436-1291
Terre Haute 47802, 110 W. Honey Creek Pkwy., 812-232-2890
West Lafayette 47906, 3851 N. River Rd., 765-464-2280 or 800-320-8387

Regional Office

Indianapolis 46204, 575 N. Pennsylvania St., statewide 800-827-1000

Vet Centers

Evansville 47711, 311 N. Weinbach Ave., 812-473-5993 or 812-473-6084
Fort Wayne 46802, 528 West Berry St., 260-460-1456
Merrillville 46410, 6505 Broadway Ave., 219-736-5633
Indianapolis 46208, 3833 N. Meridian St., Suite 120, 317-927-6440

National Cemeteries

Crown Hill NC 46208, 700 W. 38th St., Indianapolis, 765-674-0284
Marion NC 46952, 1700 E. 38th St., 765-674-0284
New Albany NC 47150, 1943 Ekin Ave., 502-893-3852

Iowa

Medical Centers

Central Iowa Health Care System:
  #Des Moines 50310, 3600 30th St., 800-294-8387
  #*Knoxville 50138, 1515 W. Pleasant St., 800-816-8878
Iowa City 52246, 601 Hwy. 6 West, 319-338-0581

Clinics

Bettendorf 52722, 2979 Victoria St., 563-332-8528
Dubuque 52001, 200 Mercy Dr., Suite 106, 563-589-8899
Fort Dodge 50501, 804 Kenyon Rd., Suite 160, 515-576-2235
Mason City 50401, 910 N. Eisenhower, 641-421-8077 or 800-351-4671
Sioux City 51104, 1551 Indian Hills Dr., Suite 206, 712-258-4700
Waterloo 50701, 1015 S. Hackett Rd., 319-235-1235

Regional Office

Des Moines 50309, 210 Walnut St., Rm. 1063, statewide 800-827-1000

Vet Centers

Cedar Rapids 52402, 1642 42nd St. NE, 319-378-0016
Des Moines 50310, 2600 Martin Luther King Jr. Pkwy., 515-284-4929
Sioux City 51104, 1551 Indian Hills Dr., Suite 204, 712-255-3808

National Cemetery

Keokuk NC 52632, 1701 J St., 309-782-2094

Kansas

Medical Centers

Eastern Kansas Health Care System:
  #*Leavenworth 66048, 4101 S. 4th St., Trafficway, 913-682-2000
  *Topeka 66622, 2200 SW Gage Blvd., 785-350-3111
  *Wichita 67218, 5500 E. Kellogg, 316-685-2221

Clinics

Abilene 67410, 510 NE 10th St., 785-263-2100, ext. 161
Chanute 66720, 629 S. Plummer, 620-431-4000, ext. 1553
Fort Dodge City 67801, 300 Custer, 620-225-7146
Emporia 66801, 1201 W. 12th St., 620-343-6800, ext. 1599
Fort Scott 66701, 710 W. 8th St., 620-223-8400
Garnett 66032, 421 S. Maple, 785-448-3131, ext. 309
Hays 67601, 207B E. 7th St., 785-625-3550
Holton 66436, 1110 Columbine Dr., 785-364-2116, ext. 115
Junction City 66441, 715 Southwind Dr., 800-574-8387, ext. 54670
Kansas City 66102, 21 N. 12th St., Suite 200, 800-952-8387, ext. 6990
Lawrence 66044, 2200 Harvard St., 800-574-8387, or 785-841-2957
Liberal 67901, 2 Rock Island Rd., Suite 200, 620-626-5574
Paola 66071, 501 S. Hospital Dr., Suite 100, 816-922-2160
Parsons 67357, 1401 N. Main St., 620-423-3858
Russell 67665, 200 South Main St., 785-483-3131
Salina 67401, 1410 East Iron, Suite 1, 785-826-1580
Seneca 66538, 1600 Community Dr., 785-336-6181, ext. 162

Regional Office

Wichita 67218, Robert J. Dole Regional Office, 5500 E. Kellogg Ave., 800-827-1000

Vet Center

Wichita 67211, 413 S. Pattie, 316-265-3260

National Cemeteries

Fort Leavenworth NC 66027, 913-758-4105
Fort Scott NC 66701, PO Box 917, 900 East National, 620-223-2840
Leavenworth NC 66048, PO Box 1694, 913-758-4105

Kentucky

Medical Centers

#*Fort Thomas 41075, 1000 S. Ft. Thomas Ave., 513-861-3100
*Lexington 40502-2236, 1101 Veterans Dr., 859-233-4511
Louisville 40206, 800 Zorn Ave., 502-287-4000

Clinics

Bellevue 41073, 103 Landmark Dr., 859-392-3840

Bowling Green 42103, 1110 Wilkinson Trace Cir., Harland Medical Plaza, 270-796-3590

Florence 41042, 7711 Ewing, 859-282-4480

Fort Campbell 42223, Desert Storm Ave., Bldg. 61639, 270-798-4118

Fort Knox 40121, 851 Ireland Loop, 502-624-9396

Hanson 42413, 926 Veterans Dr., 270-322-8019

Louisville/Dupont 40207, 4010 Dupont Circle, 502-287-6986

Louisville/Shively 40216, 3934 N. Dixie Hwy., Suite 210, 502-287-6000

Louisville/Standiford Field 40213, 1101 Grade Lane, 502-364-9635

Paducah 42001, 1800 Clark St., 270-444-8465

Prestonsburg 41653, 5230 KY Rt. 321, Suite 8, 606-886-1970

Somerset 42501, 104 Hardin Lane, 606-676-0786

Regional Office

Louisville 40202, 321 W. Main St., Suite 390, statewide 800-827-1000

Vet Centers

Lexington 40507, 301 E. Vine St., Suite C, 859-253-0717

Louisville 40208, 1347 S. 3rd St., 502-634-1916

National Cemeteries

Camp Nelson NC 40356, 6980 Danville Rd., Nicholasville, 859-885-5727

Cave Hill NC 40204, 701 Baxter Ave., Louisville, 502-893-3852

Danville NC 40442, 277 N. First St., 859-885-5727

Lebanon NC 40033, 20 Highway 208, 502-893-3852

Lexington NC 40508, 833 W. Main St., 859-885-5727

Mill Springs NC 42544, 9044 West Highway 80, Nancy, 859-885-5727

Zachary Taylor NC 40207, 4701 Brownsboro Rd., Louisville, 502-893-3852

Louisiana

Medical Centers

*Alexandria 71306, 2495 Shreveport Hwy., 318-473-0010

*New Orleans 70112, 1601 Perido St., 504-568-0811, ext. 2929, or 800-935-8387

Shreveport 71101, 510 E. Stoner Ave., 318-221-8411

Clinics

Baton Rouge 70809, 7968 Essen Park Ave., 225-761-6700
Hammond VA Mobile Clinic 70403, 1131 S. Morrison Ave., 985-340-7816
Jennings 70546, 1907 Johnson St., 337-824-1000
Lafayette 70501, 2100 Jefferson St. 337-261-0734
LaPlace 70068, 501 Rue de Sante, Suite 10, 800-935-8387
Monroe 71203, 250 DeSiard Plaza, 318-343-6100
Slidell 70461, 340 Gateway Dr., 800-935-8387

Regional Office

Gretna 70054, mailing address: PO Box 1278; physical address: 671A Whit-
ney Ave., Gretna, LA 70056, statewide 800-827-1000

Vet Centers

Kenner 70062, 2200 Veterans Blvd., Suite 114, 504-464-4743
Shreveport 71104, 2800 Youree Dr., Bldg. 1, Suite 1, 318-861-1776

National Cemeteries

Alexandria NC 71360, 209 E. Shamrock St., Pineville, 601-445-4981
Baton Rouge NC 70806, 220 N. 19th St., 225-654-3767
Port Hudson NC 70791, 20978 Port Hickey Rd., Zachary, 225-654-3767

Maine

Medical Center

*Augusta 04330, 1 VA Center, 207-623-8411

Regional Office

Togus 04330, 1 VA Center, Building 248, Room 205, 877-421-8263

Clinics

Bangor 04401, 304 Hancock St., Suite 3B, 207-561-3600
Calais 04619, 50 Union St., 207-904-3700
Caribou 04736, 163 Van Buren Dr., Suite 6, 207-493-3800
Rumford 04276, 431 Franklin St., 207-369-3200
Saco 04072, 655 Main St., 207-294-3100

Vet Centers

Bangor 04401, 352 Harlow St., 207-947-3391
Caribou 04736, 456 York St., Irving Complex, 207-496-3900
Lewiston 04240, Pkwy Complex, 29 Westminster St., 207-783-0068
Portland 04103, 475 Stevens Ave., 207-780-3584
Springvale 04083, 628 Main St., 207-490-1513

National Cemetery

Togus NC 04330, 1 VA Center, 508-563-7113

Maryland

Medical Centers

Maryland Health Care System:
 *Baltimore 21201, 10 N. Green St., 410-605-7000
 #Perry Point 21902, Bldg. 5H, 410-642-2411
Baltimore 21218, Rehab. & Extended Care, 3900 Loch Raven Blvd., 410-605-7000

Clinics

Cambridge 21613, 830 Chesapeake Dr., 410-228-6243
Charlotte Hall 20622, 29431, Charlotte Hall Rd., 301-884-7102
Cumberland 21502, 200 Glenn St., 301-724-0061
Fort Howard 21052, 9600 North Point Rd., 410-477-1800
Glen Burnie 21061, 1406 South Crain Hwy., 410-590-4140
Greenbelt 20770, 7525 Greenway Center Dr., Suite T-4, 301-345-2463
Hagerstown 21742, 1101 Opal Court, 301-665-1462
Loch Raven 21218, 3901 The Alameda, 410-605-7650
Pocomoke 21851, 101 Market St., 410-957-6718

Regional Office

Baltimore 21201, 31 Hopkins Plaza Federal Bldg., 800-827-1000

Vet Centers

Baltimore 21207, 6666 Security Blvd., Suite 2, 410-277-3600
Cambridge 21613, 5510 West Shore Dr., 410-228-6305, ext. 4123
Elkton 21921, 103 Chesapeake Blvd., Suite A, 410-392-4485
Silver Spring 20910, 1015 Spring St., Suite 101, 301-589-1073

National Cemeteries

Annapolis NC 21401, 800 West St., 410-644-9696
Baltimore NC 21228, 5501 Frederick Ave., 410-644-9696
Loudon Park NC 21228, 3445 Frederick Ave., Baltimore, 410-644-9696

Massachusetts

Medical Centers

Bedford 01730, 200 Springs Rd., 800-838-6331 or 781-275-7500
Boston 02130, 150 S. Huntington Ave., 617-232-9500
Brockton 02301, 940 Belmont St., 508-583-4500
*Northampton 01053-9764, 421 N. Main St., 413-584-4040
West Roxbury 02132, 1400 VFW Pkwy., 617-323-7700

Clinics

Boston 02114, 251 Causeway St., 617-248-1000
Dorchester 02124, 895 Blue Hill Ave., 617-822-7146
Edgartown 02539, 55 Simpson's Lane, 508-627-1044
Fitchburg 01420, 275 Nichols Rd., 978-342-9781
Framingham 01702, 61 Lincoln St., 508-628-0205
Franklin County 01301, 51 Sanderson St., Suite 9, 413-773-8428
Gloucester 01930, 298 Washington St., 978-282-0676
Haverhill 01830, 108 Merrimack St., 978-372-5207
Hyannis 02601, 145 Falmouth Rd., 508-771-3190
Lowell 01852, 130 Marshall Rd., 978-671-9000
Lynn 01904, 225 Boston St., Suite 107, 781-595-9818
Martha's Vineyard Hospital 02557, Linton Lane, Oak Bluffs, 508-693-0410
Nantucket Cottage Hospital 02554, 57 Prospect St., 508-228-1200
New Bedford 02740, 175 Elm St., 508-994-0217
Pittsfield 01201, 73 Eagle St., 413-443-4857
Quincy 02169, 114 Whitwell St., 2nd Floor, 617-376-2010
Springfield 01104, 25 Bond St., 413-731-6000
Worcester 01605, 605 Lincoln St., 508-856-0104

Regional Office

Boston 02203-0393, JFK Federal Building, Government Center, Room 1425, statewide 800-827-1000 (towns of Fall River and New Bedford, counties of Barnstable, Dukes, Nantucket, Bristol, part of Plymouth served by Providence, RI, VA Regional Office)

Vet Centers

Boston 02215, 665 Beacon St., 617-424-0665
Brockton 02401, 1041-L Pearl St., 508-580-2730
Lowell 01852, 73 East Merrimack St., 978-453-1151
New Bedford 02740, 468 North St., 508-999-6920
Springfield 01103, 1985 Main St., Northgate Plaza, 413-737-5167
Worcester 01605, 597 Lincoln St., 508-856-7428

National Cemetery

Massachusetts NC 02532, Connery Ave., Bourne, 508-563-7113

Michigan

Medical Centers

*Ann Arbor 48105, 2215 Fuller Rd., 734-769-7100
*Battle Creek 49015, 5500 Armstrong Rd., 269-966-5600
*Detroit 48201, 4646 John R. St., 313-576-1000
*Iron Mountain 49801, 325 East H St., 906-774-3300 or 800-215-8262 in
   Michigan and Wisconsin
*Saginaw 48602, 1500 Weiss St., 989-497-2500

Clinics

Benton Harbor 49022, 115 Main St., 269-934-9123
Flint 48532, G-3267 Beecher Rd., 810-720-2913
Gaylord 49735, 806 S. Otsego, 989-732-6555
Grand Rapids 49505, 3019 Coit, NE, 616-365-9575
Hancock 49930-1495, 890 Campus Dr., 906-482-7762
Ironwood 49938, 930 Cloverland Dr., 906-932-0032
Jackson 49203, 400 Hinckley Blvd., Suite 300, 517-782-7415
Lansing 48824, 2025 S. Washington Ave., 517-267-3925
Marquette 49855, 425 Fisher St., 906-226-4618
Menominee 49858, 1101 11th Ave., Suite 2, 906-863-1286
Muskegon 49442, 165 E. Apple Ave., Suite 201, 231-725-4105
Oscoda 48750, 5671 Skeel Ave., Suite 4, 989-747-0026
Pontiac 48340, 1701 Baldwin Ave., Suite 101, 248-409-0585
Sault Ste. Marie 49783, 509 Osborn Blvd., Suite 306, 906-253-9383 or 877-
   470-3811
Traverse City 49684, 3271 Racquet Club Dr., 231-932-9720
Yale 48097, 7470 Broadway Dr., 810-387-3211

Regional Office

Detroit 48226, Patrick V. McNamara Federal Bldg., 477 Michigan Ave., Rm. 1400, 800-827-1000

Vet Centers

Dearborn 48124-3438, 2881 Monroe St., Suite 100, 313-277-1428
Detroit 48201, 4161 Cass Ave., 313-831-6509
Grand Rapids 49507, 1940 Eastern SE, 616-243-0385

National Cemeteries

Fort Custer NC 49012, 15501 Dickman Rd., Augusta, 269-731-4164
Great Lakes NC 48442, 4200 Belford Rd., Holly, 866-348-8603

Minnesota

Medical Centers

*Minneapolis 55417, One Veterans Dr., 612-725-2000
#*St. Cloud 56303, 4801 Veterans Dr., 320-252-1670

Clinics

Brainerd 56401, 1777 Hwy. 18 East, 218-855-1115
Fergus Falls 56537, 1821 North Park St., 218-739-1400
Hibbing 55746, 1101 E. 37th St., Suite 220, 218-263-9698
Mankato Area, 15 sites, 612-725-1991
Maplewood 55109, 2785 White Bear Ave., Suite 210, 651-290-3040
Montevideo 56265, 1025 N. 13th St., 320-269-2222
Rochester 55902, 1617 Skyline Dr., 507-252-0885
Saint James 56081, 1205 6th Ave. South, 507-375-3391

Regional Office

St. Paul 55111, Bishop Henry Whipple Federal Bldg., 1 Federal Dr., 800-827-1000 (counties of Becker, Beltrami, Clay, Clearwater, Kittson, Lake of the Woods, Mahnomen, Marshall, Norman, Otter Tail, Pennington, Polk, Red Lake, Roseau, Wilkin served by Fargo, ND, VA Regional Office)

Vet Centers

Duluth 55802, 405 E. Superior St., 218-722-8654
St. Paul 55114, 2480 University Ave., 651-644-4022

National Cemetery

Fort Snelling NC 55450-1199, 7601 34th Ave. So., Minneapolis, 612-726-1127

Mississippi

Medical Centers

#*Biloxi 39531, 400 Veterans Ave., 228-523-5000
*Jackson 39216, 1500 E. Woodrow Wilson Dr., 601-364-7900

Clinics

Byhalia 38611, 12 East Brunswick St., 662-838-2163
Columbus 39702, 824 Alabama St., 662-244-0391
Greenville 38703, 1502 S. Colorado St., 662-332-9872
Hattiesburg 39401, 231 Methodist Blvd., 601-296-3530
Kosciusko 39090, 332 Hwy. 12 W., 662-289-8089
Meridian 39301, 2103 13th St., 601-482-3275
Natchez 39120, 46 Sgt. Prentiss Dr., Suite 16, 601-442-7141
Smithville 38870, 3 sites, 63420 Highway 25 North, for information call 901-
523-8990

Regional Office

Jackson 39216, 1600 E. Woodrow Wilson Ave., statewide 800-827-1000

Vet Centers

Biloxi 39531, 288 Veterans Ave., 228-388-9938
Jackson 39216, 1755 Lelia Dr., Suite 104, 601-965-5727

National Cemeteries

Biloxi NC 39535-4968, PO Box 4968, 400 Veterans Ave., 228-388-6668
Corinth NC 38834, 1551 Horton St., 901-386-8311
Natchez NC 39120, 41 Cemetery Rd., 601-445-4981

Missouri

Medical Centers

*Columbia 65201, 800 Hospital Dr., 573-814-6000
Kansas City 64128, 4801 Linwood Blvd., 816-861-4700
*Poplar Bluff 63901, 1500 N. Westwood Blvd., 573-686-4151

Saint Louis 63106, 915 N. Grand Blvd., 314-652-4100
*Saint Louis 63125, 1 Jefferson Barracks Dr., 314-652-4100

Clinics

Belton 64012, 17140, Bel-Ray Place, 816-922-2161 or 816-318-0251
Camdenton 65020, 246 East Hwy. 54, 573-317-1150
Cameron 64429, 1111 Euclid, 816-632-1369
Cape Girardeau 63701, 2420 Veterans Memorial Dr., 573-339-0909
Farmington 63640, 1580 W. Columbia Dr., 573-760-1365
Fort Leonard Wood 65473, 126 Missouri Ave., 573-329-8305
Kirksville 63501, 1108 East Patterson, Suite 9, 660-627-8387
Mexico 65265, One Veterans Dr., 573-581-9630
Mount Vernon 65712, 600 N. Main St., 417-466-0118 or 800-253-8387
Nevada 64772, 322 Prewitt, 417-448-8905
Salem 65560, Hwy. 72 North, 573-729-6626, ext. 5230
Saint Charles 63304, 7 Jason Court, 636-498-1113
Saint James 65559, 620 N. Jefferson, 573-265-0448
Saint Joseph 64506, 1314 N. 36th, 800-952-8387, ext. 6925
Saint Louis 63136, 10600 Lewis and Clark Blvd., 314-286-6988
Warrensburg 64093, 1300 Veterans Rd., 816-922-2500
West Plains 65775, 1211 Missouri Ave., 417-257-2454

Regional Office

Saint Louis 63103, 400 South 18th St., statewide 800-827-1000

Benefits Office

Kansas City 64128, 4801 Linwood Blvd., 816-922-2660 or 800-525-1483,
ext. 52660

Vet Centers

Kansas City 64111, 301 E. Armour Rd., 816-753-1866
Saint Louis 63103, 2345 Pine St., 314-231-1260

National Cemeteries

Jefferson Barracks NC 63125, 2900 Sheridan Rd., St. Louis, 314-260-8720
Jefferson City NC 65101, 1024 E. McCarty St., 314-260-8720
Springfield NC 65804, 1702 E. Seminole St., 417-881-9499

Montana

Medical Centers

Montana Health Care System: Fort Harrison 59636, 1892 William St., 406-442-6410
*Miles City 59301, 210 S. Winchester, 406-874-5600

Clinics

Anaconda 59711, 118 E. 7th St., 406-563-6090
Billings 59102, 2345 King Ave. W., 406-651-5670
Bozeman 59715, 300 N. Wilson, Suite 703G, 406-522-8923
Glasgow 59230, 621 3rd St. South, 406-228-3554
Great Falls 59405, 1417-9th St. South, Suite 200, 877-468-8387
Kalispell 59901, 66 Claremont St., Lower Level, Suite B, 406-751-5980
Miles City 59301, 210 S. Winchester, 406-232-3060
Missoula 59808, 2687 Palmer St., Suite C, 877-468-8387
Sidney 59270, 216 14th Ave. SW, 406-488-2307

Regional Office

Fort Harrison 59636, 1892 William St., Hwy. 12 West, statewide 800-827-1000

Vet Centers

Billings 59102, 1234 Ave., C, 406-657-6071
Missoula 59802, 500 N. Higgins Ave., 406-721-4918

Nebraska

Medical Centers

VA Nebraska–Western Iowa Health Care System:
 *Grand Island 68803, 2201 N. Broadwell Ave., 308-382-3660 or 800-451-5796
 Omaha 68105, 4101 Woolworth Ave, 402-346-8800

Clinics

Alliance 69301, 524 Box Butte Ave., 800-764-5370
Gering Scottsbluff 69341, 2540 N. 10th St., 308-220-3930
Lincoln 68510, 600 S. 70th St., 402-489-3802
Norfolk 68701, 301 N. 27th St., 402-844-8022

North Platte 69101, 600 East Francis, Suite 3, 308-532-6906 or 800-451-8796
Sidney 69162, 1116 10th Ave., 308-254-5575
Scottsbluff 69341, 1441 E. 20th St., 308-220-3930 or 800-764-5370

Regional Office

Lincoln 68516, 5631 S. 48th St., statewide 800-827-1000

Vet Centers

Lincoln 68508, 920 L St., 402-476-9736
Omaha 68131, 2428 Cuming St., 402-346-6735

National Cemetery

Fort McPherson NC 69151-1031, 12004 S. Spur 56A, Maxwell, 888-737-2800

Nevada

Medical Centers

Las Vegas Nellis Air Force Base 89191, 4700 N. Las Vegas Blvd., 702-
  653-2227
*Reno 89502, 1000 Locust St., 888-838-6256

Clinics

Carson Valley 89423, 925 Ironwood St., Suite 2102, 888-838-6256, ext. 4000
Ely 89301, 6 Steptoe Circle, 775-289-3612
Henderson 89014, 2920 N. Green Valley Pkwy., Suite 215, 702-456-3825
Las Vegas 89036, PO Box 360001, N. Las Vegas, 702-636-3000
Las Vegas 89102, Psychiatric, 1501 S. Arville, 702-259-4646
Las Vegas 89032, 2455 W. Cheyenne Ave., 702-636-6375
Las Vegas 89109, 3131 La Canada St., 702-636-6360
Las Vegas 89106, 901 Rancho Lane, 702-636-6370
Las Vegas 89106, Homeless Veterans, 405 N. Wilson, 702-386-3125
Las Vegas 89118, 4420 W. Diablo Dr., 702-636-3000, ext. 4475
Las Vegas 89106, 912 W. Owens Ave., 702-636-4077
Las Vegas 89129, 2410 Fire Mesa St., 702-636-6320
Las Vegas 89121, 4187 S Pecos Rd., 702-636-6350
Las Vegas 89103, 3880 S. Jones Blvd., 702-636-6390
Las Vegas 89030, 1841 E. Craig Rd., 702-636-3090
Las Vegas 89106, 630 S. Rancho Rd., 702-636-6355
Pahrump 89048, 2100 E. Calvada Blvd., 775-727-7535

Regional Office

Reno 89511, 5460 Reno Corporate Dr., statewide 800-827-1000

Benefits Office

Las Vegas 89107, 4800 Alpine Pl., Suite 12, 800-827-1000

Vet Centers

Las Vegas 89146, 1919 S. Jones Blvd., Suite A, 702-251-7873
Reno 89503, 1155 W. 4th St., Suite 101, 775-323-1294

New Hampshire

Medical Center

*Manchester 03104, 718 Smyth Rd., 603-624-4366 or 800-892-8384

Clinics

Conway 03818, 7 Greenwood Ave., 603-447-2555
Littleton 03561, 600 St. Johnsbury Rd., 603-444-9328
Portsmouth 03803, 302 Newmarket St., 603-624-4366, ext. 5500, or 800-892-8384
Somersworth 03878, 200 Route 108, 603-4366, ext. 5700
Tilton 03276, 139 Winter St., 603-624-4366, ext. 5600, or 800-892-8384

Regional Office

Manchester 03101, Norris Cotton Federal Bldg., 275 Chestnut St., 800-827-1000

Vet Center

Manchester 03104, 103 Liberty St., 603-668-7060/61

New Jersey

Medical Centers

New Jersey Health Care System:
    *East Orange 07018, 385 Tremont Ave., 973-676-1000
    #*Lyons 07939, 151 Knollcroft Rd., 908-647-0180

Clinics

Brick 08724, 970 Rt. 70, 732-206-8900

Cape May 08204, U.S. Coast Guard Training Center, Munro Ave., 609-898-8700

Elizabeth 07206, 654 East Jersey St., 2nd Floor, 908-994-0120

Fort Dix 08640, Marshall Hall, 8th & Alabama, 609-562-2999

Fort Monmouth 07703, Patterson Army Health Clinic, Stephenson Ave., Bldg. 1075, 732-532-4500

Hackensack 07601, 385 Prospect Ave., 201-487-1390

Jersey City 07302, 115 Christopher Columbus Dr., 201-435-3055

Morristown 07960, 340 West Hanover Ave., 973-539-9794

Newark 07102, 20 Washington Pl., 973-645-1441

New Brunswick 08901, 317 George St., 732-729-0646

Paterson 07503, 275 Getty Ave., 973-247-1666

Sewell 08080, 211 County House Rd., 856-401-7665

Trenton 08611, 171 Jersey St., Bldg. 36, 609-989-2355

Turnersville 08096, 160 Fries Mill Rd., 856-262-4140

Ventnor 08406, 6601 Ventnor Ave., Suite 302, 609-823-3122

Vineland 08360, 1051 W. Sherman Ave., 856-692-2881

Regional Office

Newark 07102, 20 Washington Pl., statewide 800-827-1000 (Philadelphia, PA, Regional Office serves counties of Atlantic, Burlington, Camden, Cape May, Cumberland, Gloucester, Salem)

Vet Centers

Bloomfield 07003, 2 Broad St., Suite 703, 973-748-0980

Jersey City 07302, 115 Christopher Columbus Dr., Suite 200, 973-645-2038

Trenton 08611, 171 Jersey St., Bldg. 36, 609-989-2260

Ventnor 08406, 6601 Ventnor Ave., Suite 105, 609-487-8387

National Cemeteries

Beverly NC 08010, 916 Bridgeboro Rd., 609-877-5460

Finn's Point NC 08079, Box 542, R.F.D. 3, Fort Mott Rd., Salem, 609-877-5460

New Mexico

Medical Center

*Albuquerque 87108, 1501 San Pedro Dr., SE., 505-265-1711 or 800-465-8262

Clinics

Alamogordo 88310, 1410 Aspen, 505-437-9195
Artesia 88210, 1700 W. Main St., 505-746-3531
Clovis 88101, 921 E. Llano Estacada St., 505-763-4335
Espanola 87532, 620 Coronado St., Suite B, 505-753-7395
Farmington 87401, 1001 W. Broadway, Suite C, 505-326-4383
Gallup 87301, 320 State Hwy. 564, 505-722-7234
Hobbs 88240, 1601 N. Turner, 505-391-0354
Las Cruces 88011, 1635 Don Roser, 505-522-1241
Las Vegas 87701, 1235 8th St., 505-425-6788
Raton 87740, 1275 S. 2nd St., 505-445-2391
Santa Fe 87507, 2213 Brothers Rd., Suite 600, 505-986-8645
Silver City 88061, 1302 32nd St., 505-538-2921
Truth or Consequences 87901, 1960 N. Date St., 505-894-7662

Regional Office

Albuquerque 87102, Dennis Chavez Federal Bldg., 500 Gold Ave. SW, statewide 800-827-1000

Vet Centers

Albuquerque 87104, 1600 Mountain Rd. NW, 505-346-6562
Farmington 87402, 4251 E. Main, Suite C, 505-327-9684
Santa Fe 87505, 2209 Brothers Rd., Suite 110, 505-988-6562

National Cemeteries

Fort Bayard NC 88036, PO Box 189, 915-564-0201
Santa Fe NC 87501, 501 N. Guadalupe St., 505-988-6400 or 877-353-6295

New York

Medical Centers

*Albany 12208, 113 Holland Ave., 518-626-5000
#*Canandaigua 14424, 400 Fort Hill Ave., 585-393-7100

#*Bath 14810, 76 Veterans Ave., 607-664-4000
*Bronx 10468, 130 W. Kingsbridge Rd., 718-584-9000
VA New York Harbor Healthcare System:
   Brooklyn 11209, 800 Poly Place, 718-836-6600
   New York 10010, 423 East 23rd St., 212-686-7500
   #*St. Albans 11425, 179 St. & Linden Blvd., 718-526-1000
VA Hudson Valley Health Care System:
   *Castle Point 12511, 845-831-2000
   #*Montrose 10548, 2094 Albany Post Rd., Route 9A/PO Box 100, 914-
      737-4400
*Northport 11768, 79 Middleville Rd., 631-261-4400
*Syracuse 13210, 800 Irving Ave., 315-425-4400
Western New York Health Care System:
   *Batavia 14020, 222 Richmond Ave., 585-297-1000
   *Buffalo 14215, 3495 Bailey Ave., 716-834-9200

Clinics

Auburn 13201, 17 Lansing St., 315-255-7002
Bainbridge 13733, 109 N. Main St., 607-967-8590
Binghamton 13001, 425 Robinson St., 607-772-9100
Brooklyn 11201, 40 Flatbush Ave. Ext., 8th Fl., 718-439-4300
Bronx 10459, 953 Southern Blvd., 718-741-4900
Buffalo 14209, Homeless Veterans, 1298 Main St., 716-881-5855
Buffalo 14214, 2963 Main St., 716-862-8865
Carmel 10512, 1875 Route 6, Warwick Savings Bank, 2nd Floor, 845-228-5291
Carthage 13619, 3 Bridge St., 315-493-4180
Catskill 12414, 159 Jefferson Heights, Columbia Greene Medical Arts Bldg.,
   Suite A102, 518-943-7515
Clifton Park 12065, 1673 Route 9, 518-383-8506
Cortland 13405, 1129 Commons Ave., 607-662-1517
Dunkirk 14048, 325 Central Ave., 716-366-2122
Elizabethtown 12932, Community Hospital, 75 Park St., 518-873-3295
Elmira 14901, 200 Madison Ave. 877-845-3247, ext. 44640
Fonda 12068, 2623 State Hwy. 30A, 518-853-1247
Glens Falls 12801, 84 Broad St., 518-798-6066
Goshen 10924, 30 Hatfield Ln., Suite 204, 845-294-6927
Islip 11751, 39 Nassau Ave., 631-581-5330
Ithaca 14850, 10 Arrowwood Dr., 607-274-4680
Jamestown 14701, 890 East 2nd St., 716-661-1447
Kingston 12401, 63 Hurley Ave., 845-331-8322
Lackawanna 14218, 227 Ridge Rd., 716-822-5944

Lindenhurst 11757, 560 N. Delaware Ave., 631-884-1133

Lockport 14094, 5875 S. Transit Rd., 716-433-2025

Malone 12953, 183 Park St., 518-481-2545

Massena 13662, 1 Hospital Dr., 315-769-4253

Monticello 12701, 461 Broadway, 845-791-4936

New City 10956, Citibank Building, Suite 400, 20 Squadron Blvd., 845-634-8942

New York 10027, Harlem Care Center, 55 W. 125th St., 11th Floor, 212-828-5265

New York 10014, Soho Center, 245 West Houston St., 212-337-2569

New York 10011, OSP Center, 437 W. 16th St., 212-462-4461

Niagara Falls 14301, 2201 Pine Ave., 800-223-4810

Olean 14760, 465 N. Union St., 716-373-7709

Oswego 13126, Seneca Hill Health Center, 105 County Rt. 45A, Suite 400, 315-343-0925

Patchogue 11772, 4 Phyllis Dr., 631-758-4419

Pine Plains 12567, 2881 Church St., Rt. 199, 518-398-9240

Plainview 11803, 1425 Old Country Rd., 516-694-6008

Plattsburgh 12901, 43 Durkee St., Suite 300, 518-561-8310

Port Jervis 12771, 150 Pike St., 845-856-5396

Poughkeepsie 12603, Freedom Exec. Park, 488 Freedom Plains Rd., Suite 120, 845-452-5151

Riverhead 11901, 89 Hubbard Ave., 631-727-7171

Rochester 14620, 465 Westfall Rd., 585-463-2600

Rome 13441, 125 Brookley Rd., Building 510, 315-334-7100

Schenectady 12308, Sheridan Plaza, 1322 Gerling St., 518-346-3334

Sidney 13733, 109 Main St., 607-967-8590

Staten Island 10314, 1150 South Ave., 3rd Fl., Suite 301, 718-761-2973

Sunnyside, 11104, 41-03 Queens Blvd., 718-741-4800

Troy 12180, 295 River St., 518-274-7707

Warsaw 14569, 400 N. Main St., 585-786-2233

Wellsville 14895, 13 Loder St., 585-596-2056

Westhampton 11978, 150 Old Riverhead Rd., 631-898-0599

White Plains 10601, 23 South Broadway, 914-421-1951

Yonkers 10701, 124 New Main St., 914-375-8055

Regional Offices

Buffalo 14202, Niagara Center, 130 S. Elmwood St., 800-827-1000 (for counties not served by New York City VA Regional Office)

New York 10014, 245 W. Houston St., statewide 800-827-1000 (serves counties of Albany, Bronx, Clinton, Columbia, Delaware, Dutchess, Essex,

Franklin, Fulton, Greene, Hamilton, Kings, Montgomery, Nassau, New York, Orange, Otsego, Putnam, Queens, Rensselaer, Richmond, Rockland, Saratoga, Schenectady, Schoharie, Suffolk, Sullivan, Ulster, Warren, Washington, Westchester)

Benefits Offices

Albany 12208, 113 Holland Ave., 800-827-1000
Rochester 14620, 465 Westfall Rd., 800-827-1000
Syracuse 13202, 344 W. Genesee St., 800-827-1000

Vet Centers

Albany 12206, 875 Central Ave., 518-438-2505
Babylon 11702, 116 West Main St., 631-661-3930
Bronx 10458, 130 West Kingsbridge Rd., Rm. 7A-13, 718-367-3500
Brooklyn 11201, 25 Chapel St., Suite 604, 718-330-2825
Buffalo 14202, 564 Franklin St., 716-882-0505
New York 10004, 32 Broadway, Suite 200, 212-742-9591
New York 10027, 55 West 125th St., 212-426-2200
Rochester 14620, 1867 Mt. Hope Ave., 585-232-5040
Staten Island 10301, 150 Richmond Terrace, 718-816-4499
Syracuse 13210, 716 E. Washington St., 315-478-7127
White Plains 10601, 300 Hamilton Ave., 914-682-6250
Woodhaven 11421, 75-10B 91st Ave., 718-296-2871

National Cemeteries

Bath NC 14810, 76 Veterans Ave., San Juan Ave., 607-664-4853
Calverton NC 11933-1031, 210 Princeton Blvd., 631-727-5410/5770
Cypress Hills NC 11208, 625 Jamaica Ave., Brooklyn, 631-454-4949
Long Island NC 11735-1211, 2040 Wellwood Ave., Farmingdale, 631-454-4949
Saratoga NC 12871-1721, 200 Duell Rd., Schuylerville, 518-581-9128
Woodlawn NC 14901, 1825 Davis St., Elmira, 607-732-5411

North Carolina

Medical Centers

*Asheville 28805, 1100 Tunnel Rd., 828-298-7911 or 800-932-6408
*Durham 27705, 508 Fulton St., 919-286-0411
*Fayetteville 28301, 2300 Ramsey St., 910-488-2120
*Salisbury 28144, 1601 Brenner Ave., 704-638-9000

Clinics

Charlotte 28262, Presb. Med. Plaza, 8401 Medical Ctr. Dr., Suite 350, 704-547-0020
Durham 27705, 1824 Hill and Dale Rd., 919-383-6107
Greenville 27858, 800 Moye Blvd., 252-830-2149
Jacksonville 28540, 1021 Hargett St., 910-219-1339
Morehead City 28557, 5420 Highway 70, 252-240-2349
Raleigh 27610, 23 Sunnybrook Rd., Suite 107, 919-212-0129
Wilmington 28401, 1606 Physicians Dr., Suite 104, 910-362-8811
Winston-Salem 27103, 190 Kimel Park Dr., 336-768-3296, ext. 1209 or 1210

Regional Office

Winston-Salem 27155, Federal Bldg., 251 N. Main St., statewide 800-827-1000, nationwide Loan Guaranty Certificate of Eligibility Center 888-244-6711

Vet Centers

Charlotte 28202, 223 S. Brevard St., Suite 103, 704-333-6107
Fayetteville 28311, 4140 Ramsey St., Suite 110, 910-488-6252
Greensboro 27406, 2009 S. Elm-Eugene St., 336-333-5366
Greenville 27858, 150 Arlington Blvd., Suite B, 252-355-7920
Raleigh 27604, 1649 Old Louisburg Rd., 919-856-4616

National Cemeteries

New Bern NC 28560, 1711 National Ave., 252-637-2912
Raleigh NC 27610-3335, 501 Rock Quarry Rd., 252-637-2912
Salisbury NC 28144, 202 Government Rd., 704-636-2661/4621
Wilmington NC 28403, 2011 Market St., 252-637-2912

North Dakota

Medical Center

*Fargo 58102, 2101 N. Elm St., 701-232-3241

Clinics

Bismarck 58503, Gateway Mall, 2700 State St., Suite 5, 701-221-9169
Grafton 58237, West 6th St., 701-352-4059
Minot 58705, 10 Missile Ave., 701-727-9800

Regional Office

Fargo 58102, 2101 Elm St., statewide 800-827-1000

Vet Centers

Bismarck 58501, 1684 Capital Way, 701-224-9751
Fargo 58103, 3310 Fiechtner Dr., Suite 100, 701-237-0942
Minot 58701, 2041 3rd St. NW, 701-852-0177

Ohio

Medical Centers

#*Brecksville 44141, 10000 Brecksville Rd., 440-526-3030
*Chillicothe 45601, 17273 State Route 104, 740-773-1141
#*Cincinnati 45220, 3200 Vine St., 513-861-3100
Cleveland 44106, 10701 East Blvd., 216-791-3800
#*Dayton 45428, 4100 W. 3rd St., 937-268-6511

Clinics

Akron 44319-1116, 55 W. Waterloo, 330-724-7715
Ashtabula 44004, 1230 Lake Ave., 440-964-6454
Athens 45701, 510 W. Union St., 740-593-7314
Cambridge 43727, 2146 Southgate Pkwy., 740-432-1963
Canton 44702, 733 Market Ave., S., 330-489-4600
Cincinnati 45245, Eastgate Prof. Bldg., 4355 Ferguson Dr., Suite 270, 513-943-3680
Cleveland/McCafferty 44113, 4242 Lorain Ave., 216-939-0699
Columbus 43203, 543 Taylor Ave., 614-257-5200
East Liverpool 43920, 332 W. 6th St., 330-386-4303
Georgetown 45121, 4903 State Route 125, 937-378-3413
Grove City 43123, 1955 Ohio Dr., 614-257-5800
Hamilton 45011, 1755C S. Erie Hwy., 513-870-9744
Lancaster 43130, Colonnade Med. Bldg, 1550 Sheridan Dr., 740-653-6145
Lima 45804, 1303 Bellefontaine Ave., 419-222-5788
Lorain 44052, 205 W. 20th St., 440-244-3833
Mansfield 44906, 1456 Park Ave. West, 419-529-4602
Marietta 45750, 418 Colegate Dr., 740-568-0412
Marion 43302, 1203 Delaware Ave., 614-257-5920
Middletown 45042, 675 N. University Blvd., 513-423-8387
New Philadelphia 44663, 1260 Monroe Ave., 15H, 330-602-5339
Newark 43055, 1912 Tamarack Rd., 740-788-8329

Painesville 44077, 7 West Jackson St., 440-357-6740
Portsmouth 45662, 621 Broadway St., 740-353-3236
Ravenna 44266, 6751 N. Chestnut St., 330-296-3641
St. Clairsville 43950, 103 Plaza Dr., Suite A, 740-695-9321
Sandusky 44870, 3416 Columbus Ave., 419-625-7350
Springfield 45505, 512 S. Burnett Rd., 937-328-3385
Toledo 43614, 3333 Glendale Ave., 419-259-2000
Warren 44485, Riverside Sq., 1400 Tod Ave. NW, 330-392-0311
Youngstown 44505, 2031 Belmont Ave., 330-740-9200
Zanesville 43701, 840 Bethesda Dr., Bldg., 3-A, 740-453-7725

Regional Office

Cleveland 44199, Anthony J. Celebrezze Federal Bldg., 1240 E. 9th St., 800-827-1000

Benefits Offices

Cincinnati 45202, 36 E. Seventh St., Suite 210, 800-827-1000
Columbus 43215, Federal Bldg., Rm. 309, 200 N. High St., 800-827-1000

Vet Centers

Cincinnati 45203, 801-B W. 8th St., 513-763-3500
Cleveland Heights 44118, 2022 Lee Rd., 216-932-8471
Columbus 43215, 30 Spruce St., 614-257-5550
Dayton 45402, 111 W 1st St., Suite 101, 937-461-9150
Parma 44129, 5700 Pearl Rd., Suite 102, 440-845-5023

National Cemeteries

Dayton NC 45428-1008, 4100 W. Third St., 937-262-2115
Ohio Western Reserve NC 44270, PO Box 8, 10175, Rawiga Rd., Rittman, 330-335-3069

Oklahoma

Medical Centers

Muskogee 74401, 1011 Honor Heights Dr., 918-683-3261
*Oklahoma City 73104, 921 NE 13th St., 405-270-0501

Clinics

Ardmore 73401, 1015 S. Commerce, 580-223-2266

Clinton 73601, 1/4 mile south of I-40 on Highway 183
Lawton/Fort Sill 73503, Bldg. 4303, 4303 Pittman and Thomas, 580-353-1131
McAlester 74501, 903 E. Monroe St., 918-423-2880
Ponca City 74601, 215 N. 3rd, 580-762-1777
Seminole Co. 74849, Konawa, 527 W. Third St., 580-925-3286
Tulsa 74145, 9322 E. 41st St., 918-764-7243

Regional Office

Muskogee 74401, Federal Bldg., 125 S. Main St., 800-827-1000

Benefits Office

Oklahoma City 73102, Federal Campus, 301 NW 6th St., Suite 113, 800-827-
1000

Vet Centers

Oklahoma City 73105, 3033 N. Walnut, Suite 101W, 405-270-5184
Tulsa 74112, 1408 S. Harvard, 918-748-5105

National Cemeteries

Fort Gibson NC 74434, 1423 Cemetery Rd., 918-478-2334
Fort Sill NC 73538, 2648 Jake Dunn Rd., 580-492-3200

Oregon

Medical Centers

#*Portland 97239, 3710 SW U.S. Veterans Hospital Rd., 503-220-8262
*Roseburg 97470, 913 NW Garden Valley Blvd., 541-440-1000

Clinics

Bandon 97411, 1010 1st St. SE, Suite 100, 541-347-4736
Bend 97701, 2115 Wyatt Court, Suite 201, 888-233-8305
Brookings 97415, 555 5th St., 541-412-1152
Eugene 97404, 100 River Ave., 541-607-0897
Klamath Falls 97601, 2819 Dahlia St, 541-273-6206/6129
Salem 97301, 1660 Oak St. SE, 888-233-8305
Warrenton 97146, Camp Rilea, 91400, Rilea Neocoxie Rd., Bldg. 7315, 888-
233-8305

Rehabilitation Center

White City 97503, 8495 Crater Lake Hwy., 541-826-2111, ext. 3210 or 3239, 800-809-8725

Regional Office

Portland 97204, Edith Green/Wendell Wyatt Federal Building, 1220 SW Third Ave., 800-827-1000

Vet Centers

Eugene 97403, 1255 Pearl St., 541-465-6918
Grants Pass 97526, 211 SE 10th St., 541-479-6912
Portland 97220, 8383 NE Sandy Blvd., Suite 110, 503-273-5370
Salem 97301, 617 Chemeketa St. NE, 503-362-9911

National Cemeteries

Eagle Point NC 97524, 2763 Riley Rd., 541-826-2511
Roseburg NC 97470, 913 Garden Valley Blvd., 541-826-2511
Willamette NC 97266-6937, 11800, SE Mt. Scott Blvd., Portland, 503-273-5250

Pennsylvania

Medical Centers

*Altoona 16602, 2907 Pleasant Valley Blvd., 814-943-8164 or 877-626-2500
#*Butler 16001, 325 New Castle Rd., 724-287-4781 or 800-362-8262
#*Coatesville 19320, 1400 Black Horse Hill Rd., 610-384-7711 or 800-290-6172
*Erie 16504-1596, 135 E. 38th St., 814-868-8661 or 800-274-8387
*Lebanon 17042, 1700 S. Lincoln Ave., 717-272-6621, 800-409-8771
*Philadelphia 19104, University & Woodland Aves., 215-823-5800 or 800-949-1001
Pittsburgh Health Care System: Pittsburgh 15240, University Dr., 412-688-6000 or 866-482-7488
*Wilkes-Barre 18711, 1111 East End Blvd., 570-824-3521 or 877-928-2621

Clinics

Aliquippa 15001, 2360 Hospital Dr., 724-857-0424
Allentown 18103, 3100 Hamilton Blvd., 610-776-4304 or 866-249-6472
Bangor 18013, 701 Slate Belt Blvd., 610-599-0127

Berwick 18603, 301 West 3rd St., 570-759-0351

Camp Hill 17011, 25 N. 32nd St., 717-730-9782

DuBois 15801, 190 West Park Ave., Suite 8, 814-375-6817 or 866-662-0447

Ellwood City 16117, Medical Arts Bldg., 304 Evans Dr., 724-285-2203

Foxburg 16049, 855 Route 58, Suite 1, 724-659-5601

Frackville 17931, 10 East Spruce St., 570-874-4289

Greensburg 15601, Hempfield Plaza, Rt. 30, 724-837-5200

Hermitage 16148, 295 N. Kerrwood Dr., Suite 110, 724-346-1569

Johnstown 15904, University Park Plaza, 1425 Scalp Ave., Suite 29, 814-266-8696

Kittanning 16201, ACMH, 1 Nolte Dr., 724-543-8711

Lancaster 17601, Greenfield Corporate Center, 1861 Charter Lane, Suite 118, 717-290-6900

Meadville 16335, 18955 Park Ave. Plaza, 814-337-0170

New Castle 16101, Jameson South Campus, 1000 S. Mercer St., 724-285-2203

Oil City 16301, 174 Bissell Ave., 814-678-2631

Pottsville 17901, 700 Schuylkill Manor Rd., 570-621-4115

Reading 19601, 145 N. Sixth St., 3rd Fl., St. Joseph Med. Comm. Camp., 610-208-4717

Sayre 18840, 1537 Elmira St., 570-888-6803 or 877-470-0920

Shippenville 16254, Marianne Family Practice, 21159 Paint Blvd., Suite 2, 814-226-6770

State College 16801-2755, 3048 Enterprise Dr., Ferguson Sq. Bldg., 1, 814-867-5415

Smethport 16749, 406 Franklin St., 814-887-5655

Spring City 19475, 11 Independence Dr., 610-948-1082

Springfield 19064, 194 W. Sproul Rd., Suite 105, Crozier Keystone Health-plex, 610-543-3246

Tobyhanna 18466, Bldg. 220, Tobyhanna Army Depot, 570-895-8341

Uniontown 15401, 404 W. Main St., 724-439-4990

Warren 16365, 3 Farm Colony Dr., 814-723-9763

Washington 15301, 100 Ridge Ave., 724-250-7790

Williamsport 17701, Divine Providence, 1705 Warren Ave., Suite 304, 570-322-4791

Willow Grove/Horsham 19044, 433 Caredean, 215-823-6050

York 17403, 1796 3rd Ave., 717-854-2481

Regional Offices

Philadelphia 19101, Regional Office and Insurance Center, PO Box 8079, 5000 Wissahickon Ave., 800-827-1000 (serves counties of Adams, Berks, Bradford, Bucks, Cameron, Carbon, Centre, Chester, Clinton, Columbia,

Dauphin, Delaware, Franklin, Juniata, Lackawanna, Lancaster, Lebanon, Lehigh, Luzerne, Lycoming, Mifflin, Monroe, Montgomery, Montour, Northampton, Northumberland, Perry, Philadelphia, Pike, Potter, Schuylkill, Snyder, Sullivan, Susquehanna, Tioga, Union, Wayne, Wyoming, York)
Pittsburgh 15222, 1000 Liberty Ave., statewide 800-827-1000 (serves remaining counties of Pennsylvania)

Benefits Office

Wilkes-Barre 18702, 1123 East End Blvd., Bldg. 35, Suite 11, 800-827-1000

Vet Centers

Erie 16501, 1000 State St., Suites 1 and 2, 814-453-7955
Harrisburg 17102, 1500 N. 2nd St., Suite 2, 717-782-3954
McKeesport 15131, 2001 Lincoln Way, 412-678-7704
Philadelphia 19107, 801 Arch St., Suite 102, 215-627-0238
Philadelphia 19120, 101 E. Olney Ave., 215-924-4670
Pittsburgh 15205, 2500 Baldwick Rd., Suite 15, 412-920-1765
Scranton 18505, 1002 Pittston Ave., 570-344-2676
Williamsport 17701, 805 Penn St., 570-327-5281

National Cemeteries

Indiantown Gap NC 17003-9618, RR 2, PO Box 484, Annville, 717-865-5254
NC of the Alleghenies 15017, 1158 Morgan Rd., Bridgeville, 724-746-4363
Philadelphia NC 19138, Haines St. & Limekiln Pike, 609-877-5460

Philippines

Regional Office

Manila 0930 1131 Roxas Blvd., 011-632-528-6300, international mailing address: PSC 501, FPO AP 96515-1100

Clinic

Manila 2201 Roxas Blvd., Pasay City, 1300 Philippines, 011-632-833-4566, international mailing address PSC 501, FPO AP 96515-1100

Puerto Rico

Medical Center

*San Juan 00921-3201, 10 Casia St., 787-641-7582 or 800-449-8729

Clinics

Arecibo 00612, Victor Rojas 2, Zona Industrial Carr 9, 787-816-1818 or 866-874-6569
Guayama 00784, FISA Building-First Floor, Paseo del Pueblo, Km. 0.3, Lote No. 6, 787-866-8766
Mayaguez 00680-1507, Avenida Hostos #345, 787-834-6900
Ponce 00716-2001, Paseo del Veterano #1010, 787-812-3163 or 800-563-5086

Regional Office

San Juan 00918-1703, 150 Carlos Chardon Ave., Suite 300, but send mail to Suite 232 (serving all Puerto Rico and the Virgin Islands, 800-827-1000)

Benefits Offices

Mayaguez 00680-1507, Ave. Hostos 345, Carretera 2, Frente al Centro Medico, 800-827-1000
Ponce 00731, 10 Paseo del Veterano, 800-827-1000
Arecibo 00612, Gonzalo Marin 50, 800-827-1000

Vet Centers

Arecibo 00612-4702, 52 Gonzalo Marin St., 787-879-4510/4581
Ponce 00731, 35 Mayo St., 787-841-3260
San Juan 00921, Condominio Med. Ctr. Plaza, Suite LC8A11, La Riviera, 787-749-4409

National Cemetery

Puerto Rico NC 00960, Ave. Cementerio Nacional 50, Barrio Hato Tejas, Bayamon, 787-798-8400

Rhode Island

Medical Center

Providence 02908, 830 Chalkstone Ave., 401-273-7100

Clinic

Middletown 02842, One Corporate Pl., West Main Rd., 401-847-6239

Regional Office

Providence 02903, 380 Westminster St., statewide, 800-827-1000

Vet Center

Warwick 02889, 2038 Warwick Ave., 401-739-0167

South Carolina

Medical Centers

*Charleston 29401, 109 Bee St., 843-577-5011
*Columbia 29209-1639, 6439 Garners Ferry Rd., 803-776-4000

Clinics

Anderson 29621, 1702 East Greenville St., 864-224-5450
Beaufort 29902, 1 Pinckney Blvd., 843-770-0444
Florence 29501, 805 Pamplico Highway, Suite 220A, 843-292-8383
Goose Creek 29406, 9237 University Blvd. North, 843-789-6400
Greenville 29605, 3510 Augusta Rd., 864-299-1600
Myrtle Beach 29577, 3381 Phillis Blvd., 843-477-0177
Orangeburg 29118, 1767 Village Park Dr., 803-533-1335
Rock Hill 29732, 205 Piedmont Blvd., 803-366-4848
Sumter 29150, 407 N. Salem St., 803-938-9901

Nursing Home

Walterboro 29488, 2461 Sidneys Rd., Veterans Victory House, 843-538-3000

Regional Office

Columbia 29201, 1801 Assembly St., statewide 800-827-1000

Vet Centers

Columbia 29201, 1513 Pickens St., 803-765-9944
Greenville 29601, 14 Lavinia Ave., 864-271-2711
North Charleston 29406, 5603-A Rivers Ave., 843-747-8387

National Cemeteries

Beaufort NC 29902-3947, 1601 Boundary St., 843-524-3925
Florence NC 29501, 803 E. National Cemetery Rd., 843-669-8783

South Dakota

Medical Centers

Black Hills Health Care System:
   *Fort Meade 57741, 113 Comanche Rd., 605-347-2511 or 800-743-1070
   #Hot Springs 57747, 500 N. 5th St., 605-745-2000 or 800-764-5370
*Sioux Falls 57105, 2501 W. 22nd St., 605-336-3230

Clinics

Aberdeen 57401, 1440 15th Ave. NW, 605-622-2640
Eagle Butte 57625, 315 Main St., 605-964-8000
Isabel 57633, 118 N. Main St., 605-466-2120
Faith 57626, 112 N. 2nd Ave., 605-967-2644
Mission/Rosebud 57570, 153 S. Main St., 605-856-2295 or 800-764-5370
Pierre 57501, 1601 N. Harrison, Suite 6, 605-945-1710
Rapid City 57701, 3625 5th St., 605-718-1095 or 800-743-1070
Winner 57580, 915 E. 8th St., 605-745-2000, ext. 2474
McLauglin TWS 57642, 302 Sale Barn Rd., 605-823-4574 or 800-743-1070

Regional Office

Sioux Falls 57117, PO Box 5046, 2501 W. 22nd St., statewide 800-827-1000

Vet Centers

Martin 57551, East Hwy 18, 605-685-1300
Rapid City 57701, 621 6th St., Suite 101, 605-348-0077
Sioux Falls 57104, 601 S. Cliff Ave., Suite C, 605-330-4552

National Cemeteries

Black Hills NC 57785, 20901, Pleasant Valley Dr., Sturgis, 605-347-3830
Fort Meade NC 57785, PO Box 640, Old Stone Rd., Sturgis, 605-347-3830
Hot Springs NC 57747, 500 N. 5th St., 605-347-3830

Tennessee

Medical Centers

*Memphis 38104, 1030 Jefferson Ave., 901-523-8990
#*Mountain Home 37684, PO Box 4000, 423-926-1171
VA Tennessee Valley Healthcare System:
  Nashville Campus 37212, 1310 24th Ave. South, 615-327-4751
  Alvin C. York Campus, Murfreesboro 37129, 3400 Lebanon Pike, 615-867-6000

Clinics

Chattanooga 37411, 150 Debra Rd., Suite 5200, Bldg 6200, 423-893-6500
Clarksville 37043, Gateway Med. Ctr., 1731 Memorial St., Suite 110, 931-221-2171
Cookeville 38501, Primary Care, 1101 Neal St., 931-525-1652
Covington 38128, 3461 Austin Peay Hwy., 901-261-4500
Dover 37058-0497, 1021 Spring St., PO Box 497, 931-232-5329
Knoxville 37923, 9031 Cross Park Dr., 865-545-4592
Memphis South 38116, 1056 East Raines Rd., 901-271-4900
Mountain City 37683, PO Box 738, 423-727-1103
Nashville/Vine Hill Clinic 37204, 601 Benton Ave., 615-292-9770
Rogersville 37857, PO Box 850, 423-272-5600
Savannah 38372, 765-A Florence Rd., 731-925-2300
Smithville 38870, 63420, Highway 25 N., 901-523-8990
Tullahoma 37389, Arnold AFB, 225 First St., 931-454-6134

Regional Office

Nashville 37203, 110 9th Ave. South, statewide 800-827-1000

Vet Centers

Chattanooga 37411, 951 Eastgate Loop Rd., Bldg. 5700, Suite 300, 423-855-6570
Johnson City 37604, 1615A W. Market St., 423-928-8387
Knoxville 37914, 2817 E. Magnolia Ave., 865-545-4680
Memphis 38104, 1835 Union, Suite 100, 901-544-0173
Nashville 37217, Airpark Bus. Cen. 1, 1420 Donelson Pike, Suite A-5, 615-366-1220

National Cemeteries

Chattanooga NC 37404, 1200 Bailey Ave., 423-855-6590

Knoxville NC 37917, 939 Tyson St. NW, 423-855-6590
Memphis NC 38122, 3568 Townes Ave., 901-386-8311
Mountain Home NC 37684, PO Box 8, VAMC, Bldg. 117, 423-979-3535
Nashville NC 37115-4619, 1420 Gallatin Rd. So., Madison, 615-860-0086

Texas

Medical Centers

*Amarillo 79106, 6010 Amarillo Blvd. West, 806-355-9703 or 800-687-8262
El Paso Health Care System: 79930, 5001 N. Piedras St., 915-564-6100, 800-672-3782
*Houston 77030, 2002 Holcombe Blvd., 713-791-1414
*West Texas Health Care System: Big Spring 79720, 300 Veterans Blvd., 432-263-7361 or 800-472-1365
Central Texas Health Care System:
  #*Temple 76504, 1901 Veterans Memorial Dr., 800-423-2111 or 254-778-4811
  Waco 76711, 4800 Memorial Dr., 254-752-6581 or 800-423-2111
North Texas Health Care System:
  #*Bonham 75418, 1201 East Ninth St., 800-924-8387
  #*Dallas 75216, 4500 S. Lancaster Rd., 800-849-3597
South Texas Health Care System:
  *San Antonio 78229-4404, 7400 Merton Minter Blvd., 210-617-5300
  *Kerrville 78028, 3600 Memorial Blvd., 830-896-2020

Clinics

Abilene 78606, 4225 Woods Place, 325-695-3252
Aledo 76008, 317 FM 1187 North, 800-924-8387
Alice/Christus Spohn San Diego 78384, 215 Dr. E.E. Dunlap St., 361-279-3378
Austin 78741, 2901 Montopolis Dr., 512-389-1010
Beaumont 77707, 3420 Veteran Circle, 409-981-8550
Beeville 78102, Family Practice, 302 South Hillside Dr., 361-358-9912
Bonham/Red River, Grayson, Delta, and Lamar Counties, 800-924-8387, ext. 36676, or 903-583-6676
Bridgeport 76426, 808 Woodrow Wilson Ray Cir., 940-683-2538
Brownwood 76801, 2600 Memorial Park Dr., 325-641-0568
Cedar Park 78613, 701 E. Whitestone Blvd., 512-260-1368
Childress 79201, Highway 83 North, 940-937-3636
Cleburne, Johnson, and Ellis Counties, 800-924-8387, ext. 36674, or 903-583-6674

College Station/Bryan 77845, 1605 Rock Prairie Rd., Suite 212, 979-680-0361
Corpus Christi 78405, 5283 Old Brownsville Rd., 361-806-5600
Decatur 76426, Wise, Jack, Clay, Archer, Baylor, Young, Throckmorton and Montague Counties, 800-924-8387, ext. 6674 or 903-583-6674
Denton 76201, 3537 Interstate 35E, 800-924-8387, x36676, or 903-583-6676
Eastland, Parker, Palo Pinto, Hood, Callahan and Stephens Counties, 800-924-8387, ext. 36674, or 903-583-6674
Fort Stockton 79735, 501 N. Main St., 432-336-0700
Fort Worth 76104, 300 W. Rosedale St., 800-443-9672
Galveston 77551, 1101 61st St., 800-310-5001
Granbury 76049, 2006 Fall Creek Hwy., 817-326-3440
Greenville 4311 Wesley St., 903-583-6674
Harlingen 78550, 1629 Treasure Hills Blvd., Suite 5-B, 956-366-4500
Kingsville/Christus Spohn Bishop 78343, 301 West Main, 361-584-2563
Laredo 78041, 6551 Star Ct., 956-523-7850
Longview 75601, 1205 E. Marshall Ave., 903-247-8262
Lubbock 79412, 6104 Ave. Q South Dr., 806-472-3400
Lufkin 75904, 1301 W. Frank Ave., 936-637-1342
Marlin 76661, 1016 Ward St., 800-423-2111
McAllen 78503, 2101 S. Colonel Rowe Blvd., 956-618-7100
New Braunfels 78130, Rural Clinic, 189 E. Austin St., Suite 106, 830-629-3614
Odessa 79761, 4241 N. Tanglewood Ln., 432-550-0152
Palestine 75801, 2000 S. Loop 256, Suite 200, 903-723-9006
Paris 75462, 635 Stone Ave., 903-583-2111
Red River County 75462, 800-924-8387, ext. 36342, or 903-583-6342
San Angelo 76905, 2018 Pulliam, 325-658-6138
San Antonio 78240, Frank M. Tejeda Clinic, 5788 Eckert Rd., 210-699-2100
San Antonio/General McMullen 78226, 1831 General McMullen, 210-434-1400
San Antonio/Greenway 78217, 2455 NE Loop 410, Suite 100, 210-599-6000
San Antonio/Northern Hills 78217, 13909 Nacogdoches, Suite 124, 210-653-8989
San Antonio/Pecan Valley 78222, 4243 E. Southcross, Suite 205, 210-304-3500
Seguin 78130, 510 E. Court St., 830-629-3614
Sherman 75090, 2612 N. Loy Lake, Suite 300, 903-891-8317
South Bexar County 78223, 1055 Ada, San Antonio, 210-358-5701
Stamford 79553, 1303 Mabee Dr., 325-773-5733
Stratford 79084, 1220 Purnell St., 806-396-5583
Tarrant County 76107, 800-924-8387, ext. 36676, or 903-583-6676
Texas City 77591, 9300 Emmett F. Lowry Expressway, Suite 206, 409-986-1129 or 800-310-5001

Tyler 75701, 3414 Golden Rd., 800-924-8387, ext. 36674, or 903-583-6674
Uvalde 78801, 137 W. Nopal, 830-279-0535
Victoria 77901, 1502 E. Airline, Suite 40, 361-582-7700
Waxahachie 75165, 201 Ferris Ave., 972-937-1613
Wichita Falls 76301, 1800 7th St., 940-723-2373

Regional Offices

Houston 77030, 6900 Almeda Rd., statewide, 800-827-1000 (serves counties of Angelina, Aransas, Atacosa, Austin, Bandera, Bee, Bexar, Blanco, Brazoria, Brewster, Brooks, Caldwell, Calhoun, Cameron, Chambers, Colorado, Comal, Crockett, DeWitt, Dimitt, Duval, Edwards, Fort Bend, Frio, Galveston, Gillespie, Goliad, Gonzales, Grimes, Guadeloupe, Hardin, Harris, Hays, Hidalgo, Houston, Jackson, Jasper, Jefferson, Jim Hogg, Jim Wells, Karnes, Kendall, Kennedy, Kerr, Kimble, Kinney, Kleberg, LaSalle, Lavaca, Liberty, Live Oak, McCulloch, McMullen, Mason, Matagorda, Maverick, Medina, Menard, Montgomery, Nacogdoches, Newton, Nueces, Orange, Pecos, Polk, Real, Refugio, Sabine, San Augustine, San Jacinto, San Patricio, Schleicher, Shelby, Starr, Sutton, Terrell, Trinity, Tyler, Uvalde, Val Verde, Victoria, Walker, Waller, Washington, Webb, Wharton, Willacy, Wilson, Zapata, Zavala)
Waco 76799, One Veterans Plaza, 701 Clay; statewide, 800- 827-1000 (serves the rest of the state. In Bowie County, the City of Texarkana is served by Little Rock, AR, VA Regional Office, 800-827-1000)

Benefits Offices

Abilene 79602, Taylor County Plaza Bldg., 400 Oak St., Suite 103, 800-827-1000
Amarillo 79106, 6010 Amarillo Blvd. W., 800-827-1000
Austin 78741, 2901 Montopolis Dr., Room 108, 800-827-1000
Corpus Christi 78405, 4646 Corona Dr., Suite 150, 800-827-1000
Dallas 75216, 4500 S. Lancaster Rd., 800-827-1000
El Paso 79930, 5001 Piedras Dr., 800-827-1000
Ft. Worth 76104-4856, 300 W. Rosedale St., 800-827-1000
Lubbock 79410, 4902 34th St., Suite 10, Rm. 134, 800-827-1000
McAllen 78503, 1901 South 1st St., Suite 400, 800-827-1000
San Antonio 78240, 5788 Eckert Rd., 800-827-1000
Temple 76504, 1901 Veterans Memorial Dr., Room 5G38 [BRB], 800-827-1000
Tyler 75701, 1700 SSE Loop 323, Suite 310, 800-827-1000

Vet Centers

Amarillo 79109, 3414 Olsen Blvd., Suite E, 806-354-9779
Austin 78745, 1110 W. Will Cannon Dr., Suite 301, 512-416-1314
Corpus Christi 78411, 4646 Corona, Suite 250, 361-854-9961
Dallas 75231, 10501 N. Central Expressway, Suite 213, 214-361-5896
El Paso 79925, 1155 Westmoreland, Suite 121, 915-772-0013
Fort Worth 76104, 1305 W. Magnolia, Suite B, 817-921-9095
Houston 77006, 503 Westheimer, 713-523-0884
Houston 77024, 701 N. Post Oak Rd., Suite 102, 713-682-2288
Laredo 78041, 6020 McPherson Rd., 1A, 956-723-4680
Lubbock 79410, 3208 34th St., 806-792-9782
McAllen 78504, 801 Nolana, Suite 140, 956-631-2147
Midland 79703, 3404 W. Illinois, Suite 1, 915-697-8222
San Antonio 78212, 231 W. Cypress St., Suite 100, 210-472-4025

Vermont

Regional Office

White River Junction 05009, 215 N. Main St., 802-296-5177 or 800-827-1000
from within Vermont

Vet Centers

South Burlington 05403, 359 Dorset St., 802-862-1806
White River Junction 05001, Gilman Office Complex 2, 802-295-2908 or
800-649-6603

Virginia

Medical Centers

#*Hampton 23667, 100 Emancipation Dr., 757-722-9961
*Richmond 23249, 1201 Broad Rock Blvd., 804-675-5000
*Salem 24153, 1970 Roanoke Blvd., 540-982-2463

Clinics

Alexandria 22309, 8796 D Sacramento Dr., 703-360-1442
Danville 24541, Southside Family Medical Center, 100 Vicar Pl., 434-836-
2100
Fredericksburg 22401, 1965 Jeff. Davis Hwy., 540-370-4468

Harrisonburg 22802, 101 North Main St., Suite 220, Harrison Plaza, 540-442-1773
Norton 24273, 340 Anderson Hollow Rd., 276-679-5880
Saltville 24370, 308 W. Main St., 276-496-4433
St. Charles 24282, PO Drawer S, 276-383-4487
Stephens City 22655, 106 Hyde Court, 540-869-0600
Tazewell 24651, Tazewell Family Physicians, PO Box 645, 276-988-2526

Regional Office

Roanoke 24011, 210 Franklin Rd., SW, statewide 800-827-1000

Vet Centers

Alexandria 22309, 8796 Sacramento Dr., Suite D&E, 703-360-8633
Norfolk 23517, 2200 Colonial Ave., Suite 3, 757-623-7584
Richmond 23230, 4902 Fitzhugh Ave., 804-353-8958
Roanoke 24016, 350 Albemarle Ave., SW, 540-342-9726

National Cemeteries

Alexandria NC 22314, 1450 Wilkes St., 703-221-2183/2184
Balls Bluff NC 22075, Rte. 7, Leesburg, 540-825-0027
City Point NC 23860, 10th Ave. & Davis St., Hopewell, 804-795-2031
Cold Harbor NC 23111, Rte. 156 North, Mechanicsville, 804-795-2031
Culpeper NC 22701, 305 U.S. Ave., 540-825-0027
Danville NC 24541, 721 Lee St., 704-636-2661
Fort Harrison NC 23231, 8620 Varina Rd., Richmond, 804-795-2031
Glendale NC 23231, 8301 Willis Church Rd., Richmond, 804-795-2031
Hampton NC 23667, Cemetery Rd. at Marshall Ave., 757-723-7104
Hampton NC 23667, VAMC, Emancipation Dr., 757-723-7104
Quantico NC 22172, PO Box 10, 18424, Joplin Rd. (Rte. 619), 703-221-2183/2184
Richmond NC 23231, 1701 Williamsburg Rd., 804-795-2031
Seven Pines NC 23150, 400 E. Williamsburg Rd., Sandston, 804-795-2031
Staunton NC, 24401, 901 Richmond Ave., 540-825-0027
Winchester NC 22601, 401 National Ave., 540-825-0027

Virgin Islands

Clinics

St. Croix 00850-4701, Village Mall #113, RR-02, Kingshill, 340-778-5553
St. Thomas 00802, Buccaneer Mall 8, 340-774-6674

Benefits

Served by San Juan, Puerto Rico, VA Regional Office, 800-827-1000

Vet Centers

St. Croix 00850, Box 12, R.R. 02, Village Mall, 113, RR2 Box 10556, Kingshill, 340-778-5553
St. Thomas 00802, 9800 Buccaneer Mall, Suite 8, 340-774-6674

Washington

Medical Centers

Puget Sound Health Care System:
  *Seattle 98108, 1660 S. Columbian Way, 206-762-1010
  #*Tacoma 98493, 9600 Veterans Dr., SW, American Lake, 253-582-8440
*Spokane 99205, 4815 N. Assembly St., 509-434-7000
*Walla Walla 99362, 77 Wainwright Dr., 509-525-5200

Clinics

Bremerton 98310, 925 Adele Ave., 360-782-0129
Factoria 98006, 13231, SE 36th St., Suite 110, 425-957-9000
Kent 98032, 23213, Pacific Hwy. South, 206-870-8880
Tri-Cities 99352, 948 Stevens Dr., Suite C, Richland, 509-946-1020
Yakima 98902, 717 Fruitvale Blvd., 509-966-0199

Regional Office

Seattle 98174, Federal Bldg., 915 2nd Ave., statewide 800-827-1000

Benefits Offices

Fort Lewis 98433, Waller Hall, Rm. 700, PO Box 331153, 253-967-7106
Bremerton 98337, W. Sound Pre-Separation Center, 262 Burwell St., 360-
782-9900

Vet Centers

Bellingham 98226, 3800 Byron Ave., Suite 124, 360-733-9226
Seattle 98121, 2030 9th Ave., Suite 210, 206-553-2706
Spokane 99206, 100 N. Mullan Rd., Suite 102, 509-444-8387
Tacoma 98409, 4916 Center St., Suite E, 253-565-7038
Yakima 98902, 1111 N. First St., 509-457-2736

National Cemetery

Tahoma NC 98042-4868, 18600, SE 240th St., Kent, 425-413-9614

West Virginia

Medical Centers

*Beckley 25801, 200 Veterans Ave., 304-255-2121
Clarksburg 26301, 1 Medical Center Dr., 304-623-3461 or 800-733-0512
Huntington 25704, 1540 Spring Valley Dr., 304-429-6741
#*Martinsburg 25401, 510 Butler Ave., 304-263-0811 or 800-817-3807

Clinics

Charleston 25304, 104 Alex Lane, 304-926-6001
Franklin 26807, Pendleton Comm. Care, 314 Pine St., 304-358-2355
Gassaway 26624, 617 River St., 304-364-5654
Logan 25601, 513 Dingess St., 304-752-8355
Parkersburg 26101, 912 Market St., 304-422-5114
Parsons 26287, 206 Spruce St., 304-478-2219
Petersburg 26847, c/o Grant Memorial Hospital, Route 55 W., 304-257-1026, ext. 120
Williamson 25661, 75 W. 4th Ave., 304-235-2187

Regional Office

Huntington 25701, 640 Fourth Ave., statewide 800-827-1000 (counties of Brooke, Hancock, Marshall, Ohio, served by Pittsburgh, PA, VA Regional Office)

Vet Centers

Beckley 25801, 101 Ellison Ave., 304-252-8220
Charleston 25302, 521 Central Ave., 304-343-3825
Huntington 25701, 3135 16th St. Rd., Suite 11, 304-523-8387
#Martinsburg 25401, 900 Winchester Ave., 304-263-6776
Morgantown 26508, 1083 Greenbag Rd., 304-291-4303
Princeton 24740, 905 Mercer St., 304-425-5653
Wheeling 26003, 1206 Chapline St., 304-232-0587

National Cemeteries

Grafton NC 26354, 431 Walnut St., 304-265-2044
West Virginia NC 26354, Rt. 2, Box 127, Grafton, 304-265-2044

Wisconsin

Medical Centers

Madison 53705, 2500 Overlook Terrace, 608-256-1901
#*Milwaukee 53295, 5000 W. National Ave., 414-384-2000
*Tomah 54660, 500 E. Veterans St., 608-372-3971

Clinics

Appleton 54914, 10 Tri-Park Way, 920-831-0070
Baraboo 53913, 626 14th St., 608-356-9318
Beaver Dam 53916, 208 LaCrosse St., 920-356-9415
Chippewa Falls 54729, 2503 County Hwy. 1, 715-720-3780
Cleveland 53015, 1205 North Ave., 920-693-3750
Green Bay 54303, 141 Siegler St., 920-497-3126
Janesville 53545, 111 N. Main St., 608-758-9300
Kenosha 53140, 800 55th St., 262-653-9286
LaCrosse 54601-3200, 2600 State Rd., 608-784-3886
Loyal 54446, PO Box 26, 141 North Main St., 715-255-9799
Rhinelander 54501, 3716 Country Dr., 6, 715-362-4080
Superior 54880, 3520 Tower Ave., 715-392-9711
Union Grove 53182, 21425 Spring St., 262-878-7000
Wausau 54401, 515 S. 32nd Ave., 715-842-2834
Wisconsin Rapids 54494, 710 E. Grand Ave., 715-424-3844

Regional Office

Milwaukee 53214, 5400 W. National Ave., statewide 800-827-1000

Vet Centers

Madison 53703, 147 S. Butler St., 608-264-5342
Milwaukee 53218, 5401 N. 76th St., 414-536-1301

National Cemetery

Wood NC 53295-4000, 5000 W. National Ave., Bldg. 1301, Milwaukee, 414-
382-5300

Wyoming

Medical Centers

*Cheyenne 82001, 2360 E. Pershing Blvd., 307-778-7550 or 888-483-9127
*Sheridan 82801, 1898 Fort Rd., 307-672-3473

Clinics

Casper 82601, 4140 S. Poplar St., 307-235-4143
Gillette 82718, 1701 Phillips Circle, Suite A, 307-685-0676
Green River 82935, 1400 Uinta Dr., 307-872-4508, ext. 4997
Newcastle 82701, 1124 Washington Blvd., 307-746-9533 or 800-764-5370
Powell 82435, 777 Ave. H, 307-754-7257
Riverton 82501, 2300 Rose Lane, 307-857-1211
Rock Springs 82901, 3000 College Dr., Suite C, 307-362-6641

Benefits Office

Cheyenne 82001, 2360 E. Pershing Blvd., statewide 800-827-1000

Vet Centers

Casper 82601, 111 S. Jefferson, Suite 100, 307-261-5355
Cheyenne 82001, 2424 Pioneer Ave., Suite 103, 307-778-7370

Appendix B

GLOSSARY

The following terms may have more than one definition, depending on the context in which they are used. The definitions provided here are for informational purposes in the use of this handbook and are not necessarily the legal definitions used for determination of benefits or application of policy.

Activities of Daily Living (ADL) The term inability to carry out activities of daily living means the inability to independently perform at least two of the six following functions: (1) bathing, (2) continence, (3) dressing, (4) eating, (5) toileting, (6) transferring in or out of a bed or chair with or without equipment.

Air Force Assistance Fund (AFAF) An aid organization that serves the Air Force.

Air Force Board of Correction of Military Records (AFBCMR) The final appeal authority for a member of the U.S. Air Force who disagrees with the findings or disposition determination of a formal PEB that has been upheld by the SAFPC.

Air Force Wounded Warrior (AFW2) Program The AFW2 Program provides personalized care and services to any airman ill or injured in support of OEF and OIF. Advocates for services on an airman's behalf, they ensure airmen have professional support and follow-up for no less than five years after separation or retirement.

America Supports You (ASY) America Supports You is a website that connects people, organizations and companies to hundreds of groups that offer a variety of support to the military community.

Americans with Disabilities Act (ADA) Signed into law in 1990, the Americans with Disabilities Act is a civil rights law that, in many cases, prohibits discrimination based on disability.

Army Board for the Correction of Military Records (ABCMR) The final appeal authority for a member of the U.S. Army who disagrees with the findings or disposition determination of a formal PEB that has been upheld by the USAPDA.

Army Career and Alumni Program (ACAP) ACAP is a world-class transition and job assistance services program for soldiers and civilian employees and their family members.

Army Emergency Relief (AER) An aid organization that serves the Army.

Army Knowledge Online (AKO) AKO is the U.S. Army's main intranet. It serves registered users to include active duty and retired service personnel and their family members, and provides single sign-on access to over 300 applications and services.

Army Wounded Warrior Program (AW2) The program's mission is to provide personalized support for severely injured soldiers, no matter where they are located or how long their recovery takes.

Basic Allowance for Subsistence (BAS) A payment to members for food. Members who are hospitalized continue receiving BAS during the hospitalization.

Board for Correction of Naval Records (BCNR) The final appeal authority for a member of the U.S. Navy or U.S. Marine Corps who disagrees with the findings or disposition determination of a formal PEB that has been upheld by the DIRSECNAVCORB.

Casual Pay Army term for an advance on a member's end of month paycheck. This payment will be automatically deducted during subsequent pay periods until paid back.

Centers for Disease Control and Prevention (CDC) The CDC is a government agency with the mission of promoting health and quality of life by preventing and controlling disease, injury, and disability. It is performing Vietnam veteran, Gulf War veteran, and Force Health Protections studies to evaluate the conditions of veterans as well as the care they receive.

Civilian Legal Counsel Members may hire, with their own funds, a civilian lawyer to represent them during formal PEB hearings.

Combat Related Injury and Rehabilitation Pay (CIP) A monthly payment for members who were evacuated from a combat zone due to an injury. This payment was replaced by PAC, but some members who were wounded before PAC was established may be eligible for back payment of the allowance.

Combat-Related Special Compensation (CRSC) A monthly compensation that is intended to replace some or all of their retired pay that is withheld due to receipt of VA compensation.

Combat Zone Tax Exclusion (CZTE) A policy that exempts a member from paying federal taxes while serving in an area designated a combat zone.

Combat/Operational Stress Injuries (COSI) Changes in mental functioning or behavior due to the challenges of combat and its aftermath; or changes in mental functioning or behavior due to the challenges of military operations other than combat.

Combined Rating The total percentage of disability for a member with more than one disability. This is not determined by adding percentages of disability for each condition. The formula for determining a combined rating can be found in Section 4.25 (Table 1) of Title 38 of the Code of Federal Regulations.

Community Based Health Care Organization (CBHCO) If you are a member of the Army National Guard and Army Reserve and require only outpatient care, you may request transfer to a CBHCO. This program allows you to live at home, receive outpatient care, and perform military duties at a local military organization such as an armory or recruiting station. You cannot work at a civilian job while you are attached to a CBHCO.

Computer/Electronic Accommodations Program (CAP) CAP is the federal government's centrally funded accommodation program.

Concurrent Retirement and Disability Payments (CRDP) A program that restores retired pay on a graduated 10-year schedule for retirees with a 50 to 90 percent VA-rated disability.

Continued Health Care Benefit Program (CHCBP) The CHCBP is a premium-based health care program similar to TRICARE Standard. It offers temporary transitional health coverage (18–36 months) and must be purchased within 60 days after your TRICARE eligibility ends.

DD Form 214—Certificate of Release or Discharge from Active Duty The Report of Separation contains information normally needed to verify military service for benefits, retirement, employment, and membership in veterans' organizations.

DD Form 2586—Verification of Military Experience and Training The DD Form 2586 is created from a service member's automated records on file. It lists military job experience and training history, recommended college credit information, and civilian equivalent job titles. This document is designed to help the member apply for jobs, but it is not a resume.

DD Form 2648 Pre-separation Counseling Checklist A form used by the DoD that helps transition assistance program employees assist members in transitioning out of the military and into civilian life.

Department of Veterans Affairs (VA) The federal agency responsible for providing a broad range of programs and services to service members and veterans as required by Title 38 of the U.S. Code.

Director, Secretary of the Navy Council of Review Boards (DIRSEC-NAVCORB) The governing body for the U.S. Navy overseeing the DES process for the service. A sailor or marine may appeal a PEB finding with the DIRSECNAVCORB, which has the authority to uphold the PEB findings, issue revised findings, or send the case back to the PEB for another review.

Disability Evaluation System (DES) Pilot A joint DoD-VA Disability Evaluation System Pilot begun in the National Capital Region in November 2007, to improve the timeliness, effectiveness and transparency of the DES review process. Under the pilot, the VA performs one medical exam and rates a member's disabilities. This examination and rating is used by the PEB to determine fitness for duty and disposition, and by VA to determine VA disability compensation.

Disability Evaluation System A system or process of the U.S. government for evaluating the nature and extent of disabilities affecting members of the Armed Forces. The DES includes medical/psychological evaluations, physical evaluations, counseling of members, and mechanisms for the final disposition of disability determinations.

Disability Retirement Pay The monthly allowance paid to members who are placed on the TDRL or PDRL. The formula for determining the amount of disability retirement pay is found in section 1 of chapter 2.

Disabled Transition Assistance Program (DTAP) DTAP works with members who may be released because of a disability or who believe they have a disability qualifying them for the VA's Vocational Rehabilitation and Employment program (VR&E).The goal of DTAP is to encourage and assist potentially eligible service members in making an informed decision about the VA's VR&E program. It is also intended to quickly deliver vocational rehabilitation services to eligible service members by assisting them in filing an application for vocational rehabilitation benefits.

Disabled Veterans Outreach Program Specialists (DVOP) A Department of Labor employee trained to help veterans make the important adjustment to the civilian job market.

DoD Job Search A website that is a part of the America's Job Bank service designed solely for service members.

DoD Suicide Prevention and Risk Reduction Committee's (SPARRC) Preventing Suicide Network The DoD SPARRC Preventing Suicide Network is a resource center aimed at providing authoritative and problem-specific information about suicide prevention.

Efficiency The measure of a member's total health minus his/her disability. A member with a 60 percent disability has only 40 percent of his/her total health that is not impacted by the disability.

Family and Medical Leave Act (FMLA) The federal law that provides unpaid leave and job protection to those who have family members with medical conditions that require their presence. The Fiscal Year 2008 National Defense Authorization Act authorized the expansion of the FMLA to support families of recovering service members.

Family Liaison Officer (FLO) An Air Force employee appointed to every airman with a combat-related injury to assist in providing support to the recovering airman's family.

Family Separation Allowance (FSA) Pay a member receives if he/she has dependents and is away from his/her permanent duty station for more than 30 days for temporary duty or on a temporary change of station, to include a deployment.

Fit/Unfit Finding of the PEB. Fitness or unfitness is solely determined by the ability of the member to perform the duties of his/her office, grade, rank or rating because of disease or injury.

Formal Physical Evaluation Board If a member disagrees with the informal PEB findings or disposition, he/she may request a formal PEB, appear before the board in person, obtain military or civilian legal counsel to represent him/her, call witnesses, present evidence, and present testimony on his/her own behalf.

GL-2005.261—Traumatic Injury Protection Payment The form used to request insurance payment for service-connected traumatic injury or loss from service in OIF/OEF.

Hardship Duty Pay Location (HDP-L) Pay a member receives while serving in a location that the Secretary of Defense identifies as a hardship duty location.

Health and Human Services (HHS) HHS is the principal agency for protecting the health of all Americans and providing essential human services, especially for those who are least able to help themselves.

Health Resources and Service Administration (HRSA) HRSA is the primary federal agency for improving access to health care services for people who are uninsured, isolated or medically vulnerable.

Hemiplegia Paralysis affecting only one side of the body.

Hospitalized For the purposes of some pay entitlements, members are considered hospitalized if they were admitted as an inpatient or were receiving extensive rehabilitation as an outpatient while living in quarters affiliated with the military health care system.

Hostile Fire Pay/Imminent Danger Pay (HFP/IDP) Pay a member receives while serving in an area the president identifies as placing him/her in imminent danger or that he/she may come under hostile fire.

Individual Transition Plan (ITP) The ITP is a framework a member can use to fulfill realistic career goals based upon his/her unique skills, knowledge, experience, and abilities. The ITP identifies actions and activities associated with a member's transition.

Informal Physical Evaluation Board The initial meeting of a PEB to determine a disposition of the member's medical case. The member will not be present at the informal PEB. The informal PEB will determine fit/unfit and the member's disposition based on the member's case file. The PEBLO counsels the member on the findings of the informal PEB and provides options for appeal of those findings.

Invitational Travel Authorizations (ITAs), Invitational Travel Orders (ITOs), or Emergency Family Member Travel (EFMT) Military travel orders that allow a recovering service member's family to travel and stay with him/her during treatment and recovery after suffering a wound, illness, or injury.

Job Accommodation Network (JAN) A free service from the Department of Labor's Office of Disability Employment Policy that provides personalized worksite accommodations, information regarding the ADA and other disability-related information, and information about self-employment.

Local Veterans Employment Representative (LVER) A Department of Labor employee trained to help veterans make the important adjustment to the civilian job market.

Medical Evaluation Board (MEB) A board, generally comprising medical officers, that determines if a member meets medical retention standards for his/her service. The board may recommend a return to duty or send the member's case to a Physical Evaluation Board.

MedlinePlus MedlinePlus is a service of the U.S. National Library of Medicine and the National Institutes of Health that provides resources regarding all aspects of veterans' health including recent news, treatments, rehabilitation and recovery programs, condition-specific information, financial issues, as well as ongoing clinical trials and research.

Mild Traumatic Brain Injury (mTBI) Mild Traumatic Brain Injury (concussion) is caused by blunt trauma to the head or acceleration/deceleration forces jogging the brain within the skull, which may or may not produce a period of unconsciousness. Mild TBI is defined as an injury to the brain as a result of any period of observed or self-reported: Confusion, disorientation, or impaired consciousness; Dysfunction of memory around the time of injury (amnesia); Loss of consciousness lasting less than 30 minutes. No other obvious neurological deficits, no intracranial complications (e.g., hematoma/blood clot) and normal computed tomography (CT) findings should be present.

Military Severely Injured Center (MSIC) A DoD call-in support program that provides information regarding medical care and rehabilitation; education, training, and job placement; personal mobility and functioning; accommodations; counseling; and financial resources.

Minority Opinion When a member of the PEB disagrees with the findings of the board, he/she will write a minority opinion outlining the areas of disagreement that become part of the board's findings.

Montgomery G.I. Bill (MGIB) The MGIB provides up to 36 months of education benefits to eligible veterans for college, technical or vocational courses, correspondence courses, apprenticeship/job training, flight training, high-tech training, licensing and certification tests, entrepreneurship training, and certain entrance examinations.

Montgomery GI Bill—Selected Reserve (MGIB-SR) The MGIB-SR program may be available to you if you are a member of the Selected Reserve. The Selected Reserve includes the Army Reserve, Navy Reserve, Air Force Reserve, Marine Corps Reserve and Coast Guard Reserve, and the Army National Guard and the Air National Guard. You may use this education assistance program for degree programs, certificate or correspondence courses, cooperative training, independent study programs, apprenticeship/ on-the-job training, and vocational flight training programs.

National Association for People of Color Against Suicide (NOPCAS) NOPCAS is a non-profit organization with the goal of stopping suicide in minority communities.

National Association of Child Care Resource and Referral Agencies (NACCRRA) NACCRRA is an organization through which you can get assistance to find and pay for safe, licensed childcare services for a period of six months during the service member's recuperation.

National Capital Region (NCR) Washington, DC, and the surrounding areas.

National Defense Authorization Act for Fiscal Year 2008 (NDAA) Public Law 110-181 that authorizes expenditures and provides guidance for the federal government concerning national defense. In the Fiscal Year 2008 version, a large section was devoted to wounded warrior issues.

National Institute of Diabetes, Digestive and Kidney Diseases (NIDDK) NIDDK supports 22 research projects related to veterans of military service.

National Institute of Mental Health (NIMH) NIMH conducts projects on trauma and post-traumatic stress disorder that involve veteran populations.

National Institute on Deafness and Other Communicative Disorders (NIDCD) The NIDCD studies the molecular mechanisms that cause the loss of hearing from exposure to loud noise.

National Institute on Dental and Craniofacial Research (NIDCR) The NIDCR conducts ongoing research in tissue engineering and regeneration for wounds to the head and face.

National Strategy for Suicide Prevention (NSSP) The NSSP is a collaborative effort between SAMSHA, CDC, NIH, HRSA and HHS and provides facts about suicide, recent publications, and resources designed to spread knowledge of the seriousness of suicides.

Navy Marine Corps Relief Society (NMCRS) An aid organization that serves the Navy and Marine Corps.

Navy Safe Harbor The Navy Safe Harbor program provides personalized assistance to severely injured sailors and their families.

Ombudsman An ombudsman is assigned to or near a major military facility or VA medical facility to further assist in the transition by helping you connect with local agencies and community groups.

Operation Enduring Freedom (OEF) OEF includes casualties that occurred: In and Around Afghanistan: Afghanistan, Pakistan, and Uzbekistan
Other Locations: Guantanamo Bay (Cuba), Djibouti, Eritrea, Ethiopia, Jordan, Kenya, Kyrgyzstan, Philippines, Seychelles, Sudan, Tajikistan, Turkey, and Yemen

Operation Iraqi Freedom (OIF) OIF includes casualties that occurred on or after March 19, 2003, in the Arabian Sea, Bahrain, Gulf of Aden, Gulf of Oman, Iraq, Kuwait, Oman, Persian Gulf, Qatar, Red Sea, Saudi Arabia, and United Arab Emirates. Prior to March 19, 2003, casualties in these countries were considered OEF.

Paraplegia Complete paralysis of the lower half of the body including both legs, usually caused by damage to the spinal cord.

Partial Pay Air Force term for an advance on a member's end of month paycheck. This payment will be automatically deducted during subsequent pay periods until paid back.

Patient Administration Team (PAT) A non-medical care organization that assists members of the military in issues related to their hospitalization and recovery.

Pay and Allowance Continuation (PAC) A new policy allowing members evacuated from a combat zone to continue receiving all combat pay and allowances they received prior to the injury for the first year they are hospitalized.

Per Diem A daily allowance paid to a person on military travel orders to cover food, lodging, and incidentals. In cases where lodging or food is provided by the government, this payment will only be for the $3.50 incidental rate.

Permanent Disabled Retirement List (PDRL) The PEB disposition finding for a member who has one or more service unfitting condition(s) with a combined rating of 30 percent or higher, was incurred in the line of duty, and is considered stable. This disposition also covers members who have served 20 or more years, have one or more service unfitting condition(s) with a combined rating of 20 percent or less, was incurred in the line of duty, and are considered stable.

Personnel Service Detachment (PSD) A military personnel office that will assist members and their families with pay and personnel problems.

Physical Evaluation Board (PEB) A board, generally comprising a senior line officer, senior personnel officer, and senior medical officer, that determines if a member is fit or unfit for continued service. This board may recommend a return to duty, separation with or without benefits, or medical retirement (temporary or permanent).

Physical Evaluation Board Disposition The findings of a PEB on a member's medical case. Member can be found fit and returned to duty, found unfit and separated with or without benefits, or medically retired on either the permanent or temporary disability retirement list.

Physical Evaluation Board Liaison Officer (PEBLO) The person assigned to assist the service member through the DES process. Duties include counseling the member on the process as well as building the case file used by the PEB to determine fitness for duty.

Post-9/11 GI Bill A new benefit providing educational assistance to individuals who have served on active duty on or after September 11, 2001. It provides additional monetary benefits for members, including a housing and book allowance, and is limited by the cost of the highest public school tuition costs in the state the member resides, rather than a set cap like the Montgomery G.I. Bill. It also allows for transfer of benefits to family members in certain instances.

Post-Traumatic Stress Disorder (PTSD) A traumatic stress injury that fails to heal such that the symptoms and behaviors it causes remain significantly troubling or disabling beyond 30 days after their onset.

Project Action Project Action maintains a national paratransit database.

Quadriplegia Paralysis of all four limbs.

REALifelines A Department of Labor program to help injured veterans return to fulfilling, productive civilian lives using federal, state, and local level efforts to create a network of resources that focus on veteran well-being and job-placement assistance.

Recovery Coordinator A person assigned to make sure your needs are being met by the right person in the right place and on time.

Recovery Plan The Recovery Coordinator prepares a Recovery Plan that lays out the path for you to meet personal and professional goals.

Reserve Components Includes the Army National Guard, the Army Reserve, the Navy Reserve, the Marine Corps Reserve, the Air National Guard, the Air Force Reserve and the Coast Guard Reserve.

Respite Care Respite care includes adult day care and home care services, as well as overnight stays in a facility, and can be provided a few hours a week or for a weekend.

Return to Duty The PEB disposition finding for a member who does not have a service unfitting condition.

Savings Deposit Program (SDP) Members deployed to combat zones may put up to $10,000 of their pay in this program and earn 10 percent interest on the money deposited.

Secretary of the Air Force Personnel Council (SAFPC) Organization that can uphold a PEB finding, revise the findings of a PEB, or return the case to the PEB for further review. Airmen may present a written rebuttal to the SAFPC if they disagree with the PEB findings.

Separate with severance pay The PEB disposition finding for a member who has a service unfitting condition, but whose combined rating is 20% or less.

Separate without benefits The PEB disposition finding for a member who has a service unfitting condition, but whose condition is not found to be in the line of duty, or is found to have existed before entry into service and not aggravated by service.

Service Members' Group Life Insurance (SGLI) SGLI is a program of low-cost group life insurance for service members on active duty, ready reservists, members of the National Guard, members of the Commissioned Corps of the National Oceanic and Atmospheric Administration and the Public Health Service, cadets and midshipmen of the four service academies, and members of the Reserve Officer Training Corps.

Severance Pay A one-time, lump-sum payment for members separated from the military for medical reasons, but who receive a combined rating of 20 percent or less for unfitting conditions. The formula for determining the amount of service pay a member will receive is found in section 1 of chapter 2.

SGL 8714—Veterans Group Life Insurance The form used to convert SGLI to VGLI.

SGLV 8715—SGLI Disability Extension The form used to request an extension of the SGLI coverage for two years from date of discharge from the military for those who are totally disabled.

Small Business Administration (SBA) Loans Business loans are available to veterans through programs of the SBA. In addition, SBA offers loans specifically to Vietnam-era and disabled veterans.

Social Security Administration (SSA) The SSA is the government agency that is charged with ensuring the economic security of Americans. While you work, you pay taxes into the Social Security system, and when you retire or become disabled you, your spouse and your dependent children receive monthly benefits that are based on your reported earnings. Also, your survivors can collect benefits if you die.

Social Security Disability Insurance Program (SSDI) SSDI pays benefits to you and certain members of your family if you are "insured," meaning that you worked long enough and paid Social Security taxes.

Special Pay Navy/Marine Corps term for an advance on a member's end of month paycheck. This payment will be automatically deducted during subsequent pay periods until paid back.

Stable A condition that, in the doctor's opinion, is unlikely to improve to the point a member can return to duty

Substance Abuse and Mental Health Services Administration SAMHSA is an agency within the DHHS that focuses on building resilience and facilitating recovery for people with or at risk for mental or substance use disorders.

Suicide Awareness Voices of Education (SAVE) SAVE is a non-profit organization with the goal of preventing suicide through public awareness and education, reducing stigma and serving as a resource to those touched by suicide.

Supplemental Security Income (SSI) SSI is a federal income supplement program funded by general tax revenues (not Social Security taxes). It is designed to help aged, blind, and disabled people, who have little or no income, and provides cash to meet basic needs for food, clothing, and shelter.

Temporary Disability Retirement List (TDRL) The PEB disposition finding for a member who has one or more service unfitting condition(s) with a combined rating of 30 percent or higher, was incurred in the line of duty, and is not considered stable.

Transition Assistance Program (TAP) TAP is a program designed to ease the transition from military service to the civilian workforce and community.

Traumatic Brain Injury (TBI) Traumatic brain injury is a neurological injury with possible physical, cognitive, behavioral, and emotional symptoms. Like all injuries, TBI is most appropriately and accurately diagnosed as soon as possible after the injury. TBI is not a mental health condition. The range of TBI includes mild, moderate, severe, and penetrating. Well after the injury event, soldiers may have residual symptoms from a TBI and new or emerging PTSD symptoms. If the TBI has not been previously identified or documented, an accurate description of the traumatic events in theater usually allows a well-trained clinician to make a distinction between TBI and PTSD or other mental health conditions.

Traumatic Event A Qualifying Traumatic Injury is an injury or loss caused by application of external force or violence (a traumatic event) OR a condition whose cause can be directly linked to a traumatic event.

Traumatic Injury Traumatic injury is derived by external force or violence or a condition that can be linked to a traumatic event.

Traumatic Service Members' Group Life Insurance (TSGLI) An insurance program related to the Service Members' Group Life Insurance that pays a member who has suffered a severe loss, such as a leg or arm amputation.

TRICARE The health care program serving eligible active duty service members, National Guard and reserve members, retirees, their families, survivors, and certain former spouses worldwide.

TRICARE Online TRICARE.mil is the entry point that offers beneficiaries access to TRICARE information about eligibility, plans, and medical, dental, vision and prescription coverage.

TRICARE Dental Program (TDP) The TRICARE Dental Program (TDP) is a voluntary dental insurance program. TDP is available to family members of all active duty service members of any of the seven uniformed services and to National Guard/reserve members and/or their families.

TRICARE Reserve Select (TRS) TRICARE Reserve Select (TRS) is a premium-based plan that qualified National Guard and reserve members may purchase. TRS, which requires a monthly premium, offers coverage similar to TRICARE Standard and Extra. For information or assistance with qualifying for and purchasing TRS, check the TRICARE website.

TRICARE Retiree Dental Program (TRDP) The TRICARE Retiree Dental Program (TRDP) is a voluntary dental insurance program for uniformed services retirees and their eligible family members.

Troops to Teachers (TTT) The TTT program is funded and overseen by the Department of Education and operated by the DoD. The TTT program helps recruit quality teachers for schools that serve students from low-income families throughout America.

U.S. Air Force Physical Disability Division Processing agency for all formal and informal PEB cases in the U.S. Air Force. This organization reviews all PEB findings and dispositions, referring those it feels need further review to the Secretary of the Air Force Personnel Council.

U.S. Army Physical Disability Agency (USAPDA) The governing body for the U.S. Army overseeing the DES process for the service. All PEB findings are sent to the USAPDA, and 20 percent of the cases are randomly reviewed for quality assurance purposes. Any case with a minority opinion will be automatically reviewed. Soldiers may appeal a PEB finding with the USAPDA, which has the authority to uphold the PEB findings, issue revised findings, or send the case back to the PEB for another review.

U.S. Public Health Service (USPHS) "Healthier Vets," the surgeon general's joint DHHS/VA initiative, is designed to help veterans and their families remain physically active after they have separated from the military.

Unemployment Compensation for Ex-Service Members Service members separating from active duty may qualify for unemployment compensation if they are unable to find a new job.

VA Form 10-8678—Clothing Allowance The form used to apply for a clothing allowance if a service-connected disability requiring a prosthetic device or orthopedic appliance (such as a wheelchair) leads to damage to a veteran's clothes.

VA Form 21-4502—Vehicle Purchase and Adaptation The form used to apply for a one-time grant toward the purchase of a vehicle with adaptive equipment approved by the VA for a veteran or service member with certain disabilities.

VA Form 21-526—Compensation and Pension The form used to request that the VA provide service-related disability compensation, or a pension for those who are wartime veterans with non-service-connected disabilities.

VA Form 21-8940—Increased Compensation Based on Unemployability The form used to request compensation based on an inability to work due to total disability from service-connected disability(ies).

VA Form 22-1990—VA Education Benefits The form used to apply for multiple education benefits, including the Montgomery GI Bill Educational Assistance Program; Montgomery GI Bill Selected Reserve Educational Assistance Program; Reserve Educational Assistance Program; Post-Vietnam Era Veterans Educational Assistance Program; National Call to Serve Program; and the Transfer of Entitlement Program.

VA Form 22-5490—Survivors and Dependents Educational Assistance The form used to apply for educational assistance to a spouse or child if the member is permanently and totally disabled as a result of a service-connected disability; dies of a service-connected disability; while rated permanently and totally disabled; or is missing in action or a prisoner of war.

VA Form 26-4555—Housing Adaptation The form used to apply for grants for constructing an adapted home or modifying an existing home to meet a disabled veteran/service member's needs.

VA Form 28-1900—Disabled Veterans Application for Vocational Rehabilitation The form used to apply for Vocational Rehabilitation and Employment benefits (Chapter 31) 196, *Wounded, Ill and Injured Compensation and Benefits Handbook.*

VA Form 28-8832—Application for Counseling The form used to apply for vocational and educational counseling.

VA Form 29-0188—Application for Supplemental Service-Disabled Veterans (RH) Life Insurance The form used to apply for Supplemental Service-Disabled Veterans Insurance.

VA Form 29-357—Claim for Disability Insurance Benefits The form used to apply for waiver of premiums on a Service-Disabled Veterans Insurance policy.

VA Form 29-4364—Application for Service-Disabled Veterans Life Insurance The form used to apply for Service-Disabled Veterans Insurance (S-DVI).

VA Form 29-8636—Veterans Mortgage Life Insurance Statement The form used to apply for Veterans Mortgage Life Insurance (VMLI).

VA Schedule for Rating Disabilities (VASRD) The document used to determine the severity of a member's disability expressed as a percentage of disability.

Vet Center program Vet Centers, run by the VA, provide free individual, group and family counseling to all veterans who served in any combat zone.

Veterans Educational Assistance Program (VEAP) VEAP is available if you elected to make contributions from your military pay to participate in this education benefit program. You may use these benefits for degree, certificate, correspondence, apprenticeship/on-the-job training programs, and vocational flight training programs. In certain circumstances, remedial, deficiency, and refresher training may also be available. Benefit entitlement is one to 36 months depending on the number of monthly contributions. You have 10 years from your release from active duty to use VEAP benefits. If there is entitlement not used after the 10-year period, your portion remaining in the fund will be automatically refunded.

Veterans' Preference (federal hiring) Veterans who are disabled, and served on active duty in the military during certain specified time periods, or in military campaigns, are entitled to preference over others in hiring for virtually all federal government jobs.

Veterans Upward Bound (VUB) program The VUB program is a free Department of Education program designed to help eligible U.S. military veterans refresh their academic skills so that they can successfully complete the post-secondary school of their choosing.

Veterans' Service Organization (VSO) Organizations that are chartered by Congress and/or recognized by VA for claims representation for today's returning service members, veterans and their families.

Vocational Rehabilitation and Employment (VR&E) VR&E delivers timely and effective vocational rehabilitation services to veterans with service-connected disabilities and to certain service members awaiting discharge due to a medical condition.

Wounded Warrior Pay Management Team (WWPMT) Highly trained finance experts whom the Defense Finance and Accounting Service have prepared to deal with the complex issues surrounding pay and allowances for recovering service members.

Wounded Warrior Project (WWP) A project offering programs and services to severely injured members during the time of active duty through transition to civilian life.

Wounded Warrior Regiment/Marine for Life Injured Support The program is to "provide information, advocacy and assistance to injured Marines, Sailors injured while serving with Marines, and their families, in order to minimize the difficulties and worries they face as they navigate the stressful and confusing process."

ABBREVIATIONS AND ACRONYMS

ACE—Automated Certificate of Eligibility

ADA—Americans with Disabilities Act: a federal law that requires employers to make reasonable accommodations for employees with disabilities and prohibits discrimination against qualified individuals with disabilities when making hiring, promotion, compensation and training decisions.

ADME—Active Duty Medical Extension: a program that allows wounded reservists to remain on active duty (and receive active duty salary) during the disability evaluation process.

AEA—Actual Expense Allowance: an allowance that, under special circumstances, permits family members to be reimbursed for actual and necessary expenses that excced the per diem allowance that otherwise serves as the maximum amount an individual will be reimbursed when traveling under an invitational travel order.

ALS—Amyotrophic lateral sclerosis

AMVETS—A service organization dedicated to working on behalf of the interests of veterans.

BVA—Board of Veterans' Appeals: a Department of Veterans Affairs (VA) panel that reviews benefit claims determinations made by local VA offices and issues decisions on appeals.

C&P—Compensation and Pension

CHAMPVA—Civilian Health and Medical Program of the Department of Veterans Affairs: a VA health benefits program that shares the costs of certain health care services and supplies for dependents of disabled veterans.

CHCBP—Continued Health Care Benefit Program: a temporary health care plan available to veterans and their families for the interim period between the end of eligibility for military health benefits and the beginning of civilian health care coverage.

COAD—Continuation on Active Duty: the program by which service members with 15-20 years of service who become disabled as a result of combat may request to remain on active duty, even if found unfit by a PEB. Service members often use COAD as a means of obtaining a longer length of service in order to receive higher retirement benefits.

CONUS—The continental United States, as opposed to OCONUS (Outside CONUS)

CRDP—Concurrent Retirement & Disability Payments: a DoD program that provides a gradual reduction, over a period of ten years, of the offset a veteran must take on his or her DoD pay when he or she is also receiving VA disability payments. CRDP is available to veterans with at least 20 years of service and at least 50% disability ratings.

CRSC—Combat-Related Special Compensation: a DoD program that restores the full amount of the VA disability compensation for a qualifying injury (e.g., a combat injury) that would otherwise be offset by DoD disability benefits. CRSC is available to veterans with least 20 years of service and a qualifying injury that is assigned a disability rating of at least 10%.

CUE—Clear and Unmistakable Error: an applicant to the Board of Veterans Appeals may make a motion for reconsideration on the basis of a clear and unmistakable error, a technical term referring to a defined set of circumstances.

CWT—Compensated Work Therapy

CZTE—Combat Zone Tax Exclusion

DAV—Disabled American Veterans: a nonprofit veterans service organization that can represent veterans and their dependents in front of the VA and is focused on building better lives for disabled veterans and their families primarily by providing free assistance in obtaining government benefits and services.

DEA—Survivors' and Dependents' Educational Assistance Program: a VA program that provides education benefits to qualified dependents and survivors.

DEERS—Defense Enrollment Eligibility System: a computerized database containing relevant personal information for military personnel, their families and others who are eligible for health care benefits from TRICARE. Service members are automatically registered in DEERS. Family members must be registered in order to receive TRICARE benefits.

DES—Disability Evaluation System: a general term applied to the entire process the military uses to determine whether injured service members are fit to continue active military service.

DIC—Dependency and Indemnity Compensation

DoD—Department of Defense: the department of the federal government responsible for coordinating and supervising all government agencies and activities directly related to the military and national security.

DSO—Department Service Officers of the American Legion: a veterans service organization that can represent veterans and dependents in front of the VA. DSO officers are available to answer questions and offer guidance to veterans filing claims with the VA.

EEOC—Equal Employment Opportunity Commission: the federal agency charged with ending employment discrimination.

ESGR—Employer Support of the Guard and Reserve: the DoD agency whose activities are aimed at promoting understanding and cooperation between reservists (and guard members) and their civilian employers. ESGR also assists in enforcing rights under USERRA and reducing and resolving conflicts between Reserve Component members and employers.

FMLA—Family and Medical Leave Act of 1993: a federal law guaranteeing certain workers unpaid leave from work in order to care for themselves or for certain family members who are seriously ill.

FSGLI—Family Service Members' Group Life Insurance

GI Bill—Montgomery GI Bill: federal programs that provides monthly educational assistance to military veterans, including reservists and members of the National Guard.

GWOT—Global War on Terror: injured Reserve Component service members mobilized in the Global War on Terrorism may be eligible to receive their regular service salary and benefits.

HUD—Department of Housing and Urban Development

IRA—Individual Retirement Account: a retirement plan account that provides certain tax advantages.

IRR—Individual Ready Reserve

ITO—Invitational Travel Order: official government orders authorizing travel by relatives of seriously ill or wounded service members to enable the relatives to visit the service member in military treatment facilities.

MEB—Medical Evaluation Board: The first formal stage of the disability evaluation process.

MGIB—Montgomery GI Bill

MMRB—MOS Medical Retention Board: an administrative board before which injured service members must appear to request a change of MOS.

MOS—Military Occupational Specialty: a service member's job classification code.

MRP—Medical Retention Processing: a program through which Reserve Component service members mobilized in support of the GWOT (Operation Enduring Freedom, Operation Iraqi Freedom, etc.) may remain on active duty pending evaluation of an injury.

NACVSO—National Association of County Veterans Service Officers: an organization made up of local government employees working in county veterans offices in 28 states.

NPRC—National Personnel Records Center

NOD—Notice of Disagreement: the means by which an applicant for VA benefits can appeal a VA decision regarding benefits.

NSLI—National Service Life Insurance

NSO—National Service Officer: a title used by both AMVETS and DAV for the officers of each organization who are dedicated to providing information, counseling on veterans' benefits and representation in front of the VA.

NVLSP—National Veterans Legal Services Program: offers training to attorneys and other veteran advocates in the area of veterans' claims.

OCONUS—Outside the continental United States (see CONUS)

OEF—Operation Enduring Freedom

OIF—Operation Iraqi Freedom

OPM—Office of Personnel Management

PDRL—Permanent Disability Retirement List: a service member will be entitled to disability retirement pay when he or she is placed on either the PDRL or the Temporary Disability Retirement List.

PEB—Physical Evaluation Board: the second formal phase of the Disability Evaluation System, the PEB evaluates a service member's physical ability to continue in the military service.

PEBLO—PEB Liaison Officer: acts as a counselor and liaison for the service member throughout the disability evaluation process.

PTSD—Post-traumatic stress disorder

PVA—Paralyzed Veterans of America: a nonprofit veterans' service organization dedicated to serving the interest of veterans with spinal cord injury or disease and authorized to represent veterans and their dependents in front of the VA.

REALifelines—Recovery and Employment Assistance Lifelines: a Department of Labor initiative that provides injured and wounded service members and their families with access to a free career assistance network.

REAP—Reserve Educational Assistance Program: a program that provides education assistance to reservists and National Guard members who were called up for at least 90 days of active duty since September 11, 2001.

SAH—Specially Adapted Housing

SBA—Small Business Administration

S-DVI—Service-Disabled Veterans Life Insurance

SCRA—Service Members Civil Relief Act: a federal law that guarantees that all service members ordered to active duty can reinstate health insurance policies that were in effect when their military service began, as long as they ended at some point during military service.

SGLI—Service Members Group Life Insurance: a government-sponsored life insurance program for service members.

SMC—Special Monthly Compensation: The additional monthly payments above and beyond the basic VA disability compensation that are provided to eligible service members who sustain particularly severe injuries, such as amputations, blindness and other severe traumas.

SOC—Statement of the Case: a response from the VA explaining its reasons for denial of benefits.

SSA—Social Security Administration: the government agency responsible for the Social Security system.

SSB—Special Separation Benefits

SSI—Supplemental Security Income

TAMP—Transitional Assistance Management Program: the temporary health care program provided through the VA after separation.

TAP—Transition Assistance Program: a program that helps service members make the initial transition from military service to the civilian workplace by providing employment and training information within 12 months of separation or 24 months of retirement.

TDRL—Temporary Disability Retirement List

TDY—Temporary Duty: A temporary assignment other than the normal billet, often at another location and frequently with additional pay during the period.

TLD—Temporary Limited Duty: TLD is a specified period of limited duty. The TLD period is normally eight months and generally will not exceed a total of 16 cumulative months.

TSGLI—Traumatic Service Members Group Life Insurance: an insurance program that provides qualified service members with up to $100,000 in the direct aftermath of a qualifying traumatic injury.

TSP–Thrift Savings Plan

USAPDA—U.S. Army Physical Disability Agency: the central agency of the Army which oversees the regional Physical Evaluation Boards.

USCAVC—U.S. Court of Appeals for Veterans Claims

USCIS—U.S. Citizenship and Immigration Services

USDA—U.S. Department of Agriculture

USERRA—Uniformed Services Employment and Reemployment Rights Act: a federal law that generally prohibits employers from discriminating against employees based on their membership or service in the armed forces.

VA—Department of Veterans Affairs (formerly Veterans Administration)

VASRD—Veterans Administration Schedule for Rating Disabilities: the VA guidelines that list various medical conditions and degrees of severity and which are used to rate service members from zero to one hundred percent disabled.

VEAP—Veterans Educational Assistance Program

VEOA—Veterans' Employment Opportunities Act

VETS—Veterans Employment and Training Services: a Department of Labor program that oversees numerous programs designed to assist veterans in seeking jobs.

VGLI—Veterans Group Life Insurance

VHA—Veterans Health Administration

VMET—Verification of Military Experience and Training

VMLI—Veterans Mortgage Life Insurance

VR&E—Vocational Rehabilitation and Employment

VSI—Voluntary Separation Incentives

Index